Concise Dermatology

T0144471

Edited by

Rashmi Sarkar, MD, MNAMS
Professor
Department of Dermatology
Lady Hardinge Medical College
and
SSK and KSCH Hospitals
New Delhi, India

Associate Editors
Anupam Das, MD
Assistant Professor
Dermatology
KPC Medical College and Hospital
Kolkata, West Bengal, India

Sumit Sethi, MBBS, MD, DNB
Consultant Dermatologist
DermaStation
Janakpuri, New Delhi, India
and
Venkateshwar Hospital
Dwarka, Delhi, India

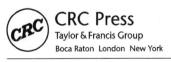

CRC Press
Taylor & Francis Group
Boca Raton London New York

CRC Press is an imprint of the
Taylor & Francis Group, an **informa** business

First edition published 2021
by CRC Press
6000 Broken Sound Parkway NW, Suite 300, Boca Raton, FL 33487-2742
and by CRC Press
2 Park Square, Milton Park, Abingdon, Oxon, OX14 4RN

© 2021 Taylor & Francis Group, LLC

We acknowledge Ronald Marks and Richard Motley's 18th Edition of *Common Skin Diseases* (By Roxburgh).

CRC Press is an imprint of Taylor & Francis Group, LLC

Library of Congress Cataloging-in-Publication Data
Names: Sarkar, Rashmi, editor. | Das, Anupam, editor. | Sethi, Sumit, editor.
Title: Concise dermatology / edited by Rashmi Sarkar, MD,MNAMS, Professor,
Department of Dermatology, Lady Hardinge Medical College and associated
SSK and KSCH Hospital, New Delhi, India, associate editors, Dr. Anupam
Das, MD, Assistant Professor, Dermatology, KPC Medical College and
Hospital, Kolkata, West Bengal, India, Dr. Sumit Sethi, MBBS, MD, DNB,
DermaStation, Janakpuri, New Delhi, India.
Description: First edition. | Boca Raton : CRC Press, 2021. | Summary:
"This concise text from an internationally respected editor presents the
most important points about the most important topics in disease of the
skin, hair, and nails; any medical professional will find here the
material for a solid grounding in the subject"-- Provided by publisher.
Identifiers: LCCN 2020049387 (print) | LCCN 2020049388 (ebook) | ISBN
9780367533656 (hardback) | ISBN 9780367533625 (paperback) | ISBN
9781003081609 (ebook)
Subjects: LCSH: Dermatology. | Skin--Diseases.
Classification: LCC RL72 .C57 2021 (print) | LCC RL72 (ebook) | DDC
616.5--dc23
LC record available at https://lccn.loc.gov/2020049387
LC ebook record available at https://lccn.loc.gov/2020049388

ISBN: 978-0-367-53365-6 (hbk)
ISBN: 978-0-367-53362-5 (pbk)
ISBN: 978-1-003-08160-9 (ebk)

Typeset in Times New Roman
by MPS Limited, Dehradun

Contents

Contributors

Dr Pooja Agarwal, MD, Assistant Professor, Department of Skin & Venereal Disease, Smt NHL Municipal Medical College, Ahmedabad, Gujarat, India

Dr Shruti Barde, MBBS, DCD, MSc (Aesthetic Medicine), Founder & CEO, Studio SkinQ, Mumbai, Maharashtra, India

Dr Yasmeen Jabeen Bhat, MD, FACP, Associate Professor Department of Dermatology, Venereology, & Leprosy Government Medical College, Srinagar J&K, India

Dr Aparajita Ghosh, MD, Associate Professor, Dermatology, KPC Medical College and Hospital, Kolkata, West Bengal, India

Dr Soumya Jagadeesan, MD, Associate Professor, Amrita Institute of Medical Sciences and Research Centre, Kochi, Kerala, India

Dr Shankila Mittal, MD, DNB, Dermatology, Senior Resident, Safdarjung Hospital, Delhi, India

Dr Isha Narang, MD, DNB, MRCP (SCE) Dermatology, Specialist Registrar, Dermatology University Hospitals of Derby and Burton, United Kingdom

Dr Shekhar Neema, MD, DNB, MRCP (SCE) Dermatology, Associate Professor, Department of Dermatology, Armed Forces Medical College, Pune, Maharashtra, India

Dr Indrashis Podder, MD, DNB, Assistant Professor, Department of Dermatology, College of Medicine and Sagore Dutta Hospital, West Bengal, India

1

An introduction to skin and skin disease

Rashmi Sarkar
Anupam Das

An overview

The skin is an extraordinary structure. It has a surface area of 2 m^2 and accounts for 16–20% of the total body weight. It is made up of several types of tissues that work in harmony with one another (Figure 1.1). The large number of cell types and functions of the skin and its proximity to numerous potentially damaging stimuli in the outside environment result in two important consequences. The first is that the skin is frequently damaged because it is right in the 'line of fire', and the second is that each of the various cell types that it contains can 'go wrong' and develop degenerative and neoplastic disorders. Knowledge of the structure and functions of the skin is important for the clinician to diagnose and treat dermatological conditions.

Skin diseases are quite common, and almost every individual suffers from skin disease at least once in his or her lifetime. Atopic dermatitis affects about 15% of the people under the age of 12, while psoriasis affects 1–2%. Other conditions that affect a significant number of people are viral warts, seborrhoeic warts, and solar keratoses. It should be noted that 10–15% of the family physician's work is with skin disorders, and that skin diseases are the second most common cause of time taken away from work. Although skin diseases are not uncommon at any age, they are particularly frequent among the elderly. The older one gets, the greater the risk of developing skin disease.

Skin disorders are not usually fatal but can cause considerable discomfort and disability. The disability caused can be physical, emotional, and socioeconomic. Patients receive help when their problems and disabilities are acknowledged and their physician makes attempts to address their various problems.

Skin structure and function

It is difficult to understand abnormal skin and its vagaries without understanding the composition and function of normal skin. Although, at the first glance, the skin may appear quite complicated, a slightly deeper look shows that there is an elegant logic behind its architecture, which helps it perform several vital functions. The skin is composed of epithelial and adipose tissues. The epithelial tissue comprises the epidermis and the dermis. The adipose tissue, on the other hand, contains the hypodermis. The accessory structures include hairs, nails, sebaceous, sweat glands, sensory receptors, etc.

The skin surface

The skin surface is a barrier between living processes and the potentially injurious outside world. Thus it plays the important role of preventing and controlling interactions between the outside and the constant

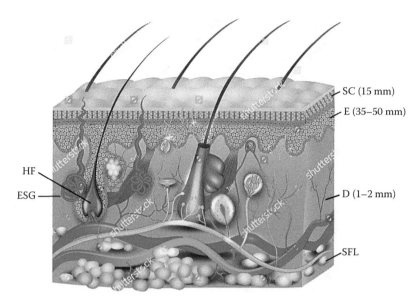

FIGURE 1.1   Structure of the skin: HF, hair follicle; ESG, eccrine sweat gland; SC, stratum corneum (15 mm); E, epidermis (35–50 mm); GCL, granular cell layer; ML, Malpighian layer; BL, basal layer; D, dermis (1–2 mm); SFL, subcutaneous fat layer.

and vulnerable inside. Its 2 m^2 area is modified regionally, which enables it to better perform particular functions. The skin on the limbs and the trunk is very much the same, but the skin on the palms and soles, facial skin, scalp skin, and genital skin differ somewhat in structure and function. The surface is thrown up into a number of intersecting ridges, which make rhomboidal patterns. There are 'pores' at regular intervals opening onto the surface – these are the openings of the eccrine sweat glands. The diameter of these openings is approximately 25 μm, and there are approximately 150–350 duct openings per square centimetre (cm^2). The hair follicle openings can also be seen at the skin surface and the diameter of these orifices and the numbers per cm^2 vary greatly between anatomical regions. A close inspection of the follicular opening reveals a distinctive arrangement of the stratum corneum cells around the orifice.

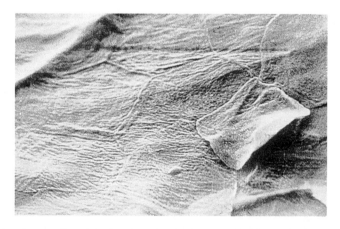

FIGURE 1.2   Scanning electron micrograph of stratum corneum shows a corneocyte in the process of desquamation (from Marks and Motley, Common Skin Diseases, 18th edition, with permission).

At magnifications of 500–1000 times, which is possible with scanning electron microscopy (SEM), individual horn cells (corneocytes) can be seen in the process of desquamation (Figure 1.2). Corneocytes are approximately 35 μm in diameter, 1 μm thick and shield-like in shape.

The stratum corneum

Also known as the horny layer, this structure is the differentiated end-product of epidermal metabolism (also known as differentiation or keratinization); the final step in differentiation is the dropping off of individual corneocytes in the process of desquamation seen in Figure 1.2. The stratum corneum is composed of 20–25 layers of cornified cells (keratinocytes), which appear as flat cells and do not possess any nuclei or cytoplasmic organelles. The keratinocytes contain soft keratin. Lamellar bodies are important structures present around these keratinocytes. Lipids are released from the lamellar bodies, and these lipids contribute to the permeability of stratum corneum.

The corneocytes are joined together by the lipid and glycoprotein of the intercellular cement material and by the vestiges of the desmosomes that are well developed in the keratinocytes of the epidermis (see later). In the stratum corneum, they are known as 'corneo-desmosomes'. The orderly release of corneocytes at the surface in the process of desquamation is not completely characterized, but it appears to depend on the dissolution of the corneo-desmosomes near the surface by a cascade of enzymes, their activators, and inhibitors, known collectively as 'chymotrypsin', which is activated by the presence of moisture. On limb and trunk skin, the stratum corneum is some 15–20 cells thick and, as each corneocyte is about 1 μm thick, it is about 15–20 μm thick in absolute terms. The stratum corneum of the palms and soles is about 0.5 μm thick and is, of course, much thicker than that on the trunk and limbs.

The stratum corneum prevents water loss, and when it is deranged, as, for example, in psoriasis or eczema, water loss is greatly increased so that severe dehydration can occur if enough skin is affected. It has been estimated that a patient with erythrodermic psoriasis (involvement of more than 90% body surface area) may lose 6 L of water per day through the disordered stratum corneum, in contrast to 0.5 L lost normally per day.

The stratum corneum also acts as a barrier to the penetration of chemical agents with which the skin comes into contact with it. It prevents systemic poisoning from skin contact, although it must be realized that it is not a complete barrier and percutaneous penetration of most agents does occur at a very slow rate. Those responsible for formulating drugs in topical formulations are well aware of this rate-limiting property for percutaneous penetration of the stratum corneum and try to find agents that accelerate the movement of drugs into the skin. In recent years, as more knowledge has been acquired about the penetrability of the stratum corneum and the pharmacokinetics of drugs, techniques have been developed for the administration of drugs systemically via the skin – the transdermal route.

The barrier properties also prevent microbial life invading into the skin; however, the barrier properties are not perfect, and, occasionally, pathogen gains entry via hair follicles or small cracks and fissures and causes infection. Antimicrobial peptides – the cathelicidins – also play an important role and some function at the stratum corneum level.

The structure of the stratum corneum is very extensible and compliant in health, permitting movement of the hands and feet, and is actually quite tough, thus providing a degree of mechanical protection against minor penetrative injury. The ability to extend is greatly aided by the system of skin surface markings (varying by the region sampled), which take the form of rectangles and behave like 'concertinas' when stretched. The various functions of the skin have been summarized in Table 1.1.

The epidermis

The epidermis mainly contains keratinocytes; but it also contains non-keratinocytes – melanocytes and Langerhans cells, both of which possess dendrites. This cellular structure is some three to five cell-layers thick, on average, 35–50 μm thick in absolute terms. Not unexpectedly, the epidermis is about two to three times thicker on the hands and feet, particularly the palms and soles. The epidermis is indented by finger-like projections from the dermis known as the dermal papillae and rests on a complex

TABLE 1.1

Functions of the skin

Barrier function

- Permeability barrier to water and electrolytes
- Prevention of entry of microbes and chemicals
- Protection from ultraviolet rays
- Prevention of injury due to blunt objects

Maintenance of body temperature

Sensory functions

- Mechanoreceptors (touch, vibration, pressure)
- Thermoreceptors (heat and cold)
- Nociceptors (pain and itch)
- Free nerve endings
- Corpuscular receptors

Immunological functions

Synthesis of vitamin D and E

Transport of nutrients and metabolites

Sexual attraction

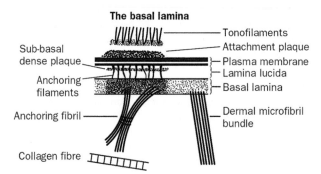

FIGURE 1.3   The junctional zone between epidermis and dermis (from Marks and Motley, Common Skin Diseases, 18E, with permission).

junctional zone that consists of a basal lamina and a condensation of dermal connective tissue (Figure 1.3).

The cells of the epidermis are mainly keratinocytes containing keratin tonofilaments, which originate in the basal generative compartment and ascend through the Malpighian layer to the granular cell layer. The keratin tonofilaments belong to the group of subcellular structures known as intermediate filaments. They consist of polypeptides and their molecular weight ranges from 40 to 65 kD. It is thought that they provide a semi-rigid endoskeleton, and because of their connection to the desmosomal apparatus, they give strength to the epidermis as a whole. They are joined to the neighbouring keratinocytes by specialized junctions known as desmosomes. These are visible as 'prickles' in formalin-fixed sections but as alternating light and dark bands when viewed by transmission electron microscopy. In the granular layer, they transform from a plump oval or rectangular shape to a more flattened profile and lose their nucleus and cytoplasmic organelles. In addition, they develop basophilic granules containing a histidine-rich protein known as filaggrin and minute, lipid-containing, membrane-bound structures known as membrane-coating granules of lamellar bodies.

These alterations are part of the process of keratinization, during which the keratinocytes differentiate into tough, disc-shaped corneocytes. Other changes include a reduction in water content from 70% in the keratinocytes to 30% in the stratum corneum, and the laying down of a chemically resistant, cross-linked protein band at the periphery of the corneocyte. This protein band is made up of the polypeptides involucrin, loricrin, and cornifin. The peptides are cross-linked by gamma-glutamyl transpeptidase. Of major importance to the barrier function of the stratum corneum is the intercellular lipid which, unlike the phospholipid of the epidermis below, is mainly polar ceramide and derives from the minute lamellar bodies of the granular cell layer.

It takes about 28 days for a new keratinocyte to ascend through the epidermis and stratum corneum and desquamate off at the skin surface. This process is greatly accelerated in some inflammatory skin disorders, notably psoriasis. Desquamation occurs by the loss of single corneocytes at the skin surface. This process depends on the dissolution of the desmosomes by the action of chymotryptases, which become activated near the surface.

Pigment-producing cells

Black pigment (melanin), a polymer synthesized by melanocytes, protects against solar ultraviolet radiation (UVR). Melanocytes, unlike keratinocytes, do not have desmosomes but have long, branching dendritic projections that transport the melanin they synthesize to the surrounding cells. They originate from the embryonic neural crest. Melanocytes account for 5–10% of cells in the basal layer of the epidermis. Melanin is a polymer that is synthesized from the amino acid tyrosine with the help of a copper-containing enzyme, tyrosinase. Other pigments contribute rarely (e.g. bilirubin in jaundice or pigments derived from drugs such as minocycline or chlorpromazine). Exposure to the sun accelerates melanin synthesis, which explains suntanning. Skin color is mainly due to melanin and blood. The number of melanocytes per unit of body surface area is variable, depending on the site of the body but the density of melanocytes is the same in all humans, irrespective of race. The racial differences in complexion are attributed to the distribution and size of melanosomes, which disperse melanin to the keratinocytes. Melanocytes are completely destroyed in vitiligo. In albinism, melanin synthesis is defective. Localized increase in the synthesis of melanin leads to the development of freckles. Melanocytes in benign proliferation are referred to as nevi, and the malignant ones are known as melanomas.

Langerhans cells

Langerhans cells are also dendritic cells but are found within the body of the epidermis in the Malpighian layer rather than in the basal layer. They constitute 2–8% of the total epidermal cell population. They derive from the reticuloendothelial system and have the function of picking up 'foreign' material and presenting it to lymphocytes in the early stages of a delayed hypersensitivity reaction. They are reduced in number after exposure to solar UVR, partially accounting for the depressed delayed hypersensitivity reaction in chronically sun-exposed skin. Additionally, the number of Langerhans cells is also reduced in psoriasis, sarcoidosis, contact dermatitis, etc.

Merkel cells

These are slow-adapting mechanoreceptors located in the basal layer of the epidermis. They are found in digits, lips, oral cavity, and hair follicles. They have important clinical bearing because of the association with the development of Merkel cell carcinoma and neuroendocrine carcinoma.

The junctional zone

The junctional zone has considerable functional importance and is vital to understanding the pathophysiology of bullous disorders and many other skin diseases. Figure 1.3 shows the main components of the junctional zone. Desmosomal processes from the basal keratinocytes, known as hemidesmosomes, are inserted into an electron-dense lamina (basal lamina). Below the electron-dense lamina, there is an electron-lucent area (lamina lucida). The dermoepidermal junction is important from the clinical point of view. When the component molecules do not function properly, the adhesive property of the junction is lost and this leads to numerous bullous diseases, including bullous pemphigoid, cicatricial pemphigoid, linear IgA disease, pemphigoid gestationis, epidermolysis bullosa acquisita, etc.

The dermis

The tissues of the dermis beneath the epidermis are important in giving mechanical protection to the underlying body parts and in binding together all the superficial structures. It is composed primarily of tough, fibrous collagen and a network of fibres of elastic tissue, as well as the vascular channels and nerve fibres of the skin. The dermis is thinnest in the eyelids and thickest on the back. It contributes to 15–20% of the total body weight. There are about 20 different types of collagen, but the adult dermis is made up mainly of types I and III, whereas type IV is a major constituent of the basal lamina of the dermoepidermal junction. Type V collagen is found in papillary dermis and periadnexal areas. Type VI collagen is present throughout the dermis and interfibrillar spaces. Type VII collagen is present in the anchoring fibrils of the dermoepidermal junction. Between the fibres of collagen is a matrix composed mainly of proteoglycan in which there are scattered fibroblasts that synthesize all the dermal components. Collagen bundles are composed of polypeptide chains arranged in a triple-helix format, in which hydroxyproline forms an important constituent amino acid. The important cells of the dermis are fibroblasts, monocytes, macrophages, dendrocytes, and mast cells.

The dermal vasculature

There are no blood vessels in the epidermis and the necessary oxygen and nutrients diffuse from the capillaries in the dermal papillae. These capillaries arise from horizontally arranged plexuses in the dermis. There are tiny arteriovenous shunts in the fingertips and other acral sites, which are referred to as glomus bodies. Their walls contain abundant plain muscle. The glomus bodies are specially designed for thermoregulation. The small lymphatic channels follow the blood capillaries but are distinguishable by the thin delicate lymphatic endothelium. Defective cutaneous vasculature is seen in Klippel–Trenaunay syndrome, Sturge–Weber syndrome, hereditary lymphedema, etc.

Nerve structures

Recently, very fine nerve fibres have been identified in the epidermis, but most of the fibres run alongside the blood vessels in the dermal papillae and deeper in the dermis. There are several types of specialized sensory receptor in the upper dermis that detect particular sensations. Free nerve endings perceive touch, temperature, pain, and itch. Pacinian corpuscles respond to deep pressure and vibrations. Other sensory receptors include Golgi-Mazzoni corpuscles, Krause end bulbs, Meissner's corpuscle (responding to dynamic pressure), Ruffini corpuscles (responding to stretching of the skin), and mucocutaneous end organs.

The adnexal structures

The skin possesses specialized epidermal structures that can be regarded as invaginations of the surface that are embedded in the dermis. These are the hair follicles and the eccrine and apocrine sweat glands.

Hair follicles

Hair follicles are arranged all over the skin surface apart from the palms and soles, the genital mucosa, and the vermilion of the lips. Hair growth is asynchronous in humans but synchronous in many other mammals. The hair follicles have a gland attached to them known as the sebaceous gland. The hair

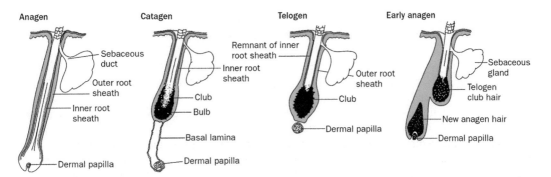

FIGURE 1.4   The hair cycle.

shaft, the canal along which the shaft tracks to the surface, the hair matrix which produces the hair shaft and sebaceous gland are together known as the pilosebaceous unit. The pilosebaceous units vary greatly in size. In some areas (e.g. the face) the hair shafts are small and the sebaceous glands quite large. These are known as sebaceous follicles and have importance in the pathogenesis of acne.

The different phases of our asynchronous hair growth occur independently in individual follicles but are timed to occur together in synchronous hair growth, accounting for the phenomenon of moulting in small, furry mammals. The phase of hair growth (anagen) is the longest phase of the hair cycle. A short transition stage (catagen) is then reached. This is followed by a resting phase (telogen), which is followed by anagen again somewhat later (Figure 1.4).

The hair shaft grows from highly active, modified epidermal tissue known as the hair matrix. The shaft traverses the hair follicle canal, which is made up of a series of investing epidermal sheaths, the most prominent of which is the external root sheath (Figure 1.5). The whole follicular structure is nourished by a small, indenting cellular and vascular connective tissue papilla, which pokes into the base of the matrix. The sebaceous gland secretes into the hair canal a lipid-rich substance known as sebum, whose function is to lubricate the hair. Sebum contains triglycerides, cholesterol esters, wax

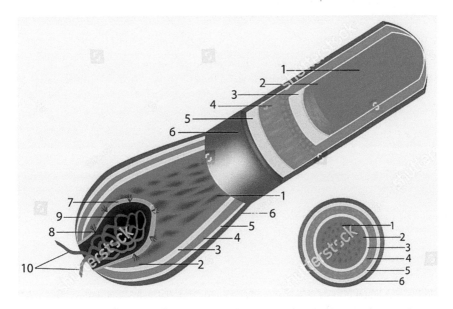

FIGURE 1.5   Components of a hair follicle: 1, medulla; 2, cortex; 3, cuticle of the hair; epithelial root sheath: 4, internal root sheath, 5, external root sheath, 6, dermal root sheath; 7, hair matrix; 8, melanocyte; 9, papilla of the hair; 10, blood vessels.

esters, and squalene. Hair growth and sebum secretion are mainly under the control of androgens, although other physiological variables may also influence these functions.

Eccrine sweat glands

The eccrine sweat glands are an extremely important part of the body's homeothermic mechanism in that the sweat secretion evaporates from the skin surface to produce a cooling effect. Apart from heat, eccrine sweat secretion may also be stimulated by emotional factors and by fear and anxiety. Certain body sites, such as the palms, soles, forehead, axillae and inguinal regions, secrete sweat selectively during emotional stimulation. They are present everywhere in the skin except vermilion border of lips, nail bed, external auditory canal, clitoris, and labia minora.

The eccrine sweat glands consist of a coiled secretory portion deep in the dermis next to the subcutaneous fat and a long, straight, tubular duct whose final portion is coiled and penetrates the epidermis to drain at the sweat pore on the surface. The gland and its duct are lined by a single layer of secretory cells and surrounded by myoepithelial cells. The secretion of eccrine sweat glands is basically an aqueous solution of electrolytes. The disturbance in basic pathophysiology of sweat formation and secretion leads to hyperhidrosis and hypohidrosis.

Apocrine sweat glands

The apocrine sweat glands drain directly into hair follicles. They are found in axillae, areolae, periumbilical areas, prepuce, mons pubis, labia minora, etc. Modified apocrine glands include ceruminous glands of the ear, Moll's glands on eyelids, and mammary glands. They are larger than eccrine sweat glands and the secretion is completely different, being semi-solid and containing odiferous materials that are thought to have the function of sexual attraction.

2

Signs and symptoms of skin disease

Anupam Das
Rashmi Sarkar

Skin disorders may be generalized, localized to one or several sites of abnormality known as 'lesions', or eruptive, in which case, many lesions appear as spots over the skin. Currently, there are no adequate explanations for the distribution of skin lesions in case of most disorders, such as psoriasis or atopic dermatitis.

Any widespread abnormality of the skin may also affect the scalp, the mucosae of the mouth, nose, eyes, and genitalia, and the nail-forming tissues, and it is important to inspect these sites whenever possible during the examination of the skin.

The examination of skin revolves around certain terms that are very distinct from one another, and the knowledge of these terms is quintessential to describing any dermatological entity. The basic lesions of the skin are classified into three categories: primary, secondary, and special lesions. Primary lesions are basically the original lesions of disease and need to be identified accurately in order to diagnose a condition. Secondary lesions are produced as a result of trauma, itching, application of topical medications, etc.

Primary lesions

- Macule: circumscribed flat lesions less than 0.5 cm in diameter, without any elevation or depression from the surrounding skin, e.g. vitiligo, leprosy, pityriasis versicolor, melasma (Figure 2.1)
- Patch: circumscribed flat lesions more than 0.5 cm in diameter, without any elevation or depression from the surrounding skin, e.g. port wine stain, leprosy, vitiligo, fixed drug rash (Figure 2.2)
- Papule: circumscribed solid elevated lesions less than 0.5 cm in diameter, e.g. acne, milium, molluscum contagiosum, lichen planus, xanthoma, angiokeratoma (Figure 2.3)
- Plaque: circumscribed solid elevated lesions more than 0.5 cm in diameter, with a width greater than the height, e.g. psoriasis, lupus vulgaris, chromoblastomycosis, cutaneous T cell lymphoma (Figure 2.4)
- Nodule: circumscribed solid lesions more than 0.5 cm in diameter, with a depth greater than the width (i.e., it has a definite palpable depth), e.g. leprosy, neurofibroma, nodulocystic acne, xanthoma disseminatum (Figure 2.5)
- Tumor: soft to firm, fixed or mobile lesion of more than 2 cm diameter, e.g. neurofibroma, lipoma, fibrolipoma (Figure 2.6)
- Vesicle: circumscribed fluid-filled lesion of less than 0.5 cm diameter, e.g. herpes simplex, varicella, herpes zoster, pompholyx, contact dermatitis (Figure 2.7)
- Bulla: circumscribed fluid-filled lesion of more than 0.5 cm diameter, e.g. pemphigus vulgaris, bullous pemphigoid, bullous drug reaction, friction blister (Figure 2.8)
- Pustule: circumscribed lesion of less than 0.5 cm diameter, containing purulent material (pus), e.g. acne, impetigo, pustular psoriasis, acropustulosis (Figure 2.9)
- Wheal: circumscribed edematous evanescent plateau-like elevations of skin, e.g. urticaria, bullous pemphigoid, urticarial vasculitis

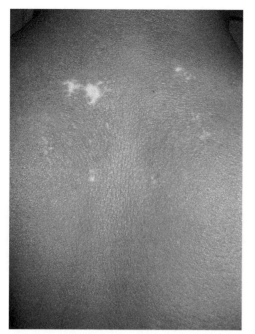

FIGURE 2.1   Macules in vitiligo.

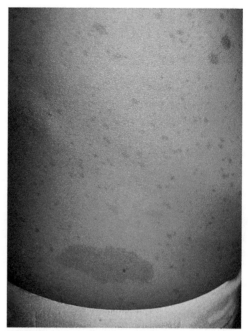

FIGURE 2.2   Café-au-lait macules and patches in neurofibromatosis.

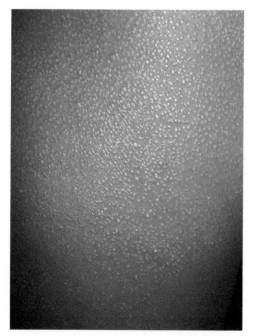

FIGURE 2.3   Discrete papules in lichen nitidus.

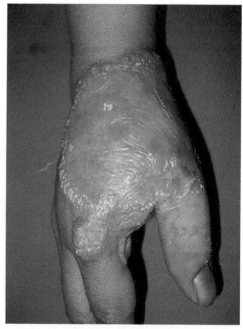

FIGURE 2.4   Plaque in lupus vulgaris.

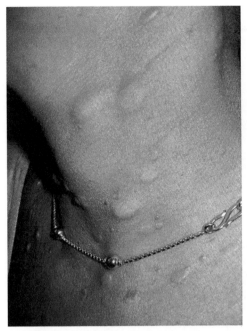

FIGURE 2.5   Nodular lesions in steatocystoma.

Secondary lesions

- Scale: visible exfoliation of the skin, e.g. psoriasis, pityriasis versicolor, exfoliative dermatitis, seborrhoeic dermatitis, ichthyosis (Figure 2.10)
- Crust: dried serum, pus, or blood admixed with epithelial debris, e.g. impetigo, favus, burns
- Excoriation: linear excavation produced as a result of severe itching and scratching, e.g. scabies, prurigo simplex, neurotic excoriation (Figure 2.11)
- Fissure: well-defined linear cleft in the epidermis, e.g. fissured sole, chapped lips (Figure 2.12)
- Erosion: loss of superficial epidermis as a result of a primary insult, heals without scarring, e.g. impetigo, herpes simples, varicella
- Ulcer: localized defect in the skin due to loss of epidermis and a part of the dermis, heals with scarring, e.g. venous ulcer, arterial ulcer, decubitus ulcer, pyoderma gangrenosum

Special lesions

- Comedone: white or black plugs of sebaceous and keratinous material impacted within the pilosebaceous follicle, e.g. acne, senile comedone (Figure 2.13)
- Burrow: serpiginous tunnel in the stratum corneum, e.g. scabies, larva migrans
- Telangiectasia: permanent superficial dilatation of capillaries, e.g. steroid abuse, discoid lupus erythematosus, scleroderma

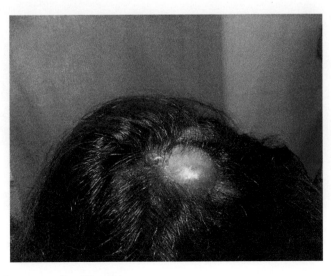

FIGURE 2.6   Tumor in cutaneous B cell lymphoma.

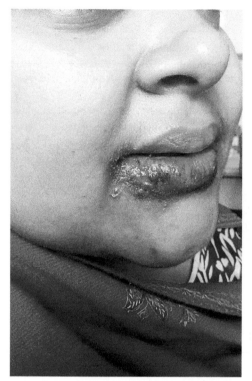

FIGURE 2.7 Grouped vesicles in herpes labialis.

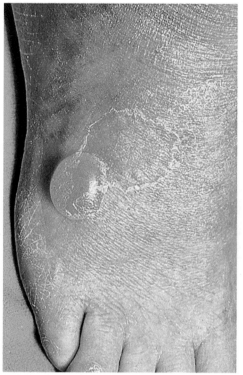

FIGURE 2.8 Bullous lesion in senile pemphigoid [from Marks and Motley, 18th edition].

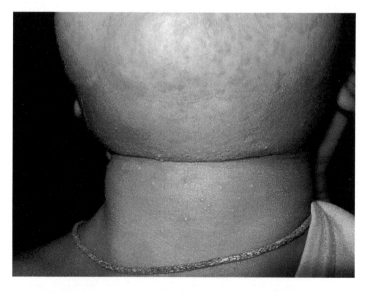

FIGURE 2.9 Pustules in miliaria pustulosa.

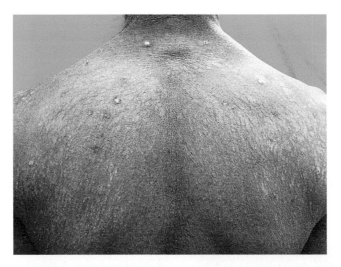

FIGURE 2.10   Furfuraceous scaling in pityriasis versicolor.

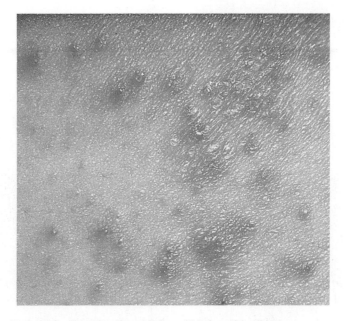

FIGURE 2.11   Excoriated papules in prurigo (from Marks and Motley, 18th edition).

- Milium: small superficial cysts with an epidermal lining, e.g. primary milia, epidermolysis bullosa dystrophica, porphyria cutanea tarda
- Lichenification: a combination of thick skin, increased skin markings, and hyperpigmentation, e.g. lichen simplex chronicus (Figure 2.14)
- Poikiloderma: combination of hypopigmentation, hyperpigmentation, telangiectasia, and atrophy, e.g. cutaneous T cell lymphoma, dermatomyositis, radiation dermatitis

Alterations in skin color

The color of normal skin is dependent on melanin pigment production and the blood supply. The color may also be altered by various exogenous or endogenous pigments. One of the most common accompaniments of skin disease is redness or erythema.

Erythema

The degree of erythema depends on the degree of oxygenation of the blood, its rate of flow and the site, and the number and size of the skin's blood vessels. Different disorders tend to be associated with particular shades of red due to characteristic alterations in the blood vessels and surrounding tissues.

- Psoriatic plaques: dark red (Figure 2.15)
- Lichen planus: mauve hue
- Dermatomyositis: the color of the heliotrope flower (Figure 2.16)

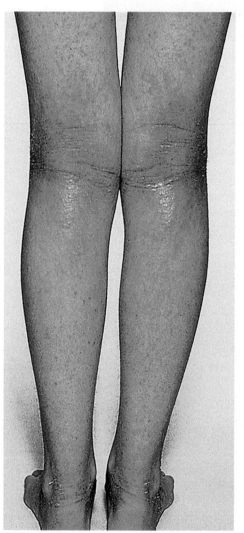

FIGURE 2.12 Painful fissures in popliteal fossa in atopic dermatitis (from Marks and Motley, 18th edition).

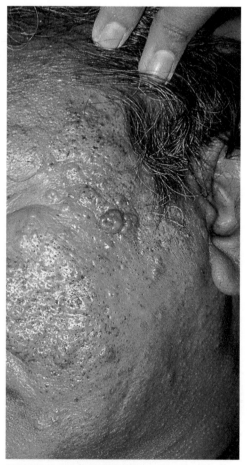

FIGURE 2.13 Senile comedones.

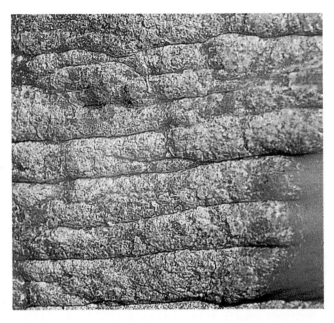

FIGURE 2.14   Lichenification with scaling and accentuation of skin markings (from Marks and Motley, 18th edition).

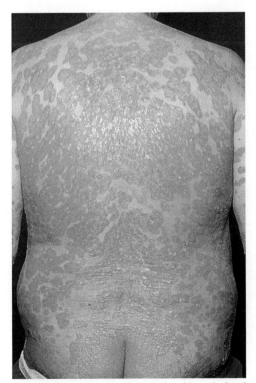

FIGURE 2.15   Plaques of psoriasis with typical red color (from Marks and Motley, 18th edition).

Brown–black pigmentation

The degree of brown–black pigmentation depends on the activity of melanocytes. It also depends on the size of the granules and the distribution of the pigment particles within the epidermal cells. Shedding of the pigment from damaged keratinocytes into the dermis is known as pigmentary incontinence and causes a kind of tattooing in which the dusky pigment produced persists for many weeks, months, or even years, usually in macrophages.

- Brown pigmentation: caused by a breakdown product of blood (haemosiderin), when this has leaked into the tissues (Figure 2.17)
- Brown–black discoloration of the skin over cartilaginous structures: alkaptonuria (Osler's sign), due to deposition of homogentisic acid
- Dark brown pigmentation of acne scars or of areas on the limbs: minocycline
- Generalized darkening of the skin: may be more pronounced in the flexures in Addison's disease, results from increased secretion of melanocyte-stimulating hormone and the consequent activation of the

melanocytes to produce more pigment; darkening of the palmar creases and mucosae may be seen as well

- White color: vitiligo, albinism, leukoderma, etc.

Symptoms of skin disease

Skin disease causes pruritus (itching), pain, soreness and discomfort, difficulty with movements of the hands and fingers, cosmetic disability, etc.

Pruritus

Itching is the classic symptom of skin disorders, but it may also occur in the apparent absence of skin disease. Any skin abnormality can give rise to irritation, but some, such as scabies, seem particularly capable of causing severe pruritus. Most scabies patients complain that their symptom of itching is much worse at night when they are warm. Itching in atopic dermatitis, senile pruritus, and senile xerosis is made worse by repeated bathing and vigorous towelling afterwards, as well as by central heating and air conditioning with low relative humidity. Clothing made from rough fabrics often aggravates itching – woollen garments are notorious for this problem and patients should be advised to wear only smooth, silky garments next to the skin. If pruritus is made worse by aspirin or food additives such as tartrazine, sodium benzoate, or cinnamates, it is quite likely that urticaria is to blame.

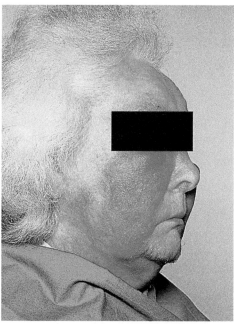

FIGURE 2.16   Reddened areas on the face in derma-tomyositis, showing typical heliotrope discoloration (from Marks and Motley, 18th edition).

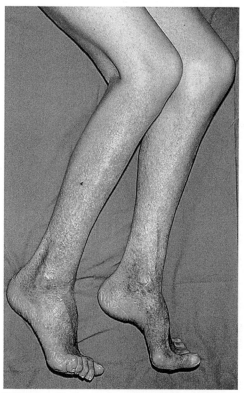

FIGURE 2.17   Lower legs of a patient with chronic venous hypertension and brown pigmentation due to hemosiderin deposits (from Marks and Motley, 18th edition).

Persistent severe pruritus can be the most disabling and distressing symptom and is quite difficult to treat. Scratching provides partial and transient relief from the symptom and it is fruitless to request that the patient stops scratching. Scratching itself causes damage to the skin surface, which is visible as scratch marks (excoriations). In some patients, the repeated scratching and rubbing cause lichenification and in others, prurigo papules occur. Occasionally, the scratch marks become infected. Uncommonly, the underlying disorder occurs at the site of the injury from the scratch. This phenomenon is found in patients with psoriasis and lichen planus and is known as the isomorphic response or the Koebner phenomenon. Uncommonly, infection may be spread by scratching and lines of viral warts or molluscum contagiosa may develop in excoriations.

Painful skin disorders

Most skin disorders do not give rise to pain. The notable exception to this is herpes zoster, which may cause pain and distorted sensations in the nerve root involved. The pain may be present before the skin lesions appear, while they are there and, occasionally, afterwards. Pain and tenderness are characteristic of acutely inflamed lesions such as boils, acne cysts, cellulitis, and erythema nodosum. Most skin tumors are not painful, at least until they enlarge and infiltrate nerves. However, there are some benign tumors that cause pain like blue rubber bleb nevus, leiomyoma, eccrine spiradenoma, neuroma, dermatofibroma, angiolipoma, neurilemmoma, endometrioma, glomus tumor, granular cell tumor, etc.

Chronic ulcers are often 'sore' and cause a variety of other discomforts, but they are not often the cause of severe pain. When they do give rise to severe pain, ischaemia is usually the cause. Painful fissures in the palms and soles develop in patches of eczema and psoriasis due to the inelastic, abnormal, horny layer in these conditions.

Disabilities from skin disease

Patients with skin disease may experience a surprising degree of disability. A very major cause of disability is the abnormal appearance of the affected skin. For reasons that are not altogether clear, there is a primitive fear of diseased skin, which even amounts to feelings of disgust and revulsion. The idea of touching skin that is scaling or exudative seems inherently distasteful and it is something that most try to avoid. It is little use pointing out that there is no rational basis for these attitudes, and all that can be hoped for is that a mixture of comprehension, compassion, and common sense, eventually tinged with pragmatism, supplants a primitive revulsion based on the contagious nature of leprosy and the infestations of scabies and lice. It is only too abundantly evident that individuals with obvious skin disease have social problems: they not only suffer more unemployment overall but also find great difficulty in obtaining positions that require any kind of interpersonal relationships.

Young patients with acne have particular problems because the disease is visible, as it usually affects the face. Psoriasis quite often affects the hands, nails, and scalp margin, also causing difficulty for those whose occupations put them into contact with the public. Numerous other skin disorders put the affected individual at an economic and social disadvantage. Vascular birthmarks and large neurofibromas are disfiguring and tend to isolate the bearers. Chronic inflammatory facial disorders, such as rosacea and discoid lupus erythematosus, also cause problems (Figure 2.18).

To summarize this point, individuals with visibly disordered skin are disabled because of society's inherent avoidance reaction. Another aspect of this problem is the sufferer's own perception of the impact they are making on all with whom they come in contact. Most individuals who have persistent, 'unsightly' skin problems become depressed and isolated. Skin problems are especially damaging for those in their late teens and twenties who are desperately trying to make relationships at a time when self-confidence is not at a high point; a disfiguring skin disorder lowers self-esteem further. Many youngsters with acne and psoriasis find it difficult to conquer their embarrassment sufficiently to have romantic partners, and that aspect of their development may become stunted. It was once thought that

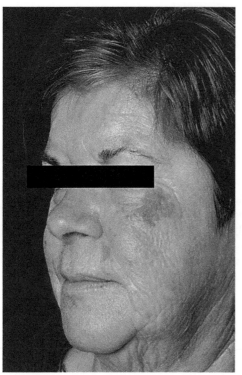

FIGURE 2.18   Plaques of erythema, scaling and hyperkeratosis in a man with discoid lupus erythematosus (from Marks and Motley, 18th edition).

many skin disorders were caused by neurotic traits, 'stress', and personality diseases; it is now increasingly appreciated that skin disorders themselves often cause depression, anxiety, and stress.

Skin disease can be enormously physically disabling when it affects the palms or soles. Although the areas affected only occupy about 1–2% of the body skin surface, disease of these sites may prevent walking or even standing and use of the hands for anything but simple tasks, i.e. they are virtually completely disabled. Psoriasis and eczema are the usual causes of this form of disablement because of the painful fissures that tend to develop in these conditions. Patients with severe atopic dermatitis may develop similar painful fissures around the popliteal and antecubital fossae, so that limb movements become extremely painful. Those with severe congenital disorders of keratinization are often severely troubled by this disordered mobility.

From what has been said so far, it will be appreciated that, contrary to popular belief, patients with skin disorders are often appreciably disabled. They are disabled on account of society's and their own reaction to the appearance of their skin disease and because of the physical limitations that the skin disease puts on them. Skin disease occasionally kills but often produces much unhappiness, usually through loss of work and social and emotional deprivation, as well as considerable physical discomfort.

To summarize, it is crucial to meticulously examine each and every patient with a dermatological problem because, in this era of technologies and investigations, dermatology is the only specialty where the clinicians rely on their eyes and examination skills to diagnose a disease and, fortunately, the need to go for investigations is negligible.

3

Skin infections

Shankila Mittal
Rashmi Sarkar

The skin surface and its adnexal structures harbor many commensal organisms, including Gram-positive cocci (*Staphylococcus epidermidis*, coagulase-negative staphylococci), Gram-positive lipophilic microaerophilic rods (*Propionibacterium acnes*), and a Gram-positive yeast-like organism (*Malassezia furfur*). However, under special conditions – e.g., excess sebum secretion, depressed immunity, and compromised stratum corneum barrier protection – they can cause disease. Additionally, various pathogenic microorganisms can cause skin infection, especially when the skin barrier is disrupted.

Fungal diseases of the skin

Superficial mycoses

Superficial mycoses are limited to the outermost layer of the skin, hair, nails, and are classified as:

* Pityriasis versicolor
* Dermatophytosis
* Tinea nigra
* Black piedra
* White piedra
* Otomycosis
* Onychomycosis
* Superficial mycosis by other non-dermatophytic moulds
* Cutaneous and mucocutaneous candidiasis

Pityriasis versicolor

Incidence

Very common in the tropics. Most commonly seen in adolescence and young adulthood.

Pathogenesis

Lipophilic yeasts, *Pityrosporum orbiculare* (round form) and *Pityrosporum ovale* (oval form) (now invalid and reclassified as *Malassezia),* are normal inhabitants of the skin. *M. sympodialis, M. globosa, M. restricta, M. slooffiae, M. furfur, M. obtusa, M. dermatis, M. japonica, M. yamotoensis, M. nana, M. caprae, M. equina,* and *M. cuniculi* are the different species identified by genetic analysis. These organisms change from the saprophytic spore form to the pathogenic hyphae form by heightened rates of sebum secretion or depressed immunity. Depigmentation is due to the azelaic acid produced by *Malassezia,* which inhibits tyrosinase activity when activated by sunlight.

Risk factors

Pregnancy, malnutrition, immunosuppression, oral contraception, excess heat, and humidity (heavy clothing with perspiration).

Clinical features

- Morphology: lesions are characterized by discrete or confluent, scaly, discolored, or depigmented areas, mainly on the upper trunk.
- Site: the trunk is the most common site; other sites include the face, upper arm, and groin (Figure 3.1). Facial lesions are more common in children.
- In the untanned white skin, the affected areas appear darker than normal, but they fail to respond to light exposure; in the suntanned subject, the affected skin is usually paler, as it usually is in black people. Lesions may sometimes show some degree of atrophy.

Differential diagnosis

Vitiligo, secondary syphilis, pityriasis alba, seborrheic dermatitis, and pityriasis rosea.

Investigations

Diagnosis is primarily clinical and is confirmed by demonstrating the hyphae and spores of *Malassezia furfur* using 10% potassium hydroxide. Large, blunt hyphae and thick-walled, budding spores forming a 'spaghetti and meatballs' appearance can be observed under the low power lens of a microscope.

Treatment

- Non-pharmacologic therapy: Sunlight accelerates pigmentation of residual hypopigmented areas after treatment.
- Acute general Rx: Topical therapy forms the mainstay of treatment and should be the first-line therapy. Oral treatment is required in cases of extensive involvement and in case recalcitrant patients do not respond to topical therapy (Table 3.1).

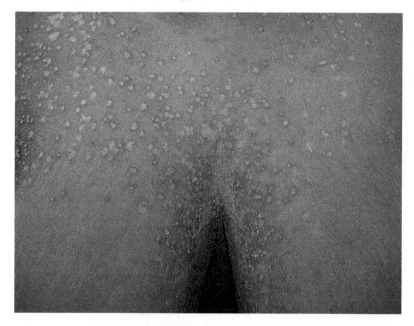

FIGURE 3.1   Hypopigmented macules with furfuraceous scaling in pityriasis versicolor.

TABLE 3.1

Treatment modalities for pityriasis versicolor

Topical	Systemic
Ketoconazole 2% shampoo for 10 min * 2 weeks	Ketoconazole 200 mg OD for 7 days, or 400-mg stat
Clotrimazole , Econazole , Miconazole BD * 2–3 weeks	Fluconazole 400 mg stat
Selenium sulfide 2.5% suspension for 15 min OD * 7 days; repeated weekly for 1 month, then monthly for maintenance	Itraconazole 200 mg/day for 5 days or 400 mg stat
Terbinafine 1% cream BD * 15 days	

- Course and complications: The prognosis is good, with the clearance of the fungus after 3–4 weeks of treatment; however, recurrence is common.

Tinea (Ringworm) infections/Dermatophytic infections

Dermatophyte infections are keratophilic fungi restricted to the stratum corneum, the hair, and the nails (i.e. horny structures).

Causative organism

Trichophyton, Microsporum, and Epidermophyton species are responsible for this group of dermatophyte infections. Microsporum affects the skin and hair; epidermophyton affects the skin and nails; trichophyton affects all three sites.

The species causing dermatophytic infection can be classified as:

- **Anthropophilic** – e.g., *Epidermophyton floccosum, Trichophyton mentagrophytes var. Interdigitale, Trichophyton rubrum, Trichophyton schoenleinii, Trichophyton soudanense, Trichophyton tonsurans, Trichophyton violaceum,* etc.
- **Zoophilic** – *Microsporum canis* (dogs, cats), *T. verrucosum* (cattle) and *T. equinum* (horses).
- **Geophilic** – *Microsporum gypseum, Microsporum praecox*

Morphology of typical lesions

Centrifugally spreading annular/circinate plaque. The centre is clear with papules, papulo-vesicles, pustules, and scaling on active margin (Figure 3.2).

Tinea infection is classified according to the site infected: the head (capitis), face (faciei), torso (corporis), hands (manuum), nails (unguium), groin (cruris), or foot (pedis).

Transmission: transmitted by human to human, animal to human, or soil to human contact through arthrospores shed by a host in skin scales.

Clinical features of ringworm infection

Tinea corporis

This is the ringworm of the skin of the body or limbs. Pruritic, round or annular, red, scaling, well-marginated patches are typical (Figure 3.3). When an animal species is involved (e.g., *T. verrucosum*), the affected skin is inflamed and pustular, and heals spontaneously after a few weeks.

Differential diagnosis: Discoid eczema, psoriasis

(a)

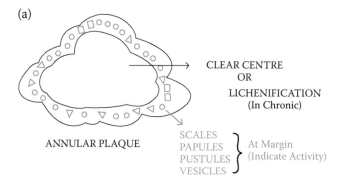

CLEAR CENTRE
OR
LICHENIFICATION
(In Chronic)

ANNULAR PLAQUE

SCALES
PAPULES   } At Margin
PUSTULES   (Indicate Activity)
VESICLES

△ PICTORIAL REPRESENTATION OF
TYPICAL LESION OF TINEA

(b)

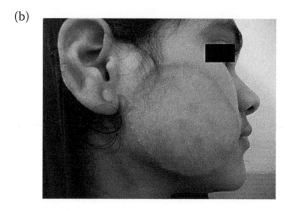

FIGURE 3.2   (a,b) Morphology of typical tinea lesion: annular plaque with papules, papulovesicles, pustules, and scaling on active margin.

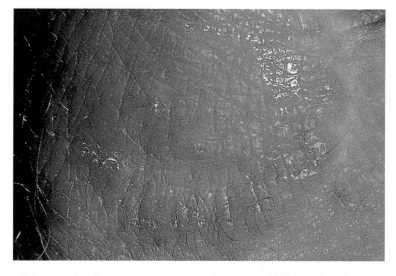

FIGURE 3.3   Well-demarcated scaling patch due to ringworm (from Marks and Motley, 18th edition, with permission).

Tinea cruris

Well-defined, itchy, red scaling patches occur asymmetrically on the medial aspects of both groins. These gradually extend down the thigh and on to the scrotum unless treated. *T. rubrum* and *E. floccosum* are the causative fungi.
- **Predisposing factors:** Summers, tight-fitting clothes
- **Differential diagnosis:** Seborrhoeic dermatitis, intertrigo, flexural psoriasis

Tinea pedis

Tinea pedis is very common and particularly so in young and middle-aged men. It tends to be itchy and persistent. *T. rubrum,* in particular, and *T. mentagrophytes* and *E. floccosum* cause the infection.
- **Predisposing factors:** Humidity, occlusive footwear, communal changing rooms, onychomycosis

Ringworm infection of the feet may be
- **Vesicular:** itchy vesicles occurring on the sides of the feet on a background of erythema
- **Dry-type infection:** the sole is red and scaly
- **Interdigital infection:** skin between the fourth and fifth toes, in particular, is scaly and macerated
- In a patient presenting with pompholyx, always examine the feet as tinea pedis may be associated with it

Tinea manuum

- **Dermatophytic infection of the palmar aspect of the hand**

This less common, chronic form mostly caused by *T. rubrum* usually involves one palm which is dull red with silvery scales in the palmar creases. *One hand–two feet syndrome* is the term used for a classic presentation involving 2 feet and 1 hand by tinea.

Tinea capitis

Ringworm of the scalp is often due to *M. canis.* In recent years, *T. tonsurans* has been increasingly seen as the cause of a subtle form of tinea capitis, particularly in those of African-Caribbean origin.
- **Age group:** Mainly children

Fungi may invade scalp stratum corneum and the hair cuticle (ectothrix infection), causing pink, scaling patches on the scalp skin and areas of hair loss due to the breakage of hair shafts (Figure 3.4) or invade the interior of the hair shaft (endothrix).

Patterns of tinea capitis are recognized as:

- **Non-inflammatory**
  - Present as patches of hair loss with scaling and easily pluckable hairs.
  - Mostly caused by anthropophilic organisms, e.g., *T. tonsurans.*
  - Can appear as black dot or grey patch with little inflammation.
- **Inflammatory (Kerion)**
  - Present as painful boggy swelling with loss of hairs, studded with pustules with sinus formation, matted hairs may be present (Figure 3.5).
  - Mostly caused by zoophilic species but rarely by anthropophilic if a high degree of hypersensitivity develops.

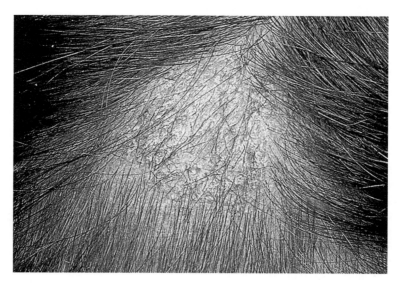

FIGURE 3.4   Scaling area with hair loss in tinea capitis (from Marks and Motley 18th edition, with permission).

- **Favus**
  - ○ Caused by *T. schoenleinii*.
  - ○ Presents with yellowish cup-shaped crusts developing round the hairs (scutula).
  - ○ May develop scarring alopecia.

Tinea unguium

Ringworm infection of the nail plate and the nail bed.
- **Causative organism:** Dermatophytes associated with hand and foot infections (*T. rubrum*, *T. mentagrophytes* or *E. floccosum*) or scalp infections (*T. tonsurans, T. violaceum, T. soudanensei*).
- **Predisposing factors:** Walking barefoot, wearing ill-fitting shoes, poor peripheral circulation, trauma to nails.

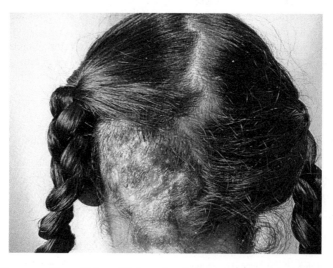

FIGURE 3.5   Painful boggy swelling with loss of hairs and pustules.

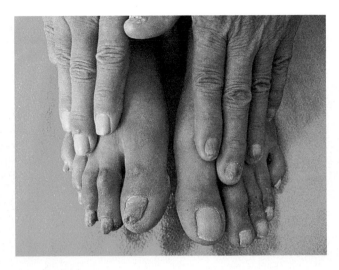

FIGURE 3.6 *Tinea unguium* and pedis.

- **Clinical features:** It is seen more commonly in the toenails than in the fingernails. Infected nail plates are discolored yellowish or white and thickened. Onycholysis occurs and subungual debris collects (subungual hyperkeratosis, Figure 3.6). *Tinea unguium* has to be distinguished from psoriasis of the nails.

Tinea incognito

This is extensive ringworm with an atypical appearance due to the inappropriate use of topical corticosteroids (Figure 3.7). The corticosteroids suppress the protective inflammatory response of the skin to the ringworm fungus, allowing it to spread with absence of typical annular configuration and scaling. Fungal infection should always be ruled out if a suspected eczematous lesion is not responding to treatment with steroids.

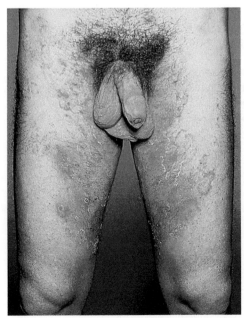

FIGURE 3.7 Tinea cruris showing extensive and unusual-looking infection due to tinea incognito (from Marks and Motley, 18th edition, with permission).

Diagnosis

Sample collection:

a. **Skin:** with scalpel blades from the active margin. If there is no margin, then scales/generalized scraping taken.

b. **Hair:** Dermatophytosis: remove hairs with the roots intact, brush samples can be taken.

c. **Nails:**

   i. Distal lateral subungual onychomycosis: debride from the most proximally involved part of the nail (undersurface of nails).

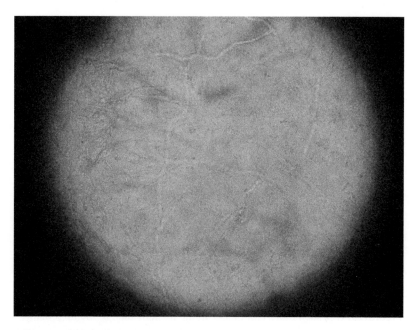

FIGURE 3.8   KOH hair mount showing branching fungal hyphae.

ii. Superficial white onychomycosis: superficial scrapings from nail plate.

iii. Proximal subungual onychomycosis: proximal nail plate (undersurface).

- **Microscopy:** mounted in 10–30% KOH and branching fungal hyphae identified (Figure 3.8). Use of fluorescent markers like acridine orange, Calcofluor white, or Blankophor in some laboratories has improved the diagnostic sensitivity of direct microscopy for the identification of fungal hyphae.
- **Culture:** culture may be positive when direct microscopy is not, but it takes 2–3 weeks or longer before the culture is ready to read. Glucose/peptone agar, or Sabouraud's dextrose agar may be used. Antibacterial antibiotics like gentamycin (0.0025%) and cycloheximide may be added to reduce contamination. Avoid cycloheximide if non-dermatophyte moulds are suspected.
- **Wood's lamp examination:** helps in diagnosis of tinea capitis as some fungal infections especially some ectothrix and favus fluoresce green under Wood's light. It may serve as an important tool for screening asymptomatic family members and school children during epidemics.

Treatment

Key points for management for tinea infections:

- Avoid excessive heat and moisture
- Wear loose-fitted cotton clothes
- Weight reduction for obese patients
- Avoid sharing of clothes, towel, and combs
- Treat all affected family members
- Treat concomitant onychomycosis or tinea pedis
- Examine pets for focus of fungal infection
- Continue topical management for at least 2 more weeks after resolution of lesions (Table 3.2)

TABLE 3.2

Treatment of different types of dermatophytic infections

Infection	Drug	Dose	Duration	Others
Tinea capitis	Griseofulvin (DOC)	10–20 mg/kg/d	6–8 wks	• Avoid sharing of hairbrushes • Add ketoconazole shampoo to reduce transmission
	Terbinafine	10–20kg to 62.5 mg 20–40kg to 125 mg >40kg to 250 mg	6 wks	
Tinea cruris/ corporis	Terbinafine	250 mg OD	1–2 wks	Topical therapy preferred Topical Terbinafine or imidazoles BD for 2 wks Systemic therapy when multiple areas are affected and topical treatment has failed
	Itraconazole	100 mg OD	1–2 wks	
	Fluconazole	150 mg/wks	2–4 wks	
	Griseofulvin	500 mg BD	4 wks	
Tinea mannum/ pedis	Terbinafine	250 mg OD	2 wks	Keep feet dry Topical therapy Terbinafine or imidazoles BD for 4 wks
	Itraconazole	200 mg BD	1–2 wks	
Tinea unguium	Terbinafine	250 mg OD	6 wks for fingernails 12 wks for toenails	Topical therapy like amorolfine nail lacquer and ciclopirox olamine nail lacquer may be added
	Itraconazole	100 mg BD	6 wks for fingernails 12 wks for toenails	
		200 mg BD (pulse for one week for each month)	2 pulses for fingernails 3 pulses for toenails	

Candidiasis (Moniliasis, Thrush)

- **Causative organism:** Yeast pathogen (*Candida albicans*) that also resides in the gastrointestinal tract as a commensal.
- **Predisposing factors:** Moisture, immunosuppression, pregnancy, oral contraceptives, broad-spectrum antibiotics for acne, obesity, diabetes mellitus.

Cutaneous candidiasis can present as
- Stomatitis
- Angular cheilitis
- Intertrigo
- Napkin candidiasis in infancy
- Vulvovaginal candidiasis
- Candidal balanitis
- Candidal paronychia

Candidal intertrigo presents with erythema of skin folds with subcorneal pustules and satellite lesions (Figure 3.9).
- **Diagnosis:** Potassium hydroxide (KOH) mount showing budding yeast and pseudohyphae. Always rule out diabetes or immunosuppression in case of recurrent infection.

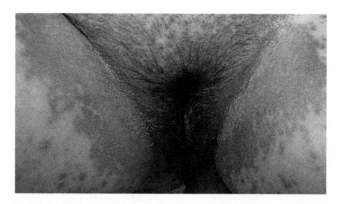

FIGURE 3.9 Candidiasis showing satellite lesions

- **Treatment:** Eliminate the predisposing factor and avoid moisture. Topical therapy such as polyenes (nystatin) and imidazole preparations (miconazole, clotrimazole, and econazole) is effective. Systemic therapy in various forms of candidiasis is as shown in Table 3.3.

Deep fungul infection

There are several fungal species that cause deep and sometimes life-threatening infection. They can be subcutaneous (involving dermis, subcutaneous tissue, adjacent bone) or systemic (originate in lungs, spread to other organs).

Subcutaneous fungal infections include:

- Mycetoma/Madura foot
- Chromoblastomycosis
- Sporotrichosis
- Rhinosporidiosis
- Lobomycosis
- Phaeohyphomycotic cyst

Sporotrichosis may produce a series of inflamed nodules along the line of lymphatic drainage. Deep fungul infections of this type produce a granulomatous type of inflammation, with many giant cells and histiocytes as well as polymorphs and lymphocytes. Madura foot is a deep fungul infection of the foot and is seen in various countries of the African continent and India. The affected foot is swollen and infiltrated by inflammatory tissue, with many sinuses (Figure 3.10). The infection spreads throughout the foot, invades bone, and is very destructive and disabling.

TABLE 3.3

Systemic therapy for various forms of candidiasis

Infection	Drug	Dose	Duration
Oropharyngeal candidiasis	Fluconazole	100–200 mg OD	7 days
	Itraconazole	100 mg OD	7 days
Vulvovaginal candidiasis	Fluconazole	150 mg	Stat
Candidal onychomycosis	Fluconazole	300 mg/wk	4 wks for fingernails 12 wks for toenails
	Itraconazole	200 mg BD for 7 days/month	2–3 cycles

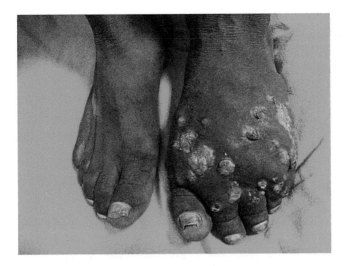

FIGURE 3.10   Mycetoma with swelling of foot and discharging sinuses.

Systemic fungal infections include

- Aspergillosis
- Blastomycosis
- Candidiasis
- Cryptococcosis
- Coccidioidomycosis
- Cerebral chromomycosis
- Histoplasmosis
- Mucormycosis
- Paracoccidioidomycosis
- Penicilliosis

They are much more common in immunocompromised patients, including those with acquired immune deficiency syndrome (AIDS), transplant recipients, those on corticosteroids or immunosuppressive agents, and those with congenital immunodeficiencies. Some, such as histoplasmosis, cryptococcosis, and coccidioidomycosis, are widespread systemic infections, which only occasionally involve the skin.

Bacterial infection of the skin

Most skin infections are caused by Gram-positive organisms – staphylococci and streptococci. The primary skin infections caused by them may or may not be purulent and can be classified as follows.

Direct infection of the skin

- Impetigo
- Folliculitis
- Furunculosis
- Carbuncle
- Ecthyma
- Sycosis
- Cellulitis (occasionally)
- Damage from *bacterial toxin*
- Toxic shock syndrome
- Staphylococcal scalded skin syndrome
- Staphylococcal scarlatina
- Recurrent toxin-mediated perineal erythema

Predisposing factors: scabies, atopic dermatitis, overcrowding, poor personal hygiene, insect bite, diabetes, malnutrition.

Impetigo contagiosa

- **Causative organism:** *Staphylococcus aureus* in most instances or β-haemolytic streptococci in few.
- **Age group:** preschool and young children

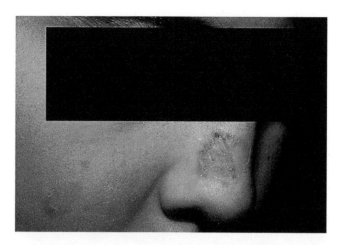

FIGURE 3.11   Patch of impetigo on the nose (from Marks and Motley, 18th edition, with permission).

- **Clinical features:** Red, sore areas, which may blister, appear on the exposed skin surface (Figure 3.11). A yellowish-gold crust surmounts the lesions that appear and spreads within a few days with peripheral extension without central healing (Figure 3.12). It is, however, not uncommon for the signs of the lesions to appear over an area of eczema. The condition is then said to be 'impetiginized'.

Bullous impetigo

- **Causative organism:** *Staphylococcus aureus*
- **Age group:** All ages (common in children)
- **Clinical features:** Present with bulla lasting about 2–3 days which rupture and thin brownish crust forms. Lesions spread with peripheral extension and central healing forming circinate lesions

Ecthyma

- **Causative organism:** β-haemolytic streptococci (mostly) or staphylococci
- **Clinical features:** pustule forms on erythematous skin followed by adherent crusting which on removal with difficulty reveals underlying ulcer.
- **Complication:** risk of post-streptococcal glomerulonephritis in cases of streptococcal infection. However, it does not predispose to rheumatic fever.
- **Investigation:** routine investigation is not needed. However, if the infection is recurrent/resistant to treatment or MRSA is suspected, then a pus culture and sensitivity should be sent.

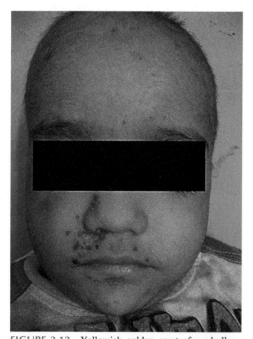

FIGURE 3.12   Yellowish golden crust of nonbullous impetigo.

TABLE 3.4

TABLE 3.4

Treatments for bullous impetigo

Specific Management	
Topical (for limited disease)	Mupirocin (1st line) Retapamulin Fusidic acid Neomycin (staphylococci > streptococci) Gentian violet
Systemic (ideally 7-day course)	Dicloxacillin (250 mg qid) Cephalexin (250 mg qid) Amoxyxilllin-clavulanate (500 mg/125 mg tds) Erythromycin (250 mg qid)
	If MRSA suspected:
	Cotrimoxazole (800/160 mg bd) Clindamycin (300–400 mg qid) Doxycycline (100 mg bd) Minocycline (100 mg bd) Linezolid (600 mg bd)

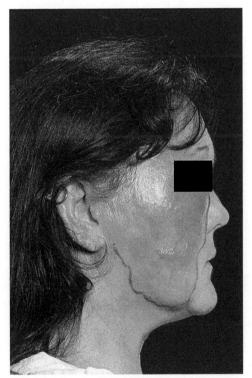

FIGURE 3.13 Erysipelas of the right cheek; the area of erythema has been outlined in order to monitor the response to treatment (from Marks and Motley, 18th edition, with permission).

Treatment

General measures

- Clean the area with soap and wash/antiseptic washes like povidone iodine, chlorhexidine
- Avoid sharing of towels, maintain personal hygiene
- Treat any underlying skin condition like eczema, scabies, pediculosis

Specific management

Some treatment approaches for bullous impetigo are presented in Table 3.4.

Topical therapy is effective for limited disease.

Indications for systemic therapy include

- Extensive skin involvement
- Fever, lymph node enlargement
- Suspected infection by nephritogenic streptococcal strains

Erysipelas (St. Anthony's Fire)

Erysipelas is a bacterial infection of the dermis and upper subcutaneous tissue.

- **Causative organism:** β-haemolytic streptococcus.
- **Clinical features:** Characterized by sudden onset of a well-marginated, painful, and swollen erythematous area, usually on the face

(a)

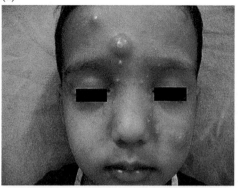

(b)

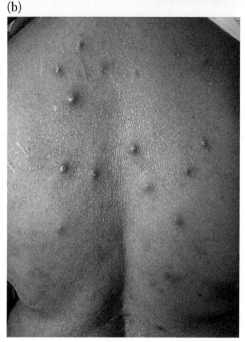

FIGURE 3.14   (a,b) Folliculitis.

or lower limbs (Figure 3.13). The inflammation may be very intense and the area may become haemorrhagic and even blister. There is usually accompanying pyrexia and malaise.

Cellulitis

This is a diffuse, inflammatory disorder of the subcutis and skin.

- **Causative organism:** this is caused most commonly by β-haemolytic streptococci; occasionally, S. areus also implicated. H. influenza B may be responsible for facial cellulitis in children

Clinical features

It is relatively common, particularly on the limbs, and often occurs on legs affected by venous ulceration or by lymphoedema. There is pain, tenderness, slight swelling, and a variable degree of diffuse erythema. There is often a breach in the skin surface – frequently fissuring in the toe webs due to intertrigo – as the portal of entry of the infection.

Treatment of erysipelas and cellulitis

- Rest, elevation of the affected part
- Treating predisposing factors
- Patient has to be admitted if associated with comorbidities or severe involvement (skin blistering, necrosis)
- Mild cases: oral antibiotics
  - Penicillin V, 250 mg qid daily
  - Dicloxacillin 250 mg qid daily
  - Amoxicillin-clavulanate 625mg TDS
  - Cephalexin 250 mg qid

- If MRSA is suspected:
  - Linezolid 600 mg bd
  - Cotrimoxazole, doxycycline or minocycline along with a β-lactam antibiotic to cover streptococci.

- Severe cases: parenteral antibiotics (ceftriaxone/penicillin/clindamycin/vancomycin) required followed by oral therapy after clinical improvement.

Folliculitis, furuncles (boils), and carbuncles

- **Causative organism**: *S. aureus*

Folliculitis is inflammation of the hair follicle with changes confined to follicular infundibulum (Figure 3.14).

A furuncle is an infection of the hair follicle and perifollicular tissue, which presents as a follicular, inflammatory nodule with pus formation.

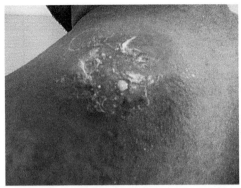

A carbuncle is an infection of contiguous hair follicles presenting as painful red swelling with pus discharging from multiple follicular orifices (Figure 3.15). Patients with impaired blood sugar are particularly at risk.

Treatment

- Gram stain and culture of pus recommended from carbuncles and furuncle
- Maintain good personal hygiene
- Clean site and hands with soap and water
- Avoid sharing towels, clothes, razors
- Incision and drainage
- Topical antibiotics
- Systemic antibiotics based on sensitivity pattern

FIGURE 3.15 Painful red swelling with pus discharging from multiple follicular orifices.

may be needed, if abscess is difficult to drain, there is no response to treatment, the patient is immunocompromised, or there are accompanying cellulitis or systemic symptoms

Antibiotics are effective in various skin and soft tissue infections by staphylococcus and streptococci are shown in Table 3.5.

Management of recurrent staphylococcal infections

- Send pus culture sensitivity and prescribe antibiotics accordingly.
- Promote regular handwashing with soap and water by the patient as well as the caregivers.
- Regular decontamination of towels and clothes.
- Decolonization
  - Nasal decolonization may be done with twice daily application of mupirocin for 10 days.
  - Body decolonization with antiseptic solutions like chlorhexidine (5–14 days) or dilute bleach baths (1 teaspoon of bleaching powder in 1 gallon of water or ¼ cup of bleaching powder per ¼ tub of water or 13 gallons of water) twice a week for 15 minutes for 3 months.
  - All carriage sites like nasal, axilla, and perineum should be treated.
  - Oral rifampicin 600 mg daily for 7–10 days may be used with due caution to the risk of resistance.

TABLE 3.5

Antibiotic treatments for staphylococcal and streptococcal soft tissue infections (1,2)

Sensitivity	Antibiotic
MSSA	Dicloxacillin Amoxicillin Cephalexin Erythromycin azithromycin
MRSA	Topical drugs: mupirocin, retapamulin
	Oral drugs: clindamycin, trimethoprim-sulfamethoxazole (TMP-SMX), tetracycline (doxycycline or minocycline), linezolid, rifampicin
	IV drugs: intravenous (IV) vancomycin (A-I), oral (PO) or IV linezolid 600 mg twice daily (A-I), daptomycin 4 mg/kg/dose IV once daily (A-I), telavancin 10 mg/kg/dose IV once daily (A-I), and clindamycin 600 mg IV or PO 3 times a day, ceftaroline fosamil, quinupristin-dalfopristin
	Newer drugs: tedizolid, dalbavancin, oritavancin

1 Practice Guidelines for the Diagnosis and Management of Skin and Soft Tissue Infections: 2014 Update by the Infectious Diseases Society of America.

2 Clinical Practice Guidelines by the Infectious Diseases Society of America for the Treatment of Methicillin-Resistant *Staphylococcus aureus* Infections in Adults and Children.

TABLE 3.6

Classification of cutaneous tuberculosis

Immunity of host	Multi/Paucibacillary (M/P)	Inoculation	Disease
Naïve host	M	Direct inoculation	Tuberculosis chancre (primary inoculation)
Low host immunity	M	Contiguous spread	Scrofuloderma
		Autoinoculation	Orificial tuberculosis
		Haematogenous spread	Acute Miliary tuberculosis Tuberculous gumma (abscess)
High host immunity	P	Direct inoculation	Warty tuberculosis (verruca cutis)
		Direct inoculation Haematogenous spread	Lupus vulgaris
Tuberculids			Lichen scrofulosorum Papulonecrotic tuberculid Erythema induratum (Bazin) Nodular tuberculid

Anthrax

- **Causative organism:** Gram-positive bacillus (*Bacillus anthracis*)

Anthrax is due to a rare, potentially fatal infection-causing black, scabbed sores and septicaemia. It is spread by farm animals and because the microorganism has a resistant spore form, it can stay on infected land for years. It has assumed major importance because of its potential for use in bioterrorism.

Tuberculosis

Tuberculosis is a multi-system disease caused by varieties of the waxy-enveloped bacterium *Mycobacterium tuberculosis*. Tuberculosis is, unfortunately, now once again becoming common and multiple-drug resistant strains of *M. tuberculosis* are becoming a major problem in communities with a high prevalence of HIV infection. Cutaneous tuberculosis has been classified as shown in Table 3.6.

- **Diagnosis:** The bacillus can be cultured in special media in vitro, but grows very slowly. Special stains are needed to detect it in tissue.

Lupus vulgaris

Lupus vulgaris presents as a slowly progressive, granulomatous plaque on the skin, head and neck followed by arms and legs (buttocks in developing countries) caused by the tubercle bacillus. It slowly increases in size, over one to three decades. It often has a thickened psoriasiform appearance, grows by peripheral extension with areas of atrophy and scarring.

Blanching with a glass microscope slide (diascopy) will reveal 'apple jelly nodules' due to the underlying granulomatous inflammation. Diagnosis can be confirmed with biopsy showing tuberculoid granulomas.

Tuberculosis verrucosa Cutis (warty tuberculosis)

This is commonly seen on the back of the hands, knees, elbows, and buttocks whenever abrasive contact with the earth and expectorated tubercle bacilli occurs. Thickened, warty plaques are present, which are sometimes misdiagnosed as viral warts. Diagnosis is confirmed by biopsy samples showing tuberculoid granulomata and caseation necrosis.

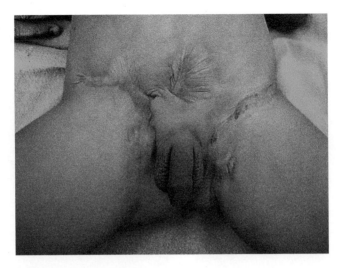

FIGURE 3.16   Puckered scarring of scrofuloderma.

Scrofuloderma

An eroded, weeping area with bluish margins often develops where a tuberculous sinus drains onto the skin from an underlying focus of tuberculosis infection which heals with puckered scarring (Figure 3.16).

Other forms of cutaneous tuberculosis

Tuberculous chancre: a persistent ulcer may arise at the site of inoculation as a 'primary' infection. Tuberculides may develop as hypersensitivity to the tubercle bacillus.

- **Lichen scrofulosorum:** lichenoid eruptions of papules predominantly in children often peri-follicular develop on abdomen, chest, and back (Figure 3.17).
- **Papulonecrotic tuberculide:** papules arise and develop central necrosis with a black crust.
- **Erythema induratum:** uncommon disorder, which in many cases appears to fulfil the criterion of being a response to tuberculous infection. It is characterized by the development of plaque-like areas of induration and necrosis on the lower calves and occurs predominantly in young women.

Treatment of cutaneous tuberculosis

Intensive phase: isoniazid, rifampicin, ethambutol, and pyrazinamide for 2 months
Continuation phase: isoniazid and rifampicin for 4 months

Some other mycobacterial infections

Swimming pool granuloma

Mycobacterium marinum, which lives in water, is sometimes caught from swimming pools and fish tanks. It has a 3-week incubation period and causes plaques, abscesses, and erosions on the elbows and knees, in particular (Figure 3.18).

The condition usually responds to minocycline, although occasionally other antibiotic combinations are required, as determined by the sensitivity of the cultured organism.

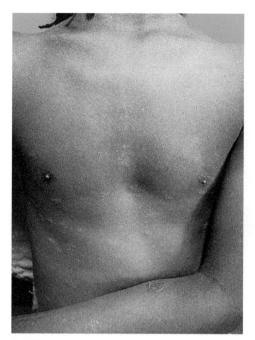

FIGURE 3.17   Lichen scrofulosorum

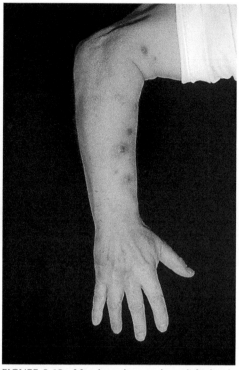

FIGURE 3.18   Mycobacterium marinum infection in the dorsum of the hand with 'sporotrichoid' spread into the forearm (from Marks and Motley, 18th edition, with permission).

Buruli ulcer

Mycobacterium ulcerans is responsible for this disorder occurring in Uganda and south-east Asia. Large, undermined ulcers form quite rapidly and persist. Surgical removal is currently the best treatment.

Leprosy (Hansen's disease)

- **Causative organism:** Slow-growing bacillus, *Mycobacterium leprae*, which cannot be grown in vitro, although it can be passaged in armadillos and small rodents. As with the tubercle bacillus, it is detected in tissue by the Ziehl–Nielsen stain or by an immunocytochemical test.
- **Transmission:** The disease is spread by droplet infection and by close contact with an infected individual.

It is still a serious problem globally, with one to two million people affected, mostly in the poor and underprivileged countries of Africa and Asia.

Clinical features

The pattern of involvement is highly dependent on the immune status of the individual.

It shows involvement of skin and nerve characterized by hypopigmented lesions and peripheral nerve thickening. The two extremes are the lepromatous form seen in anergic individuals and the tuberculoid form seen in individuals with a high resistance. Because there are many gradations between these polar types, the range of clinical signs and the corresponding nomenclature have become very complicated.

Where the changes are near tuberculoid, the term 'borderline tuberculoid' is used; similarly, 'borderline lepromatous' is used for lesions that are close to the other type. 'Dimorphic' refers to characteristics of both types of lesion being present. In tuberculoid lesions, nerves are infected, which become thickened. The affected areas are well defined, macular and hypopigmented, as well as anaesthetic because of the nerve involvement. The anaesthesia results in injury, deformity, and disability. In lepromatous leprosy, the infection is much more extensive, with thickening of the affected tissue as well as surface changes, with some hypopigmentation. On the face, the thickening gives rise to the characteristic leonine facies, with accentuation of the soft tissues of the nose and supraorbital areas.

In general, the disease can produce dreadful deformity and disability unless skilfully treated, and it still evokes great fear in traditional communities. Because the disorder causes patchy hypopigmentation, the differential diagnosis includes vitiligo, pityriasis versicolor, and pityriasis alba.

In tuberculoid types, there is a striking granulomatous inflammation with many giant cells and only a few *M. leprae* to be found. In the lepromatous types, there are many macrophages stuffed with *M. leprae* (causing the appearance of foamy macrophages).

Treatment

See Table 3.7.

Lyme disease

- **Causative organism:** *Borrelia burgdorferi*
- **Spread by (vector):** Bite of a tick

This has been described in several areas of Europe, including the UK, and in the United States. It is a multi-system disease with arthropathy, cardiovascular, and central nervous components, as well as systemic upset. The skin may be involved in the early stages and show an erythematous ring that expands outwards (erythema chronicum migrans). In late stages, skin atrophy may be seen (acrodermatitis chronica atrophicans), or fibrosis in a morphoea-like condition. Diagnosis is made by identification of the organism in the tissues or by detection of antibodies in the blood.

- **Treatment:** Doxycycline, 200 mg/day for 3 weeks

Leishmaniasis

This term refers to a group of diseases caused by a genus of closely related protozoal parasites with complex lifecycles, which include time spent in small rodents. These diseases are spread by biting arthropods (mostly sandflies) in tropical and subtropical areas. Some forms cause severe systemic disease and are prevalent in some areas of Africa and South America and the Indian subcontinent; others cause predominantly cutaneous or mucocutaneous disease.

- **Cutaneous forms** are found around the Mediterranean littoral and North Africa and in South America. The 'Mediterranean' type is caused by *Leishmania major* and *L. tropica*. After an incubation period of about 2 months, a boil-like lesion appears, usually on an exposed site ('Baghdad boil'). Later, this breaks down to produce a sloughy ulcer ('oriental sore':

TABLE 3.7

Multidrug therapy for leprosy (WHO regimen)

Type	Drug	Frequency	Adult dose
Paucibacillary (total duration—6 months)	Rifampicin	Monthly	600 mg
	Dapsone	Daily	100 mg
Multibacillary (total duration—12 months)	Rifampicin	Monthly	600 mg
	Dapsone	Daily	100 mg
	Clofazimine	Monthly	300 mg
		Daily	50 mg

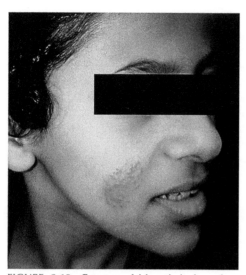

FIGURE 3.19 Cutaneous leishmaniasis in a boy, showing persistent plaque and papules on the skin of the cheek (from Marks and Motley, 18th edition, with permission).

Figure 3.19), which persists for some months before healing spontaneously, with scarring and the development of immunity.

- **Mucocutaneous forms** occur mainly in South America (New World leishmaniasis) and are due to *L. mexicana* and *L. brasiliensis*. Small ulcers develop (Chiclero's ulcer) that seem more destructive than the Old World types but also more persistent, and later in the disease destructive lesions appear, affecting the nasal mucosa in about half of patients. A cutaneous component to visceral forms is less common, but more extensive, and includes a diffuse cutaneous form with many plaques and nodules resembling lepromatous leprosy, a recidivans form with persistent plaques resembling lupus vulgaris, and post kala-azar (dermal leishmaniasis), occurring after the visceral disease and marked by the appearance of numerous small papules.

Biopsy sections show mixed granulomatous inflammation. The parasites can be identified by special stains and can also be cultured in specialized media. There is also an intracutaneous test (Leishmanin test) which is positive if the skin becomes inflamed and indurated 48–72 hours after injection of a measured amount of Leishmanin antigen, which indicates present or previous infection.

Treatment

The localized small ulcers heal spontaneously but can be treated by freezing or curettage. Infiltration with sodium stibogluconate has been used. Amphotericin B deoxycholate, Miltefosine, Liposomal amphotericin B, Pentavalent antimonial are used in management.

Viral infections of the skin

Herpesviruses

Herpesviruses are enveloped DNA viruses producing typical intranuclear inclusion bodies. They are classified into α, β, and γ (Table 3.8).

TABLE 3.8

Classification of herpesviruses

Subgroup	Virus
α	Human simplex virus 1 (HSV1)
	Human simplex virus 2 (HSV2)
	Varicella zoster virus (VZV)
β	Cytomegalovirus (CMV)
	Human herpesvirus 6 (HHV6)
	Human-herpesvirus 7 (HHV 7)
γ	Epstein-Barr virus (EBV)
	Human herpesvirus 8 (HHV 8)

(a)

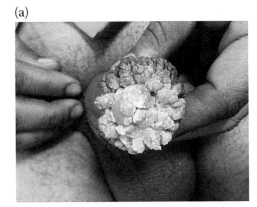

(b)

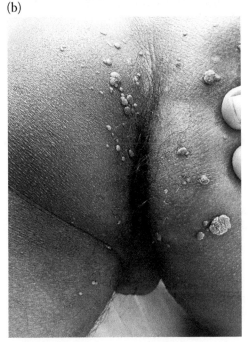

FIGURE 3.20 (a,b) Anogenital warts

Herpes simplex

Causative organism: HSV-1, HSV-2

- Herpes labialis: HSV-1 >HSV-2
- Herpes genitalis: HSV-2 >HSV-1

Mode of transmission: Direct contact of skin or mucosa.

Clinical features

Primary infection has greater severity than recurrent episodes.

- **Herpetic gingivostomatitis:** Commonly, the lesions occur around the mouth or on the lip. They start as grouped, tender and/or painful papules or papulovesicles (Figure 3.20) and then coalesce to form a crusted erosion. The sequence takes about 7–14 days from initial discomfort to the final pink macule, marking where lesions have been. The initial infection may be quite unpleasant, with severe stomatitis, systemic upset and pyrexia. Resolution takes place in about 10 days. Reactivation of the herpes infection occurs in some cases, at varying intervals. Up to 20% of the population develops recurrent 'cold sores', so named because the disorder is often precipitated by minor pyrexial episodes.
- **Herpes genitalis:** Genital herpes in males affects the glans penis and the shaft of the penis. In females, the vulval region or labia minora is usually involved, but lesions may occur elsewhere on the buttocks or mons pubis. The disorder is sexually transmitted and has become extremely common. Recurrences are more common with HSV-2 with recurrent episodes being less painful and of shorter duration.
- **Herpes gladiatorum:** Crops of vesicles and pustules on face, scalp, and upper trunk transmitted by skin-to-skin contact, common in wrestlers.
- **Precipitating factors for recurrences:** Minor trauma, febrile illnesses, upper respiratory tract infections, trigeminal neuralgia, laser resurfacing, menstruation.

Diagnosis

- Direct microscopy: Tzanck Smear-acantholytic cells or multinucleated giant cells on giemsa stain
- Immunofluorescent method with antibodies to the herpesvirus
- Viral culture
- Polymerase chain reaction

TABLE 3.9

Treatment of herpes infections

Disease	Treatment		
	First episode	**Recurrent disease**	
		Episodic disease	**Suppressive therapy**
Herpes labialis	Acyclovir 400 mg tds * 10 days	Acyclovir 400 mg tds * 5 days	Acyclovir 400 mg bd
	Acyclovir 200 mg 5 times a day * 10 days	Valcyclovir 2 g bd * 1 day	
	Valcyclovir 1 g bd * 10 days		
Herpes genitalis	Acyclovir 400 mg tds * 10 days	Acyclovir 400 mg tds * 5 days	Acyclovir 400 mg bd
	Famciclovir 250 mg tds * 10 days	Valacyclovir 500 mg bd * 3 days	Valacyclovir 500 mg od OR Valacyclovir 1 g od (>10 episode/yr)
	Valcyclovir 1 g bd * 10 days	Famciclovir 500 mg od, followed by 250 mg bd * 2 days	Famiciclovir 250 mg bd
Varicella & Herpes zoster	Oral Acyclovir 800 mg 5 times a day		

Treatment

Most patients do not require treatment. Treatment may be needed for severe episodes and is effective only if initiated early (Table 3.9).

Herpes zoster (shingles) and chicken pox (varicella)

- **Causative organism:** Varicella zoster virus is a small DNA virus causing both zoster and chicken pox, which differ only in the extent of the disease, the symptoms caused, and the immune status of the individual affected.

Varicella

- **Transmission:** Highly contagious. Spread by droplets and debris from the lesions. Infectious for 1–2 days before rash to 4–5 days after until all the vesicles crust.
- **Incubation period:** 4–21 days
- **Age group:** Childhood, rarely adults

Clinical features

- **Prodrome:** Fever and malaise
- **Rash:** Begins on the face and trunk relatively spare extremities (centripetal). Pleomorphic lesions with macules, papules, papulovesicles which crust, the crust dropping off after some 7–14 days, leaving pock-type scars in many instances. Oral mucosa may be involved.

Complications

Rarely complicated in children. Secondary bacterial infection, secondary bacterial pneumonia, and otitis media may occur rarely. Complications are more frequent in adults.

Treatment

For most people, no specific treatment is required apart from keeping the lesions clean and, if necessary, the application of antimicrobial preparations to prevent or combat secondary infection.

Oral acyclovir 800 mg five times a day within 24 hrs of the onset of rash shortens the duration of disease and decreases its severity.

Prevention

Live attenuated (oka strain) VZV vaccines.

Herpes zoster (shingles)

- **Transmission:** Due to the reactivation of latent virus in a posterior root ganglion of a spinal nerve. In immunosuppressed individuals, the disorder is often very severe and may involve several dermatomes.
- **Age group:** Mostly affects individuals over the age of 50 years, but it also affects im munosuppressed individuals, such as patients with AIDS or lymphomas.
- **Sites of predilection:** Branches of the trigeminal ganglion, dermatomes of the cervical and thoracic regions.

Clinical features

The disorder often starts with paraesthesias or pain in the distribution of one or more dermatomes. Erythema followed by vesicles appears in segmental distribution (Figure 3.21). Later, the vesicles become pustular and then crust.

- **Complications**
  - Post-herpetic neuralgia: about 25–30% of patients with shingles continue to have pain and paraesthesiae in the affected dermatome long after the skin lesions have disappeared.
  - Secondary bacterial infection
- **Treatment:** Acyclovir reduces duration and severity of pain and healing time for rash if started within 72 hrs of onset of rash (same dose as varicella).
- **Prevention:** FDA has approved zoster vaccine in 2006 for adults over 60 years of age.

Viral warts

- **Causative organism:** Human papillomavirus (a small DNA virus) which has many antigenic types (Table 3.1). Particular clinical types of wart are caused by particular antigenic types.
- **Transmission:** Direct contact of skin with wart virus-containing horny debris. Genital warts are caught mostly (but not exclusively) by venereal contact. Some perianal warts may be transmitted by homosexual contact or by 'child abuse'. Vertical transmission can rarely occur from mother to infant presenting as laryngeal papilloma or genital warts.

Clinical types

- Verruca vulgaris: single/multiple papules with verrucous surface
- Periungual warts
- Verruca plana: multiple flat smooth papules with pseudokoebnerization
- Filiform warts: thin elongated projections
- Palmoplantar warts
- Anogenital warts

The different varieties are illustrated in Figures 3.20, 3.22, and 3.23.
- **Histopathology:** Epidermal thickening, with acanthosis and koilocytes in upper layers, granular layer shows a characteristic basophilic, stippled appearance (Figure 3.24).

(a)

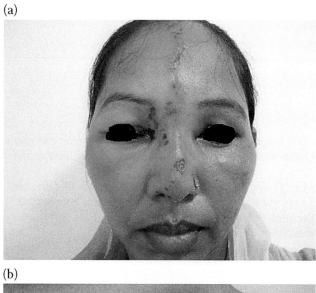

(b)

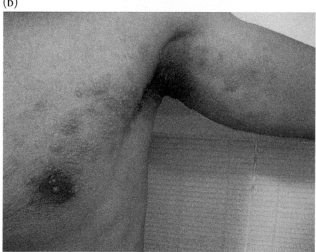

FIGURE 3.21   (a,b) Herpes zoster in dermatomal distribution.

- **Course of disease:** All warts disappear spontaneously but may persist for many months or some years.

Treatment

Treatment is not very satisfactory and includes:

- Local tissue destruction
  - Cryotherapy (tissue freezing with liquid nitrogen or solid carbon dioxide)
  - Curettage
  - Cautery
  - Chemical destruction with topical preparations containing salicylic acid, lactic acid, podophyllin, or glutaraldehyde. Popular preparations contain high concentrations of salicylic acid (12–20%) and lactic acid (4–20%) or podophyllin 10–25% (for genital warts)
- Other methods—intracutaneous injections of cytotoxics such as bleomycin, injections of recombinant interferon, and use of vesicants such as cantharidin, CO_2 laser.

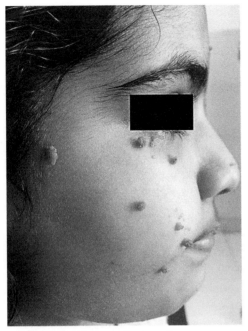

FIGURE 3.22　Verruca vulgaris on face.

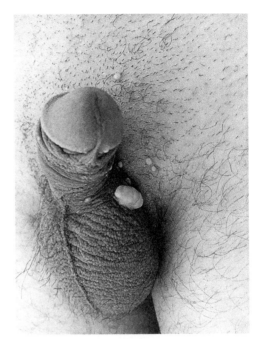

FIGURE 3.23　Giant molluscum contagiosum.

Molluscum contagiosum

- **Causative organism:** pox virus group (molluscum contagiosum virus)
- **Transmission:** skin-to-skin contact
- **Age group:** schoolchildren, immunosuppressed
- **Incubation period:** 14 days to 6 months

Clinical features

The typical molluscum lesion is a pink-colored or pearly white umbilicated papule (Figure 3.23). There may be one or many lesions. Pseudokoebnerization is observed. The face and genital regions (Figure 3.24) are commonly involved.

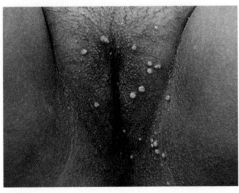

FIGURE 3.24　Genital molluscum contagiosum.

Pathology

Cells proliferate to form lobulated pear-shaped epidermal growths separated by fibrous septa. Cells at the centre show characteristic degenerative change and appear as globular eosinophilic bodies in the cytoplasm (molluscum bodies).

Treatment

Mollusca may resolve spontaneously. Treatment modalities include curettage and cautery, salicylic acid preparations, brief applications of cantharidin, or mechanical removal.

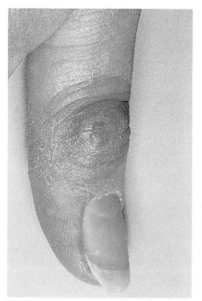

FIGURE 3.25   Area of orf infection on the thumb (from Marks and Motley, 18th edition, with permission).

Orf (contagious pustular dermatitis of sheep)

- **Casuative organism:** Parapox virus that mostly affects sheep, but also cattle.
- **Transmission:** Direct inoculation with infected material. Seen in butchers, meat porters, and cooks.
- **Clinical features:** The lesions are solitary, acute, inflammatory, and blistering and are mostly on the fingers (Figure 3.25). Following the attack, a surprisingly high proportion of patients develop erythema multiforme.

Treatment

Spontaneous recovery occurs. Treat secondary infection.

4

Infestations, insect bites, and stings

Sumit Sethi

The way that the skin reacts to the attacks of arthropods and small invertebrates depends partly on the extent and severity of the attack and, particularly, on the immune status of the individual attacked.

Each geographical region has its own spectrum of skin problems due to the local fauna. Although some disorders, such as scabies, are the same the world over, the pattern and incidence of infestations and bites differ markedly from place to place. In general, the extent of skin problems due to arthropods is directly related to the sophistication and wealth of the society in question, because of the effects of personal hygiene, education, effective waste disposal, and prophylaxis.

Scabies

Scabies is caused by infestation with the human scabies mite (*Sarcoptes scabiei var. homini*). The mite is a host-specific, obligate parasite and has no separate existence off the human body. The key presenting features are intense pruritus and a similar history in close contact. The diagnosis is confirmed by demonstrating the scabies mite in the patient's skin.

Aetiology and epidemiology

The female mite burrows into the human stratum corneum and lays eggs within this very superficial layer. (The male is smaller than the female and dies shortly after impregnating the female.) The characteristic intense pruritus and eczematous rash in scabies are a result of the affected individual becoming sensitive to the waste products of the mites within the intra-corneal burrows. This generally takes 4–6 weeks from the initial invasion of the mite; but subsequent re-infestations cause signs and symptoms within 24–48 hours, as the individual is already sensitized.

Infestation occurs after close skin-to-skin contact with an infected individual. Fomite transmission is also possible in case of crusted scabies. In most adults with symptoms, there are no more than 10–15 mites within the skin; however, the number may reach millions in crusted scabies.

There have been several notable pandemics of scabies in recent history, making it notorious as the '7-year itch'. The most recent of these started in the mid-1960s and ended in the early 1970s, although between peaks of incidence, the disorder continues to appear sporadically and in localized mini-epidemics – such as within families or in nursing homes.

Clinical features

The diagnosis of scabies is based on a history of pruritus associated with a characteristic distribution of lesions and epidemiologic pattern (e.g. pruritus in close contacts). The pruritus is intense and is classically accentuated at night, or after a hot bath, and might be present before any overt physical signs. Cutaneous lesions comprise small erythematous papules associated with a variable degree of excoriation (Figure 4.1). They are symmetrically distributed, typically involving the interdigital webs, sides of fingers, volar aspect of the wrists, lateral palms, axillae, posterior

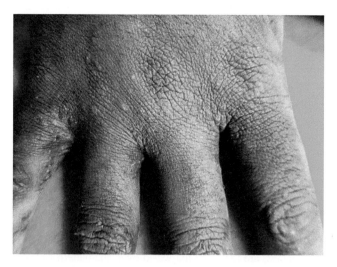

FIGURE 4.1   Papules and excoriations in scabies.

auricular area, elbows, waist (including the umbilicus), ankles, feet, and buttocks. In men, penis and scrotum are commonly involved, while the areolae, nipples, and vulvar areas are most often affected in women. The lesions tend to avoid areas with a high density of pilosebaceous follicles; thus, the head and neck are usually spared in adults while the involvement of these areas is frequent in infants, the elderly, and the immunocompromised. Eczematous dermatitis, vesicles, indurated nodules and secondary bacterial infection with *Streptococcus pyogenes* or *Staphylococcus aureus* is commonly seen. The pathognomonic sign of scabies is the burrow, which represents the tunnel excavated by the female mite while laying eggs. The burrow is a wavy, thread-like, greyish-white lesion 1–10 mm in length (Figure 4.2). Acral vesiculopustules can represent a clue to the diagnosis of scabies in infants.

The severity of the eruption depends on the number of mites present on cutaneous surface and the immune status of the patient. In individuals with defective immunologic or sensory response – such as human immunodeficiency virus (HIV) infection, patients receiving immunosuppressive drugs, frail elderly, and those who unable to respond to itch by scratching, due to paralysis or mental retardation – the infestation is very severe, known as Norwegian or crusted scabies.

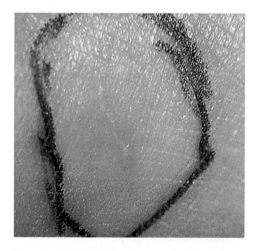

FIGURE 4.2   Scabies burrow on the foot (from Marks and Motley, 18th edition, with permission).

Diagnosis

The burrows of the female scabies mite are pathognomonic of the disease, and diagnostic of infection. The burrows are grey-white, linear, slightly raised marks, 1–8 mm long, and present on the favored sites such as hands, finger webs, wrists, the instep of feet, and male genitalia (Figure 4.3). A dermatoscope characteristically illuminates the burrow and shows the female mite at one end as a small dark semicircular spot with a triangular point 'jet with contrail' sign. A definitive diagnosis can also be made by microscopic identification of the scabies mites, eggs, or fecal pellets (scybala).

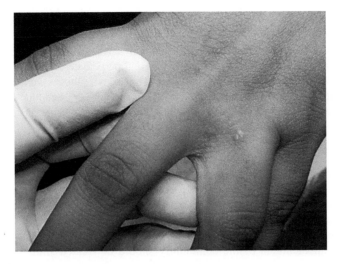

FIGURE 4.3   Scabies burrow in the interdigital space of the hand.

For patients in whom burrows cannot be identified, a positive family or social history with itching contacts is helpful evidence and, in the presence of a compatible clinical picture, treatment may be instituted by the experienced clinician. Unfortunately, it is all too common for patients to be suspected of having scabies and to be prescribed treatment by inexperienced clinicians when the underlying diagnosis is, in fact, eczema, and the patient's skin deteriorates further as a result. The differential diagnosis is set out in Table 4.1.

Treatment

Treatment should be instituted as soon as the diagnosis has been made to prevent the infestation from spreading. It should also be offered to everyone who lives with the patient and to all his or her sexual contacts, who should use the treatment at the same time as the patient. The 5% permethrin lotion or cream employed are applied to the whole skin surface below the neck and ears. Treatment should be in contact with the skin for a minimum of 12 hours or overnight. All contacts of index case should be treated simultaneously, and the treatment should be repeated 7 days later to kill any new mites that might have emerged from eggs. The particular agents used are set out in Table 4.2.

Community outbreaks and crusted (Norwegian) scabies

Crusted scabies has a different clinical presentation from sporadic scabies and represents an altered host response to the infestation; the mite is no different. The term 'Norwegian' scabies should be discarded in favor of 'crusted' scabies, which more accurately reflects the clinical presentation. It manifests as

TABLE 4.1

Differential diagnosis of scabies

Disorder	Comment
Canine scabies	Different distribution – self-limited – not transmitted between humans
Eczematous diseases	Particularly atopic dermatitis – usually a history of eczema is present in the patient or family
Dermatitis herpetiformis	different distribution; vesicles and urticarial lesions more prominent – biopsy discriminates
Pediculosis	Presence of lice and nits

hyperkeratotic crusted plaques developing diffusely on the palmar and plantar surfaces, with thickening and dystrophy of the fingernails and toenails.

Whenever there is an outbreak of scabies in a community, it is essential to look for patients with crusted scabies, who act as a reservoir for the condition and perpetuate the outbreak.

Individuals with crusted scabies should be isolated. They may require several repeated courses of topical permethrin treatment or oral ivermectin and their clothing and bedding should be treated as infectious and washed at a high temperature.

Community treatment of scabies

When scabies is identified within a community it is important to ensure thorough treatment of all affected individuals and their contacts to eliminate the condition. Because of the common occurrence of asymptomatic mite carriers in the household, all family members and close contacts of the index case should be treated simultaneously. No individual should be permitted to re-enter the 'community' until they have been treated (whether for the condition or as a contact), and wherever possible, all members of the community should be treated simultaneously to prevent re-infestation.

Animal scabies

The species of mite that causes scabies in animals is similar to the one that causes human scabies but does not give rise to scabies infestation in humans. Contact with infested animals may cause transient lesions in humans skin at the sites of contact, and, occasionally, living animal scabies mites have been found in human skin but burrows have not been. Sarcoptic mange may be seen in horses, cattle, pigs, monkeys, guinea pigs, sheep, and goats, but the most common animal scabies to cause problems is that found in dogs or cats. The correct management approach is to treat the animal appropriately on veterinary advice and to give any topical anti-itch preparation to the human patient for the affected site. With proven human scabies infestation, it is important to look for the human contacts, not the animal contacts.

Pediculosis

Pediculosis is the result of infestation with one of the varieties of the human louse: (1) *Pediculus humanus capitis*, the head louse; (2) *Pediculus humanus humanus*, the body or clothing louse; and (3) *Phthirus pubis*, the pubic, or crab, louse.

TABLE 4.2

Treatments used for scabies

Agent	Percentage	Comment
Permethrin	5%	Treatment of choice
Benzyl benzoate	25%	Apply twice in 24 hours and repeat on the third day, very irritant
6–10% Sulphur in petrolatum ointment		A traditional treatment, irritant but inexpensive
Oral ivermectin		Single dose of 200 micrograms/kg: repeated after 7–10 days
For crusted scabies combination of oral with topical treatments is preferred.		

Pediculosis capitis (head lice)

Infestation with *P. capitis* is extremely common and is most frequently seen in children between the ages of 3 and 12. Although once more often seen in the poorer sections of society, the head louse is now seen in long-haired schoolchildren, regardless of their social background. It is more common during times of social upheaval, such as war. The louse is transmitted among children by close head-to-head contact or by fomites through brushes, combs, blow dryers, hair accessories, pillows, upholstery, helmets, bedding, or other headgear.

Clinical features

The average incubation period is 4–6 weeks. Itching is the predominant complaint. Some individuals are asymptomatic, despite infestation and considered to be 'carriers'. The scratching that results can cause secondary infection with exudation and crusting, but if this does not occur, all that may be seen are excoriations, erythema, scaling, and red papules on the skin surface. Other clinical findings include a low-grade fever and regional lymphadenopathy. Examination of the hair will reveal the louse eggs (nits) stuck to the hair shaft (Figure 4.4). Careful inspection will also detect the adult louse itself, which is less than 1 mm long and greyish or, after feeding, reddish in hue. When it moves, it deserves the description of 'mobile dandruff'. Infestations are diagnosed by demonstrating egg capsules (nits) and live lice. Nits are readily seen by the naked eye, most commonly in the occipital and retroauricular regions, and are an efficient marker of past or present infestation. They need to be differentiated from dandruff, hair casts, as nits are not easily dislodged from the hair shaft. Newly laid or viable eggs are tan to brown in color while the remains of hatched eggs are clear, white, or light in color. The presence of adult lice or viable nits within 1 inch of the scalp is confirmatory of active infestation.

Differential diagnosis

seborrhoeic dermatitis (dandruff), insect bites, eczema, psoriasis, hair gel spray, pseudonits, piedra.

Treatment

The treatments used are set out in Table 4.3. 1% permethrin cream rinse is recommended as first line therapy. Ivermectin lotion is approved for children 6 months or older for head lice. Care must be taken to ensure that all close friends and family are also treated. A further treatment 7 days later is also

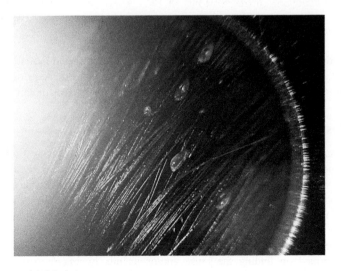

FIGURE 4.4   Louse eggs (nits) in hair.

TABLE 4.3

Treatments for pediculosis

Agent	Percentage	Comment
Malathion	0.5%	Both lotion (aqueous and alcoholic) and shampoo
Spinosad	0.9%	Topical suspension
Dimethicone	4.0%	Asphyxiating agent
Ulesfia	5%	Containing benzyl alcohol
Permethrin	1.0%	Creamy rinse for head lice
Permethrin	5.0%	Dermal crème, for crab lice, not recommended for head lice
Because no treatment is reliably ovicidal, retreatment after 1 week is reasonable.		

necessary to kill off all the young lice that may have hatched from the nits that remained alive after the initial treatment.

Pediculosis corporis (body lice)

Infestation with body lice is common in homeless individuals, victims of war, refugees and natural disasters, or those forced into crowded living conditions and socially deprived communities with poor hygiene. Transmission is via infested clothes or bedding or by close contact with the infected subject. The failure to wash or change clothes after exposure allows the infestation to persist. The body louse is responsible for the transmission of epidemic typhus, which is due to *Rickettsia prowazekii,* as well as trench fever (caused by *B. quintana*), and relapsing fever due to *Borrelia recurrentis*. The body louse spends most of its time attached to the seams of clothing, where the nits should be sought if the disorder is suspected.

Clinical features

Itching, without a great deal to see to account for the symptom, is usual in the early stages. Some excoriations mostly linear and primarily on the back, neck, shoulders, and waist; blood crusts and bluish marks on the skin where the louse has fed may also be seen. Later in the disease, lichenification, and eczema complete the picture of 'vagabond's disease'.

Treatment

Destruction and/or disinfestation of all clothes and bedding of the infested individual, the individual's family, friends, and close contacts are necessary. The patient should be treated from head to toe with a pediculicide (Table 4.3) or given oral ivermectin. Repeat treatment after 1 month is advised.

Pediculosis pubis (pubic lice, crab lice)

The pubic louse (*Phthirus pubis*) looks different from the head and body lice, as it is broader, with crab-like rear legs. It is mostly spread by sexual contact. The crab lice cling tenaciously to pubic hair, nipping down to skin level every so often to have a blood meal. In heavy infestations, the lice spread to body hair and even to the eyebrows and eyelashes. Sometimes they are found in moustache, beard, axillae, and scalp hair. Slate grey to bluish, irregular shaped macules about 1 cm in diameter representing haemorrhage from louse bite named maculae cerulea can be seen. *Pediculosis palpebrarum*, or phthiriasis palpebrarum, is the infestation of the eyelashes with crab lice.

Diagnosis is confirmed on finding the louse and/or its nits by microscopic examination of the plucked hair.

Treatment

A pediculicide (see Table 4.3) should be used, with repeat treatment after 1 month. Ivermectin is the first-line therapy for phthiriasis palpebrarum. Shaving of pubic hair is sometimes advised but is not necessary. All sexual contacts should be treated.

Insect bites and stings

A vast number of flying, jumping, and crawling arthropods are capable of causing injury in a variety of ways to human skin. Some are capable of transmitting disease, and a few important examples of this are given in Table 4.4 (see also Table 4.5).

Mosquitoes

Mosquito bites tend to be in exposed areas. Some varieties of mosquito (e.g. the culicine mosquitoes) can cause blisters when they bite. The bites may be extremely itchy and prominent (Figure 4.5) and may become infected after being scratched.

Fleas

Flea bites are mainly sustained from cat and dog fleas, which occasionally temporarily 'visit' a human host. They drop off their original hosts and live on carpets and rugs, as do their young, and jump up when they feel the vibration of footsteps. The bites, which are small and itchy, are often, but not exclusively, on the legs and usually distributed in a linear fashion. Unfed, fleas can enter a state of hibernation and remain

TABLE 4.4

Examples of important arthropod-spread diseases

Disease	Arthropod	Microorganism
Malaria	Mosquitoes (*Anopheles* species)	*Malaria parasitea* (*Plasmodium* species)
Trypanosomiasis (sleeping sickness)	Tsetse fly	*Trypanosoma bruceia*
Leishmaniasis	Sandfly (*Phlebotomus* species)	
Visceral		*Leishmania donovania*
Cutaneous		*Leishmania tropica*
Mucocutaneous		*Leishmania braziliensisa*
Onchocerciasis	Blackfly (*Similium* species)	Onchocerca volvulus
Bubonic plague	Rat flea	*Yersinia pestis* (formerly *Pasteurella pestis*)

TABLE 4.5

Examples of methods of injury to the skin by arthropods

Mechanism	Arthropod
Bites from piercing and cutting mouthpieces – injection of saliva	Mosquitoes, ticks, sandflies, blackflies
Stings from 'purpose-built' structures with an injection of toxic materials	Wasps, bees, scorpions, jellyfish
Release of toxic body fluids after being on the skin surface, causing blistering crushed	'Blister beetles' – cantharidin (Figure 4.10)

dormant in soft furnishings for up to 2 years, awakening in the presence of a new potential host. As a result, it is possible for humans to get flea bites long after the departure of the host animal.

Ticks

Ticks stay stuck to the skin for some time after biting and are found mainly in agricultural communities, as the principal host is mostly sheep. They may be the vector for a variety of infectious conditions, such as typhus and Lyme disease (Figure 4.6).

Mites

There is a large variety of mites that occasionally may bite humans. Most of these, such as bird mites or Cheyletellia mites living on cats, dogs, and rabbits (among others) cause small, red, itchy papules and are quite difficult to identify (Figure 4.7).

FIGURE 4.5 Mosquito bites on the leg (from Marks and Motley, 18th edition, with permission).

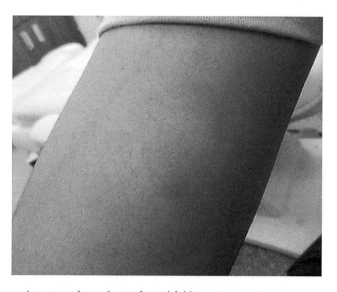

FIGURE 4.6 Erythema migrans: annular erythema after a tick bite.

Bedbugs (*Cimex lectularius*)

This primitive creature lives in the woodwork of old houses and comes out at night to bite its sleeping victims. The bites are often quite large and inflamed and arranged in straight lines where the creature has taken a 'stroll' over the skin surface. In recent years, bedbug bites have become more frequent and a problem for hotels.

Wasps and bees

The stings of wasps and bees are usually quite painful. The stung part may become very swollen a short time after the sting and when hypersensitivity is present, the individual may develop a widespread reaction. Rarely, such a reaction can cause anaphylactic shock and even death.

Papular urticaria

Papular urticaria is a term used to describe a recurrent, disseminated, itchy papular eruption due to either insect bites or hypersensitivity to them.

Diagnosis

The lesions themselves should be compatible, i.e., they should be papules or, less commonly, blisters, and it helps if puncture marks can be found in the lesion. It is commonplace for the patients (or their parents) to deny the possibility of insect bites being responsible for the lesions, as there seems to be a social stigma attached to being the recipient of them. A detailed history is necessary, with particular attention being given to the presence of domestic animals, proximity to farms, the occurrence of similar lesions in other family members, and the periodicity of lesions.

Biopsy may occasionally be helpful in that it may well rule out other disorders. The presence of a mixed inflammatory cell infiltrate in the upper and mid-dermis is typical, but the pattern and density of cellular infiltrate **are variable.**

Searching for the biting arthropod in the home may be fruitless unless the assistance of trained personnel is sought. Examination of 'brushings' from the coats of dogs by veterinarians may be successful in identifying the culprit – cheyletellia, for example. Some types of insect bite reaction can be unusually long-lived and may take many months to resolve.

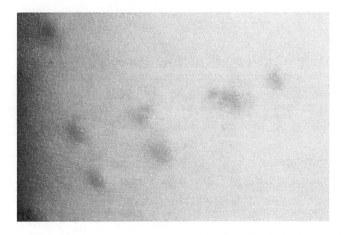

FIGURE 4.7   Multiple small papules due to mite bites (from Marks and Motley, 18th edition, with permission).

Treatment

Identification of the creature responsible and prevention of further attacks is important. Uncommonly, when there is evidence of hypersensitivity (as in a bee or wasp sting), systemic antihistamines may be required and, when there is a severe systemic reaction, systemic steroids and even adrenaline may be needed.

A major problem with insect bites is their intense itchiness. Occasionally, this may result in infection in the excoriated skin, when treatment is required for this complication. Topical antihistamines (e.g. diphenhydramine, promethazine) are often prescribed and may have a slight antipruritic effect, but all that is usually required is calamine or mentholated calamine preparation. Where insect levels are high, appropriate use of an insect repellent and insect nets is helpful.

Helminthic infestations of the skin

Onchocerciasis

This is caused by the parasite *Onchocerca volvulus* and is found in equatorial West Africa. The disorder is spread by the bite of the blackfly *Simulium damnosum*, which is found around rivers. The larval forms, known as microfilariae, are injected into the skin by the blackfly and develop after some years into adult onchocercal worms. These are extremely long (up to 1 m) but very thin (1–2 mm in diameter) creatures that live curled up in the subcutis surrounded by a palpable, host-supplied fibrous capsule. The adult worm procreates by producing enormous numbers of microfilariae, which invade the subcutis of large areas of truncal skin.

Clinical features

The disorder is characterized by severe and persistent irritation of the affected skin. Affected areas become thickened, lichenified, slightly scaly, and often hyperpigmented (Figure 4.8). The microfilariae may also invade the superficial tissues of the eye and cause blindness ('river blindness').

Diagnosis

Biopsies show non-specific inflammation, but occasionally demonstrate portions of the microfilariae. A more successful way of identifying the larval forms is by taking a series of skin 'snips' with a needle and scalpel. The tiny portions of the skin are then immersed in saline and observed microscopically to watch for the emergence of microfilariae. There is usually marked eosinophilia and a complement-fixation test for antibodies is also available in some centres.

Treatment

The pruritus is much improved by Hetrazan® (diethyl carbamazine). The drug must be given cautiously because of the possibility of a severe systemic reaction due to the liberation of toxic products from the dying microfilariae. Hetrazan has no effect on the adult worm and it is necessary to treat with the potentially toxic drug suramin to kill off the worm and prevent further production of microfilariae. Ivermectin is also helpful.

Cutaneous larva migrans

This is a distinctive migrating eruption caused by larvae from animal species which temporarily grow within human skin but cannot complete their life cycle in the human host. It is most commonly caused by the larvae of *Ancylostoma caninum*, which are excreted in dog feces and contaminate sandy beaches (particularly above the high-water line where the sand is never washed). Visitors sitting or standing on the beach may develop a creeping eruption on the affected skin as the larva moves slowly

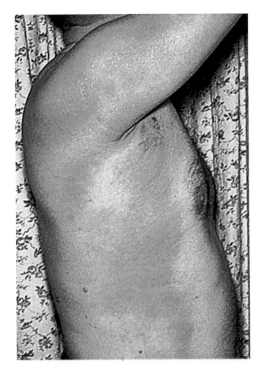

FIGURE 4.8 Skin changes of onchocerciasis, with marked thickening and discoloration (from Marks and Motley, 18th edition, with permission).

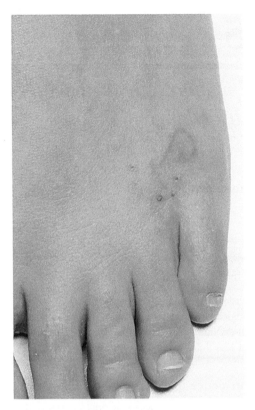

FIGURE 4.9 Serpiginous track of cutaneous larva migrans on the dorsum of the foot (from Marks and Motley, 18th edition, with permission).

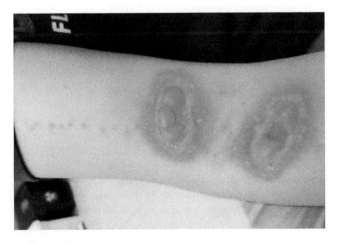

FIGURE 4.10 Kissing lesions – blister beetle dermatitis.

within the skin, advancing 1–2 mm per day (Figure 4.9). This creates a dramatic clinical picture and some irritation of the host skin. The condition may be treated with topical thiabendazole, or oral ivermectin; untreated, it usually resolves spontaneously after several weeks.

5

Immunologically mediated skin disorders

Yasmeen Jabeen Bhat

Urticaria and angioedema

Urticaria is characterized by transient, superficial well-defined pruritic wheals of the skin, whereas angioedema involves oedema of the dermis and subcutaneous or submucosal tissue that is deep and ill-defined. Urticaria can be acute or chronic. Acute urticaria has a sudden onset and recurs over a period of less than 6 weeks.

Incidence

Acutely urticaria occurs in 20% of the population, whereas chronic urticaria and angioedema occur in 0.5%.

Pathogenesis

Both immunologic and non-immunologic mechanisms lead to mast cell activation and release of mediators like histamine, prostaglandins, and cytokines. Non-immunological activation occurs with substances like neuropeptides, drugs, opiate derivatives, radiocontrast media, and foods. In immunologic activation, linkage of two α-subunits of IgE receptors (FcεRIα) of mast cells leads to the release of histamine, proteases, PGD2, and cytokines. Various bacterial and helminthic infections have been associated with chronic urticaria.

Clinical features

Urticarias can be classified clinically as:

a. **Ordinary urticaria:** may be acute, episodic, or chronic. Erythematous wheals occur anywhere on the body, including scalp, palms, and soles (Figure 5.1). Wheals generally last a few hours and resolve within 24 hours, leaving the skin with a normal appearance. Patients tend to rub rather than scratch, so excoriation marks are unusual. Angioedema may be found in 50% of patients. Urticaria may be associated with systemic symptoms like malaise, vomiting, arthralgia, dizziness, syncope, and rarely anaphylaxis. The duration of chronic urticaria is more than 6 weeks, and 50% of patients have an idiopathic type with no recognized cause. Pruritic wheals can occur on an almost daily basis and may greatly impair the patient's quality of life.

b. **Physical and cholinergic urticarias:** reproducible wheals induced by a physical stimulus form the basis of diagnosis. Wheals caused by physical stimuli occur within minutes and persist for

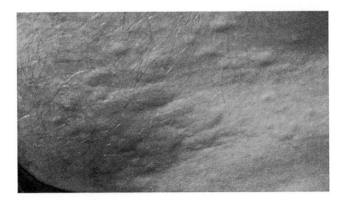

FIGURE 5.1   Erythematous wheals on the trunk of a man.

less than 30–60 min. In many forms of physical urticaria, if the stimulus is sufficiently great, angioedema may occur upon mediator release. Physical urticarias may be

 i) **Dermographism**: means skin writing. In symptomatic dermographism, patients complain of whealing and itching at sites of friction with clothing or scratching the skin.

 ii) **Delayed pressure urticaria**: whealing occurs at sites of sustained pressure applied to the skin after a delay of 30 min to 9 hours and lasts 12–72 hours.

 iii) **Vibratory urticaria**: any vibratory stimulus induces a localized, red, itchy swelling within minutes and lasting less than a few hours.

 iv) **Heat or cholinergic urticaria**: due to stimulation of the cholinergic postganglionic sympathetic nerve supply to the sweat glands. The patient complains of itching wheals that appear within minutes of exertion, when they are hot, experience emotional disturbances, or eat spicy food.

 v) **Cold urticaria**: includes a variety of syndromes in which cold induces urticaria. Idiopathic cold urticaria may be immediate, delayed, localized, familial, or acquired. It may also occur secondary to serum cryoproteins.

 vi) **Solar urticaria**: wheals develop at the site of exposure within minutes of visible, long or short-wave ultraviolet radiation and usually fade within 2 hours.

 vii) **Aquagenic urticaria**: contact with water at any temperature induces wheals resembling cholinergic urticaria.

 c. **Urticarial vasculitis:** In urticarial vasculitis, the cutaneous lesions resemble urticaria but histology demonstrates vasculitis. The lesions persist for more than 24 hours, have burning or itching sensation, are tender or painful, and resolve with bruising or staining. Systemic involvement is common.

 d. **Contact urticaria:** results from skin or mucosal contact with provoking substance.

 e. **Angioedema without wheals:**

 i) Idiopathic angioedema (angioneurotic or Quinke's oedema): a variant of urticaria in which subcutaneous tissues, rather than dermis, are involved. Common sites involved are lips, eyelids, and genitalia. Itching is often absent. The lesions last for a few hours or persist for 2–3 days (Figure 5.2)

 ii) Drug-induced angioedema: ACE inhibitors and NSAIDs may cause angioedema, which affects the face, and oral mucosa, and symptoms may be severe. The ACE inhibitors prolong bradykinin survival and potentiate its effects by inhibiting ACE. Most cases develop within 3 weeks of commencing the treatment.

iii) Hereditary angioedema: a rare disorder with autosomal dominant inheritance. Over 75% present before puberty, but the onset may be delayed into late adult life. There are recurrent swellings of the skin and mucous membranes throughout life, associated with nausea, vomiting, colic, and urinary symptoms. These patients have deficiency of a natural inhibitor of C1 esterase.

Investigations of urticaria

A comprehensive history is of utmost importance. It includes the type of lesions, duration, pruritus, systemic symptoms (like hoarseness, dyspnea, abdominal pain, and arthralgia), and medications. ASST (autologous serum skin test) and anti FcεRIα antibody determination can be done for autoimmune urticaria. Dermographism is evoked by skin stroking; pressure urticaria by application of weight to the skin; vibratory angioedema by a vibratory stimulus; cholinergic urticaria can be diagnosed by exercise to sweating; solar urticaria by testing with UVB, UVA, and visible light; cold urticaria by application of ice cube to skin. Urticarial vasculitis can be diagnosed by histopathology showing features of vasculitis. Complement levels can also be helpful.

Differential diagnosis

Papular urticaria, systemic capillary leak syndrome, erythema multiforme.

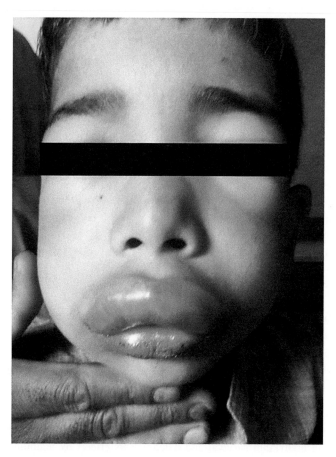

FIGURE 5.2   Marked swelling of the upper lip and eyelids in angioedema.

Angioedema: cellulitis, contact dermatitis, lymphoedema, connective tissue diseases like dermatomyositis.

Course and complications

In 50% of patients, urticaria resolves within 1 year but 20% have lesions for >10 years. Prognosis is good in most syndromes except hereditary angioedema, which may be fatal if untreated.

Treatment

Elimination of the suspected etiological agent or precipitating factor is important. Antihistamines with selective H_1 receptor blocking activity are the first-line treatment of urticaria. Low-sedating anti-histamines, e.g., cetirizine (10 mg/day), levocetirizine (5 mg/day), loratadine (10 mg/day), fexofenadine (180 mg/day), etc., are used to reduce urticarial activity with minimal side effects. H_2 antihistamines, such as ranitidine, can be combined with an H_1 blocker for a more effective response.

Second-line therapies (targeted therapy) could involve a short course of oral systemic corticosteroids (in doses of 0.5–1 mg prednisolone/kg/day) for severe urticaria and urticarial vasculitis. For severe angioedema, epinephrine must be injected intramuscularly. Danazol and stanozolol can be given for hereditary angioedema.

Third-line therapies (immunomodulatory) could include ciclosporin (2.5–3.5 mg/kg/day), methotrexate (7.5 mg/week), cyclophosphamide (50 mg/day), omalizumab (anti IgE), IvIg infusion (0.4 g/kg/day for 5 days), plasmapheresis, etc.

Erythema multiforme

Erythema multiforme (EM) is a cutaneous reaction to a variety of stimuli characterized by classical 'target lesions' on the skin and involvement of mucous membranes.

Incidence

EM can occur at any age. It is more frequent in males than in females.

Pathogenesis

It is a reaction pattern to many triggering factors due to immune mechanisms. It has an HLA association, and immune complexes and autoantibodies have been demonstrated. Delayed hypersensitivity also plays a role with the predominance of T lymphocytes in the lesions. Infections such as herpes simplex virus, orf, mycoplasma, coccidioidomycosis, and histoplasmosis; drugs such as sulphonamides and penicillin; and vaccination may trigger it.

Clinical features

The eruption develops over a few days and resolves in 2–3 weeks. Repeated attacks are associated with recurrent herpes simplex. In the more common mild form, EM minor, macules, papules or wheals, and classical 'target or iris' lesions are seen symmetrically on the distal extremities (Figure 5.3). A target lesion has three zones – a central area of dusky erythema or purpura, a middle paler zone, and an outer well-defined ring of erythema. Mucous membranes may show erosions or bullae. In the less common severe form, EM major, a more extensive skin and mucosal involvement with systemic symptoms may be seen.

Investigations

Pathology: The lower epidermis shows vacuolar degeneration and necrotic epidermal cells. The upper dermis shows oedema and perivascular mononuclear inflammation.

Differential diagnosis

Acute exanthematic eruptions following drugs and infections; autoimmune bullous disorders; vasculitis.

Course and complications

EM minor resolves in 2–3 weeks. EM major may lead to extensive cutaneous involvement, keratitis, and systemic symptoms.

Treatment

Symptomatic treatment is helpful. Antiviral therapy with acyclovir for recurrent EM following herpes simplex infection prevents relapse. For more severe cases, prednisolone (30–60 mg/day), decreasing over a period of 1–4 weeks, is given. Other immunosuppressants may be tried.

Erythema nodosum

A painful inflammatory disorder in which crops of tender nodules occur in response to antigenic stimuli.

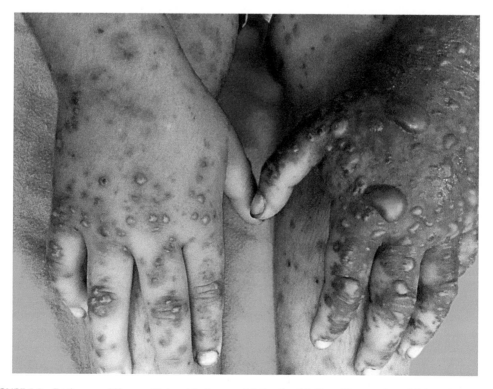

FIGURE 5.3 Erythema multiforme with target lesions on right hand and bullae with necrosis on left hand in a child.

Incidence

1–5 in 100,000 people per year, four times more common in women aged 15–40 years.

Pathogenesis

It is a cutaneous reaction pattern (panniculitis) to various infections, drugs like penicillins, inflammatory diseases like connective tissue diseases, granulomatous diseases like sarcoidosis, and malignancies like lymphoma.

Clinical features

Crops of painful, bright red, tender nodules, 1–3 cm in size, occur on the shins and rarely arms, bilaterally. They take 2–6 weeks to resolve and leave a bruised appearance. This is accompanied by fever, malaise, and arthralgias (Figure 5.4).

Investigations

Hematologic: Elevated ESR, CRP, leucocytosis, ASO titer, throat swab for bacterial culture, X-ray chest. Pathology shows the septal type of panniculitis.

Differential diagnosis

Other forms of panniculitis, polyarteritis nodosa, nodular vasculitis, pretibial myxedema.

Course

Spontaneous resolution occurs in 6 weeks. Lesions never ulcerate and heal without scarring.

Treatment

Bed rest, elevation of limbs, and NSAIDs. Antibiotics in case of infection and systemic steroids may be indicated.

Annular erythemas

There are several disorders that are marked by the appearance of erythematous rings, which usually gradually enlarge and then disappear. Various annular erythemas are granuloma annulare, erythema annulare centrifugum, erythema gyratum repens, and erythema migrans. Granuloma annulare is the common type.

Pathogenesis

Immunologically mediated inflammation surrounding the blood vessels and altering collagen and elastic tissue.

Clinical features

Usually asymptomatic, occurs from months to years, firm, smooth, shiny, skin-colored to erythematous beaded annular plaques on the body. Single lesions may be seen on dorsum of hand while as multiple lesions on extremities and trunk (Figure 5.5).

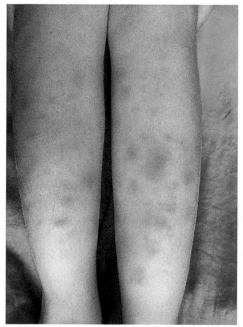

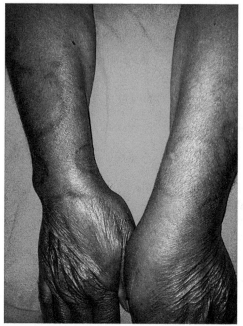

FIGURE 5.4 Erythematous tender nodules distributed bilaterally on the shins in erythema nodosum.

FIGURE 5.5 Multiple annular plaques with erythematous raised margins and clear centre in granuloma annulare.

Investigations

Pathology-necrobiosis of connective tissue surrounded by a wall of palisading histiocytes and multi-nucleated giant cells.

Differential Diagnosis

Other annular lesions.

Treatment

Topical and intralesional steroids, topical calcineurin inhibitors like tacrolimus. In generalized type, phototherapy and systemic steroids may be tried.

Course and complications

Generally, their significance is uncertain, but erythema gyratum repens, signifies the presence of an underlying visceral neoplasm and erythema chronicum migrans indicates the presence of Lyme disease.

Autoimmune disorders

These disorders are also known as the collagen vascular disorders and the connective tissue diseases. They arise in the context of a break in the immune tolerance to self where the immune system fails to 'recognize' the individual's own tissues and mounts an attack on them. In most of the disorders in this group, the inflammatory process seems to involve the small blood vessels in particular (vasculitis).

a. **Lupus erythematosus**: comprises a spectrum ranging from cutaneous disease only in chronic cutaneous lupus erythematosus to systemic disease only in acute cutaneous lupus.

Systemic lupus erythematosus

Incidence

1–12.5 in 100,000 per year. It is 3 times more common in blacks and much more common in women than men (9:1).

Pathogenesis

Genetic predisposition with susceptibility genes on the major histocompatibility complex (MHC) loci HLA-B8, -DR3, A1 and –DR2, autoantibodies, ultraviolet radiation, infections, stress, hormonal factors, and drugs are implicated.

Clinical features

Include arthralgias or arthritis, renal disease, inflammatory disorder of the pulmonary and cardiovascular systems, a polyserositis, central nervous system involvement, and skin disorder. Skin lesions of SLE include facial erythema across the cheeks and nose (butterfly rash or malar rash) (Figure 5.6). Subacute SLE, a type of SLE, predominantly affects the skin and presents with annular and psoriasiform lesions on the face and exposed parts.

Investigations

Pathology—atrophy of the epidermis, degeneration of the basal epidermal cells, oedema of dermis, mononuclear infiltrate around the small blood vessels. Direct immunofluorescence of unexposed, uninvolved skin has granular deposits of immune reactants IgG, IgA, IgM, and C3 at the dermo-epidermal junction in about 60% of the patients.

Serology—Antinuclear antibodies (>80%), anti-double-stranded DNA antibodies, anti-Sm antibodies, increase in the level of serum gamma globulins, decreased levels of complement.

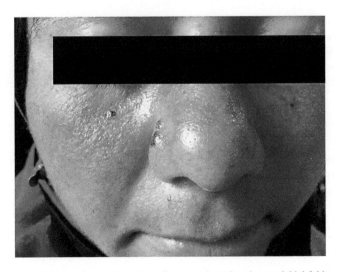

FIGURE 5.6   Malar rash involving both cheeks, bridge of nose, and sparing the nasolabial folds.

Hematological—a normocytic normochromic anaemia, neutropenia, lymphopenia, thrombocytopenia, and elevated ESR. Urinalysis shows persistent proteinuria and casts.

Differential diagnosis

Mixed connective tissue disease, drug hypersensitivity reaction, viral exanthems, photoallergic or phototoxic reactions.

Treatment

In addition to the general measures like rest and sun-protection, patients require systemic steroids to suppress the inflammatory process. Immunosuppressants such as azathioprine, methotrexate, mycophenolate mofetil, ciclosporin, cyclophosphamide, and biological therapies may be needed.

Course and complications

The 5-year survival rate (80–95%) has progressively improved. Poor prognostic signs are hypertension, nephritis, systemic vasculitis, and CNS disease.

Discoid lupus erythematosus (DLE)

Incidence

4 or 5 in 1000, twice as many females as males affected, common in the fourth decade and severe in blacks.

Pathogenesis

Genetic factors with environmental factors like UV radiation, viral infection, drugs, and stress may be responsible. Lesions of DLE can occur in the course of SLE or may be the only manifestation of the disorder.

Clinical features

Slightly pruritic, sharply marginated red scaly plaques appear on sun-exposed skin of the face and neck (localized DLE), hands, or arms (disseminated DLE) (Figure 5.7). Follicular involvement is a permanent feature and the lifted adherent scales show the 'Carpet tack' sign. The plaques develop hyperpigmentation at the periphery leaving atrophic central scarring, telangiectasia, and hypopigmentation. On the scalp, scarring alopecia occurs in the affected areas. Mucous membranes may be involved in 25% of patients.

Investigations

Pathology – the changes are similar to those described for SLE but there is hyperkeratosis with marked atrophy and epidermal degenerative changes. Also perifollicular and periappendageal lymphocytic infiltrate can be seen (Figure 5.8).

Differential diagnosis

Lupus vulgaris, hypertrophic lichen planus, sarcoidosis, panniculitis.

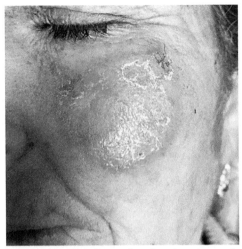

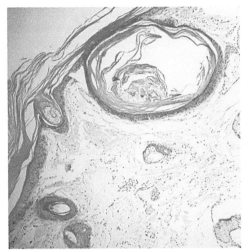

FIGURE 5.7 Sharply marginated erythematous scaly plaque on exposed surface in DLE.

FIGURE 5.8 HPE image (100×) showing thinning

Treatment

Sun protection with sunscreens is important. Topical corticosteroids and calcineurin inhibitors are used for localized lesions. Antimalarials like hydroxychloroquin (200–400 mg per day) are given with monitoring of ocular side effects. Systemic steroids, immunosuppresants, acitretin, and biological therapies have been used.

Course and complications

Five per cent patients develop SLE, the risk being higher in patients with disseminated DLE (22%). Squamous cell carcinoma occasionally occurs in the scars of DLE (Figure 5.9).

Systemic sclerosis

Incidence

A rare disorder with an incidence between 2.3 and 10 per million population, four times more common in females.

Pathogenesis

Autoimmunity in the presence of genetic factors leads to inflammation, vascular abnormalities, and deposition of fibrous connective tissue in specialized organs. Depending on the extent of cutaneous involvement, systemic sclerosis can be divided into diffuse cutaneous systemic sclerosis (dSSc) and limited cutaneous systemic sclerosis (lSSc).

Clinical features

The disease starts insidiously over years. The earliest feature is Raynaud's phenomenon and non-pitting edema of hands and feet with painful ulcerations at fingertips (rat bite necrosis) (Figure 5.10). Fibrosis of the face results in characteristic mask-like facial appearance, thinning of lips, microstomia, beak-like nose (Figure 5.11). Macular mat-like telangiectasia appear over the face and deposits of calcium

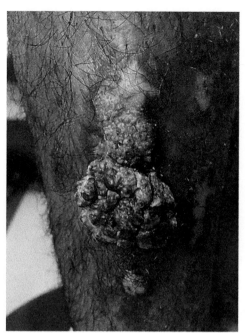

FIGURE 5.9   Squamous cell carcinoma developing on the scar of DLE.

develop in the skin. The term CREST syndrome – i.e. calcinosis cutis, Raynaud's phenomenon, esophageal dysfunction, sclerodactyly, and telangiectasia – is used. In diffuse cutaneous systemic sclerosis, involvement of the skin of upper arms, thigh, chest, and abdomen occurs. High frequency of pulmonary fibrosis, cardiac involvement, and scleroderma renal crisis may occur.

Investigations

Pathology – thickening of dermis with hyalinized collagen and paucity of blood vessels with thickening and hyalinization of vessel walls. Anticentomere autoantibodies occur in 71% of CREST and DNA topoisomerase I (Scl-70) antibodies in 30% of dSSc.

Differential diagnosis

Morphea, scleromyxoedema, mixed connective tissue disease, eosinophilic fasciitis, porphyria cutanea tarda.

Treatment

There is no specific treatment. Symptomatic management of the patient is very important. Vasodilators for Raynaud's phenomenon, penicillamine (750 mg/day), and immunosuppressants like low dose corticosteroids, cyclosporin, and azathioprine appear to help. ACE inhibitors for renal involvement and cyclophosphamide for pulmonary involvement are useful.

Course and complications

In more rapidly progressive systemic sclerosis, there may be more serious vascular disease affecting the fingers, resulting in tissue necrosis and even the loss of portions of the digits (Figure 5.12). Renal or pulmonary disease may eventually cause the death of the patient – the 5-year mortality rate of this disease is 30% or more.

Morphoea

Morphoea is a localized scleroderma.

Incidence

2.7% in 10,000 with female-to-male ratio of 2.5:1, peak occurrence between 20 and 40 years of age.

Pathogenesis

Unknown; however, infection with borrelial organisms and irradiation may be implicated.

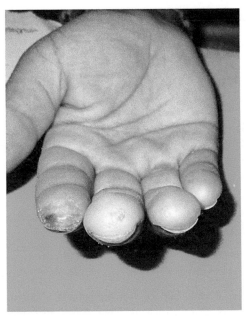

FIGURE 5.10   Finger tip ulcers in scleroderma.

Clinical features

One or more thickened, variably sized sclerotic plaques develop over the trunk or limbs. Initially purplish or mauve, they become smooth and shiny brownish plaques with a lilac-colored edge (Figure 5.13). The lesions can be linear (en coup de sabre when present on scalp and face), guttate, bullous, subcutaneous, or disabling pansclerotic.

Investigations

Pathology – there is marked replacement of the subcutaneous fat with new collagen which has pale, homogenized appearance.

Differential diagnosis

Systemic sclerosis, eosinophilic fasciitis, scleroedema, Parry Romberg's syndrome.

Treatment

There is no effective treatment. Topical calcipotriol and topical tacrolimus are beneficial in localized type.

Course and complications

Linear morphea may affect the limbs in children and lead to atrophy and restricted movement. Generalized morphea leads to a considerable limitation of movement and impedes breathing.

Variants of morphoea
   i. **Generalized mophoea**: A rare type in which widespread idiopathic sclerosis of the skin occurs, causing considerable limitation of movement without any systemic disturbances.

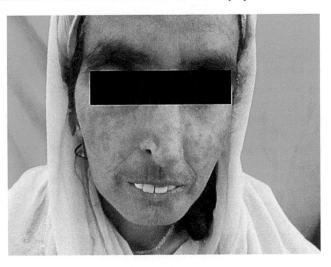

FIGURE 5.11   Beaked nose, thinning of lips, microstomia, mask-like facies, and mat telangiectasia in dSSc.

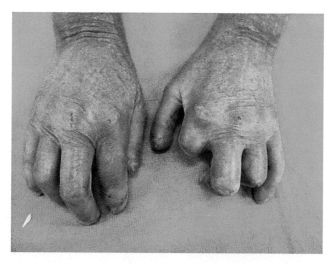

FIGURE 5.12   Loss of digits, sclerodactyly, and calcinosis cutis in SSc.

ii. **Lichen sclerosus et atrophicus (LSA):** Is a disease of adults but occurs in pre-pubertal children. Females are ten times more affected than men. Aetiology of LSA is unknown. Small, irritating, whitish, or ivory, sharply demarcated plaques occur on genitalia, around anus, or less commonly, elsewhere on skin. Dilated pilosebaceous or sweat duct orifices filled with keratin plugs (dells) and bullae, erosions and telangiectasia may be seen (Figure 5.14). In females, vulva may become atrophic and in males, it may lead to phimosis.

Topical agents like potent steroids and calcineurin inhibitors have shown good results. Circumcision may be helpful in males.

Dermatomyositis

Both muscle and skin are affected in this disabling disorder. The skin manifestations may precede, or occur in isolation from, the muscle inflammation.

Incidence

A rare disease with an incidence of 1.9 per million, occurring twice as frequently in females as in males. Occurs predominantly between the ages of 40 and 60 years but may occur in children under 16 years (juvenile).

Pathogenesis

Evolves through multiple phases – a genetically determined susceptibility phase, an induction phase triggered by environmental stimulus (infection, malignancy, drugs), an autoimmune expansion phase, and an injury phase involving multiple immunologic effector mechanisms.

Clinical features

Dull red to mauve areas develop over the face, back of the neck, backs of the hands, elbows, knees, and elsewhere. A particularly characteristic sign is the presence of violaceus erythema and oedema around the eyes (heliotrope rash, Figure 5.15). Small violaceus flat papules (Gottron's papules) over knuckles

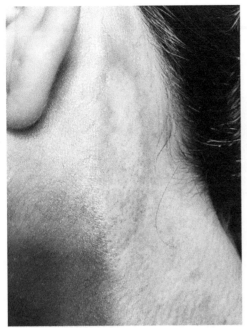

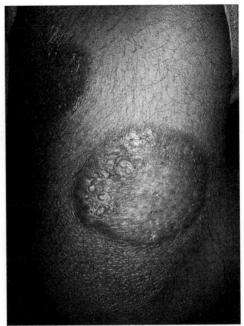

FIGURE 5.13 Atrophic indurated hypopigmented plaque with voilaceous margins. Bhat YJ, Akhtar S, Hassan I. Dermoscopy of morphea. *Indian Dermatol Online J* 2019;10:92-3. Reproduced with permission.

FIGURE 5.14 Sclerotic plaque with follicular plugs in LSA.

and interphalangeal joints with linear erythema on the dorsa of fingers can be seen (Figure 5.16). Small areas of necrosis may appear and long-lasting lesions may evolve into poikiloderma and calcification in subcutaneous tissue. Progressive muscle weakness, pain, and tenderness affecting proximal muscles of limbs also occur.

Investigations

Muscle enzymes such as creatine kinase, aldolase, and lactate dehydrogenase are increased in the blood. Urine creatinine is also a good indicator of disease activity. Muscle damage can be assessed by muscle biopsy and electromyography. Pathology – in the skin, interface dermatitis with mucin accumulation and in muscles, a characteristic pattern of inflammatory myositis is seen.

Differential diagnosis

Seborrheic dermatitis, lupus erythematosus, steroid myopathy.

Treatment

Rest is essential in acute pain. Oral corticosteroids (prednisolone 60 mg/day) clinically and bio-chemically improve. Immunosuppressive drugs are sometimes required to achieve or maintain remission.

Course and complications

If progressive, pharyngeal and respiratory muscles are affected. With treatment, the 8-year survival rate is 70–80%. Poor prognosis is seen in patients with malignancy and pulmonary involvement.

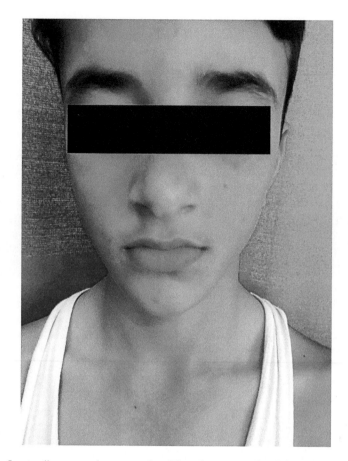

FIGURE 5.15   Confluent voilaceous erythema around eyelids and on v-area of neck in childhood dermatomyositis.

The vasculitis group of diseases

The term 'vasculitis' is applied to inflammation and necrosis of blood vessels (small, medium-sized, and large vessels). Systemic vascular involvement occurs mainly in kidneys, muscles, joints, respiratory system, skin, gut, and nervous system.

Cutaneous small-vessel vasculitis (CSVV): It is the most common type of vasculitis seen in dermatology.

Incidence

All ages may be involved, with equal incidence in males and females.

Pathogenesis

A history of drug exposure or recent infection is frequently present. Circulating immune complexes are deposited in the endothelium of postcapillary venules, leading to activation of the complement system with activation of inflammatory cascade damaging the vascular tissue.

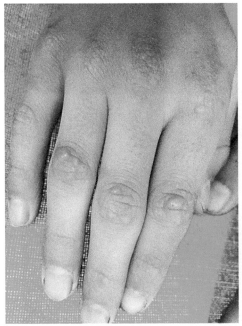

FIGURE 5.16 Gottron's papules on knuckles and interphalangeal joints of hands.

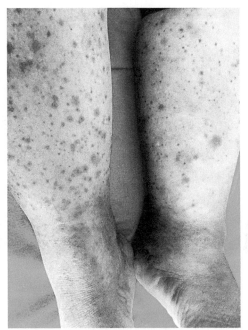

FIGURE 5.17 Palpable purpura on the legs in a patient of cutaneous small cell vasculitis.

Clinical features

The asymptomatic skin lesions typically arrive as a simultaneous 'crop of palpable purpura', primarily localized to legs (Figure 5.17). Mild systemic symptoms including fever, arthralgia, myalgia, and anorexia may be present.

Investigations

Pathology – deposition of eosinophilic material in the walls of postcapillary venules, extravasation of erythrocytes, infiltrate of neutrophils with karyorrhexis of nuclei (i.e. leukocytoclasia) are seen. The endothelium is swollen and shows degenerative changes. Figure 5.18 shows leukocytoclastic vasculitis.

Differential diagnosis

Thrombocytopenic purpura, meningococcemia, pigmented purpuric dermatosis.

Treatment

Disease is usually self-limiting.

Henoch Schönlein purpura (HSP)

Incidence

Although any age group can be affected, children are mainly affected.

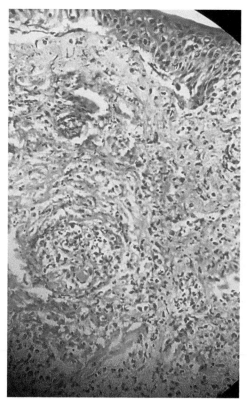

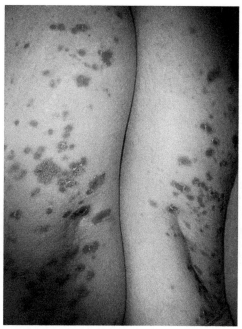

FIGURE 5.19 Crops of palpable purpura involving thighs and buttocks in HSP.

FIGURE 5.18 HPE image (400×) showing perivascular neutrophilic infiltrate, eosinophilic fibrinoid change of vessel walls, and nuclear debris (leukocytoclasia).

Pathogenesis

Hypersensitivity to streptococcal antigens may play a role as patients have a history of upper respiratory tract infection.

Clinical features

Classic findings of purpura, arthralgia, and abdominal pain are seen (Figure 5.19). Renal involvement with HSP is common, presenting as hematuria and proteinuria. Gastrointestinal bleeding may occur. Painful arthritis affects knees and ankles.

Investigations

HSP is a clinical diagnosis, confirmed by routine histology showing necrotizing vasculitis. In direct immunofluorescence, perivascular IgA deposits are characteristic.

Treatment

It is mainly supportive. Oral corticosteroids are given to patients with systemic involvement.

Course and complications

Long-term morbidity results from progressive renal disease (5%).

Polyarteritis nodosa

This is a multisystem, necrotizing vasculitis of medium-sized or small arteries.

Incidence

More common in adult males with a ratio of 2.5:1, with an incidence of 4.6–9 per million per year.

Pathogenesis

About 30% of cases are associated with hepatitis B and C antigenemia. Immune complexes lead to necrotizing inflammation of small and medium-sized arteries, with segmental lesions and involvement of bifurcations, leading to aneurysmal dilatation, rupture, and ischemic changes.

Clinical features

Cardiovascular, neurological, gastrointestinal, renal, and ocular involvement may be seen in this potentially fatal disease. Bright red to bluish nodules, ulcers, and livedo-reticularis occur in the skin.

Investigations

Fibrinoid necrosis of vessel wall with thrombosis and infarction of tissues supplied and neutrophilic infiltrate in all layers of muscular vessel wall and perivascular areas.

Differential diagnosis

Other types of vasculitis and panniculitis.

Treatment

NSAIDs, systemic corticosteroids, and cyclophosphamide are helpful. Surgery may be needed for complications.

Course and complications

Death from renal failure, bowel infarction, and cardiovascular complications may occur if untreated.

a. Giant cell arteritis

It is a systemic vasculitis of medium and large-sized arteries, notably temporal artery. It is characterized by headaches, fatigue, fever, high ESR, with necrosis and ulceration on the scalp.

b. Other types of cutaneous vasculitis

The development of crops of purple purpuric papules with darker and occasionally crusted central areas and sometimes pustules occur in the course of subacute bacterial endocarditis, gonococcaemia, and meningococcaemia. Drugs such as the thiazides may also cause a vasculitis. Renal involvement sometimes accompanies skin lesions. The importance of such lesions is that they are signs of an underlying systemic disorder, demanding rapid diagnosis and treatment.

c. Capillaritis

This is a group of benign, persistent, mildly inflammatory skin disorders in which the focus of the abnormality appears to be in the papillary dermis and the immediately subepidermal capillary vasculature. The term 'persistent pigmented purpuric eruption' seems appropriate, as they are persistent and because of the damage to capillaries, causing leakage of blood and pigmentation from haemosiderin staining. The lesions mostly occur on the lower legs and vary from a macular, spattered appearance (Schamberg's disease; Figure 5.20) to an itchy, papular eruption (lichenoid purpuric eruption) or a macular golden eruption (lichen aureus). These disorders generally cause little disability and remit spontaneously after a variable period.

Drug eruptions

Drug eruptions are skin disorders resulting from drug side effects, ranging from common skin eruptions to rare or life-threatening drug-induced diseases.

Incidence

The incidence of cutaneous adverse drug reactions (CADRs) is 5.5 per 100,000 of the population.

Pathogenesis

New drugs started within the preceding 6 weeks are potential causative agents. Both immunological and non-immunological mechanisms are involved. They may be provoked by systemic or topical administration of a drug. Variation in drug-metabolizing enzymes and HLA associations are the constitutional factors. Acquired facts like active viral infection and concurrent use of other medications also alter the frequency of drug-associated eruptions.

Clinical features

There are various patterns of cutaneous adverse drug reactions.

- Exanthematic (maculopapular) reactions: Most frequent of all cutaneous reactions to drugs, usually within 2 weeks after administration. The lesions may be scarlatiniform, rubelliform, morbilliform, or profuse eruption of small macules and papules. The distribution is generally symmetrical. The trunk and extremities are usually involved in comparison to viral rashes which may start on the face and progress to involve trunk, accompanied by conjunctivitis, lymphadenopathy, and fever. Maculopapular drug eruption usually fades with desquamation (Figure 5.21). Ampicillin, the psychotropic drugs, and the non-steroidal anti-inflammatory agents commonly cause this type of rash.

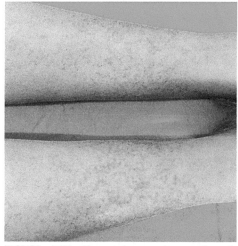

FIGURE 5.20 Pigmented purpuric eruption in Schamberg's disease.

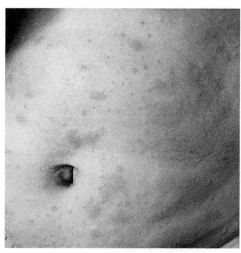

FIGURE 5.21 Exanthematic drug eruption.

- Exfoliative dermatitis: is one of the most dangerous patterns of CADR, characterized by generalized uniform redness and scaling of entire skin usually associated with fever, malaise, and lymphadenopathy.
- Urticaria, angioedema, and anaphylaxis: this systemic reaction may have constitutional symptoms in addition to cutaneous lesions and in severe cases, hypotension, bronchospasm, and laryngeal oedema.
- Erythema multiforme, Stevens–Johnson syndrome (SJS) and toxic epidermal necrolysis: (TEN) Characterized by target lesions in EM, involvement of skin as well as mucous membranes in SJS by bullae and erosions, and necrosis of sheets of the epidermis in case of TEN (Figure 5.22). SJS and TEN have immunologic pathogenesis. Genetic differences in the metabolism of some drugs may lead to idiosyncratic toxicity. Drugs causing SJS and TEN include sulphonamides, tetracycline, penicillins, and NSAIDs.
- Drug rash with eosinophilia and systemic symptoms (DRESS syndrome): Also known as drug hypersensitivity syndrome. It begins within 3–8 weeks of drug intake (mostly anticonvulsant drugs). It presents with constitutional symptoms, maculopapular exanthema, lymphadenopathy, eosinophilia, and multiple organ involvement.
- Acute generalized exanthematous pustulosis (AGEP or toxic pustuloderma): is characterized by sudden onset of multiple sterile non-follicular pustules on the background of diffuse erythema, starting in the flexural areas and face. Fever and neutrophilia are associated. Drugs causing AGEP include penicillins and NSAIDs.
- Fixed drug eruption: characterized by the repeated onset of a single (occasionally multiple) erythematous plaque at the same site. The skin lesion can be bullous or erosive and heals with hyperpigmentation. Numerous drugs – including dapsone, the sulfonamides, tetracycline, and mefenamic acid – may be responsible.
- Photosensitivity reactions to drugs (phototoxic dermatitis): results from exposure to certain drugs by ingestion or topical application and to UV radiation or visible light. It presents as an exaggerated sunburn response – erythema, oedema, vesicles, and bullae. Tetracyclines and sulfonamides may cause a phototoxic response. The phenothiazines may cause either a phototoxic or a photoallergic reaction.

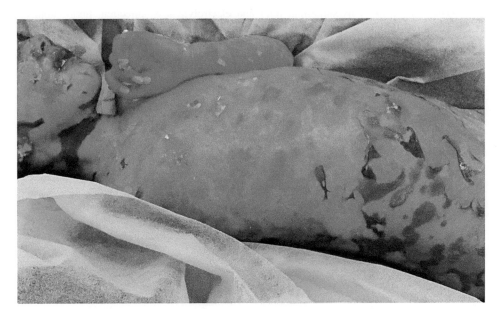

FIGURE 5.22   Denudation of the skin in toxic epidermal necrolysis.

- Drug-induced pigmentation: drug-induced alterations in pigmentation may occur from the deposition of a variety of endogenous and exogenous pigments in the skin. The pigmentation usually has a slate-grey hue on sun-exposed sites.
- Lichenoid drug eruption: Lichenoid drug eruption can be seen with many medications, including hydrochlorothiazide, NSAIDs, furosemide, antihypertensives (ACE inhibitors, β-blockers, CCBs), proton pump inhibitors, phenothiazines, anticonvulsants, antituberculous drugs, sildenafil, imatinib, and antimalarials. Lichenoid drug reactions may be photodistributed (lichenoid photoeruption) or generalized.
- Symmetrical drug-related intertriginous and flexural exanthema (SDRIFE): It is a delayed hypersensitivity immune response to drugs like antibiotics, characterised by well demarcated symmetrical erythema of intertriginous areas without systemic symptoms.

Investigations

History of drug exposure, the interval between the introduction of a drug, and onset of rash and improvement after drug withdrawal may give a clue. Skin testing, radioallergosorbent test, and patch test can be done.

Differential diagnosis

Viral exanthems.

Treatment

Drugs implicated in a previous reaction should be avoided. For minor conditions, withdrawal of the suspected drug and symptomatic therapy with emollients, topical steroids, and systemic antihistamines may help. For severe reactions, maintenance of body temperature, fluid and electrolyte balance, prednisolone 40–60 mg/day should be given.

Course and complications

Severe CADRs may lead to hypothermia, fluid and electrolyte loss, infection, high-output cardiac failure, stress ulceration, malabsorption, and venous thrombosis.

6

Blistering skin disorders

Pooja Agarwal
Rashmi Sarkar

Many inflammatory skin disorders can produce blistering at some stage in their natural history. In primary blistering diseases, blistering, a direct result of the initial pathological process, is a major feature. The different primary blistering diseases are listed in Table 6.1.

Bullous pemphigoid (senile pemphigoid)

Bullous pemphigoid (BP) is an uncommon blistering disease that occurs mainly in people over 60 years of age. Large, tense, often bloodstained blisters develop over a few days anywhere on the skin surface (Figure 6.1). A history of skin lesions like urticaria, papules, or pruritus can be found in many cases. Mucosal lesions can be seen in 10–30% of patients. New crops of blisters continue to appear for many months without adequate treatment, and the disease is painful and disabling. Rarely, the disorder is a sign of an underlying malignancy and can be associated with some neurological disorders (Table 6.2).

Laboratory findings

There is a circulating antibody directed to the epidermal basement membrane zone in 85–90% of patients, which can be detected using the immunofluorescence method. The titre of this antibody is to, some extent, a reflection of the activity of the disease. Antibodies of the IgG type and the complement component C3 are also deposited in the subepidermal zone around the lesions in the majority of patients and can also be detected using the direct immunofluorescence technique. Biopsy reveals that there is subepidermal fluid, with polymorphs and eosinophils, present in the infiltrate subepidermally.

Treatment

Patients with widespread blistering may need to be hospitalized and treated as though they had severe burns. Milder cases may be treated with potent topical corticosteroid ointments, and many patients respond, albeit slowly, over several weeks, to doxycycline. High doses of corticosteroids (40 mg per day of prednisone, or more) may be needed to control the disease, and immunosuppressive treatment with azathioprine, methotrexate, or mycophenolate mofetil may be used to allow a reduced dose of systemic steroids. Anti-inflammatory agents administered with dapsone or nicotinamide may also be beneficial.

Mucous membrane pemphigoid

It is not a single disease, but a group of heterogeneous, chronic blistering diseases primarily affecting mucosal surfaces. It is the second most common autoimmune blistering disorder in central Europe. Historically, because of the scarring complications that may develop clinically, it was described as cicatricial pemphigoid but is now categorized as mucous membrane pemphigoid. Cicatricial pemphigoid is

TABLE 6.1

The 'primary' blistering disorders

Subepidermal	Intraepidermal
Bullous pemphigoid	Pemphigus and its variants
Mucous membrane pemphigoid	Pemphigus vulgaris
Dermatitis herpetiformis	Pemphigus vegetans
Linear IgA disease and chronic bullous disorder of childhood	Pemphigus foliaceus
Anti-p200 pemphigoid	Endemic pemphigus foliaceus
Epidermolysis bullosa	Intercelluar IgA Dermatosis
Epidermolysis bullosa acquisita	Paraneoplastic pemphigus
Pemphigoid gestationis	
Bullous systemic lupus erythematosus	

TABLE 6.2

Diseases associated with bullous pemphigoid

Malignancy	Neurologic disorder
Gastric cancer	Parkinson's disease
Renal cancer	Dementia
Leukemia	Unipolar or bipolar disorder
Lymphoma	Multiple scelrosis

now used for blistering disorders where skin lesions heal with scarring, but mucosal lesions are absent. The mucous membranes that are most frequently affected are the oral cavity, the eyes, and nasopharynx.

MMP typically presents as remitting and relapsing mucosal inflammation and erosions. Intact vesicles or bullae are seen less frequently. Cutaneous lesions may resemble pemphigoid but are differentiated as they heal with scarring.

Dermatitis herpetiformis

Intensely itchy vesicles, papulovesicles, and urticarial papules appear in crops over the knees, elbows, scalp, buttocks, and around the axillae (Figure 6.2). Most patients with dermatitis herpetiformis (DH) have a mild, asymptomatic gastrointestinal absorptive defect due to gluten enteropathy, as in patients with coeliac disease. Some diseases with an immunopathogenetic component are more common in patients with DH, including thyrotoxicosis, rheumatoid arthritis, myasthenia gravis, and ulcerative colitis. The disorder is persistent but fluctuates in intensity.

Laboratory findings

Small-bowel mucosal biopsy reveals partial villous atrophy in 70–80% of patients with DH. Minor abnormalities of small-bowel absorptive function are also common. Biopsy of new cutaneous lesions demonstrates that the vesicle forms subepidermally and develops from collections of neutrophils in the papillary tips (the papillary tip abscess). Direct immunofluorescent examination from perilesional skin reveals the presence of IgA in the papillary tips in the skin around the lesions in all patients.

Treatment

The most important therapeutic interventions include a gluten-free diet and oral dapsone therapy.

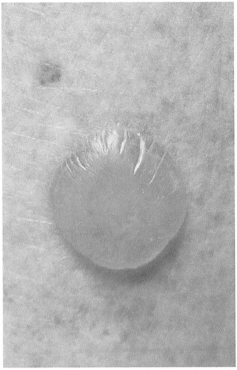

FIGURE 6.1   Tense blister due to bullous pemphigoid (from Marks and Motley, 18th edition with permission).

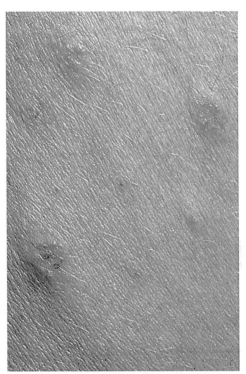

FIGURE 6.2   Vesiculopapules in dermatitis herpetiformis (from Marks and Motley, 18th edition with permission).

Skin lesions respond rapidly to the drug dapsone (50–200 mg per day) in most patients. However, dapsone has several potential toxic side effects, including haemolysis, methaemoglobinaemia, and sulfaemoglobinaemia, and may itself cause rashes such as fixed drug eruption. It should not be given to patients with glucose 6-phosphate dehydrogenase deficiency. A gluten-free diet will improve the gastrointestinal lesion and skin disorder in many patients after some months. Topical superpotent corticosteroids, though not useful alone, may help alleviate pruritus when given along with dapsone.

Linear IgA disease

This is an interesting condition, which may present with clinical features mimicking both bullous pemphigoid and dermatitis herpetiformis. It was recognized by the characteristic findings on direct immunofluorescent examination of the skin, which reveal a linear deposition of IgA antibodies at the dermoepidermal junction. In children, it is seen as a condition known as 'chronic bullous disease of childhood'. In adults, it may occur spontaneously or occasionally be induced by drugs such as nonsteroidal anti-inflammatory drugs or vancomycin. Clinically, there are vesicles or bullae on normal skin. New blisters form at the periphery of healing lesions, resulting in an annular appearance frequently described as strings of pearls or crowns of jewels. Common sites of affliction are the trunk, buttocks, extensor extremities, and the perioral area. Treatment is outlined in Table 6.3.

Epidermolysis bullosa

This is not a single disorder, but a group of similar, inherited blistering diseases. The blistering is caused by various congenital structural and metabolic defects. It can be present since birth as a result of

TABLE 6.3

Subepidermal blistering disorders

Disease	Bullous pemphigoid	Mucous membrane pemphigoid	Linear IgA disease and chronic bullous disorder of childhood	Dermatitis herpetiformis	Anti-p200/Laminin γ1 pemphigoid	Epidermolysis bullosa acquisita	Bullous systemic lupus erythematosus (SLE)	Pemphigoid gestationis
Clinical features	Old age (>75 years); tense blisters, erosions, intense pruritus, mucosal involvement rare	Erosions with predominant mucosal involvement, scarring in severe cases	Tense blisters, erosions, mucosal involvement rare, blisters arranged in annular pattern like 'string of pearls'	Intensely pruritic grouped vesicles on extensor sites	<75 years of age; tense blisters, erosions; mucosal involvement rare	Erosions, blisters, and scars on trauma-prone areas in mechanobullous variant. Lesions resembling BP in inflammatory variant	SLE patient, tense blisters, erosions; photoexposed areas	Pregnancy or postpartum period; erythemia, papules, bullae, intense pruritus
Special features	Association with neurologic disorders and rarely malignant	Ocular, laryngeal complications due to scarring	Can be drug-induced, most commonly vancomycin, NSAIDs, and penicillin	Association with celiac disease	Rare association with psoriasis	Rare association with inflammatory bowel disease, haematological malignancies	Precipitating drugs include hydralazine, penicillamine	Recurrence with pregnancy or with hydatidiform mole
1st line	Potent topical steroid Prednisolone Dapsone	Potent topical steroid Dapsone Cyclophosphamide	Oral dapsone Potent topical corticosteroids Oral prednisolone	Gluten-free diet Dapsone Potent topical steroid	Potent topical steroid Prednisolone Dapsone	Prednisolone Colchicines Dapsone	Dapsone	Topical steroids Oral antihistaminics
2nd Line	Azathioprine, Doxycycline, Methotrexate, Mycophenolate	Mycophenolate mofeil	Tetracycline ± nicotinamide	Other sulfa drugs	Doxycycline, azathioprine	Mycophenolate Cyclosporine	Azathioprine Prednisolone Mycophenolate	Prednisolone
3rd line	Immunoglobulins Immunoadsorption Rituximab	Immunoglobulins Immunoadsorption Rituximab	Mycophenolate mofetil Immunoglobulins		Immunoglobulins Immunoadsorption	Immunoglobulins Immunoadsorption Rituximab	Methotrexate Rituximab	Azathioprine Immunoglobulins

Treatment

mutations in genes coding for structural elements in the basement membrane, or can present later in life as a result of antibodies produced against collagen VII. The various forms of epidermolysis bullosa are summarized in Table 6.4.

There is no effective treatment other than to avoid trauma and to keep the blistered areas clean and dry.

Epidermolysis bullosa acquisita

This condition has only been recognized in the last 25 years. As the name implies, it is an acquired blistering disorder, often affecting middle-aged to elderly individuals, which, at the first sight, resembles bullous pemphigoid. It has two variants – mechanobullous type which resembles epidermolysis bullosa and an inflammatory variant resembling pemphigoid. It is more resistant to treatment than pemphigoid and many cases originally diagnosed as pemphigoid, which were thought to be resistant to treatment, were most probably epidermolysis bullosa acquisita. Confirmation of the diagnosis is made by immunofluorescent tests on salt-split skin (skin which is incubated in hypertonic saline to induce a split at the dermoepidermal junction). The antibodies in epidermolysis bullosa acquisita bind to the dermal side of the split; in bullous pemphigoid, they bind to the epidermal side.

Anti-p200 pemphigoid

It is a distinct bullous skin disorder characterized by autoantibodies against p200 protein at the dermoepidermal junction. Clinically, the disease resembles pemphigoid with tense cutaneous blisters.

TABLE 6.4

Major variants of epidermolysis bullosa

Variant	Cleavage plane	Clinical features
Epidermolysis bullosa simplex	Intraepidermal	Most common subtype
		Friction-induced blistering
		Palms and soles most commonly affected
		Blisters in herpetiform pattern in severe disease
		Erosions heal without scarring
		Residual pigmentary changes may remain
		Milia and atrophy can occur after healing
Junctional epidermolysis bullosa	At the level of lamina lucida	Extensive mucocuatneous blistering at birth
		Nails and hair are affected frequently, resulting in complete loss
		Scarring, webbing, milia, and atrophy occur commonly after healing
Dystrophic epidermolysis bullosa	Dermal	Extensive mucocutaneous blistering, severe skin fragility
		Nail dystrophy, alopecia common
		Pseudosyndactyly is characteristic
		Oral, esophageal, anal mucosa also affected
Kindler syndrome	Mixed	Trauma induced blistering in childhood
		Poikiloderma and atrophy seen in adults
		Photosensitivity
		Gingivitis and periodontitis common

Diagnosis can be made only by detecting antibodies against p200 by Western blot against an extract of the upper dermis.

The subepidermal blistering disorders are summarized in Table 6.3.

Pemphigus

Pemphigus is a group of blistering disorders, which is characterized by acantholysis, i.e. loss of keratinocyte to keratinocyte adhesion, which results in the formation of epidermal blisters in mucosae and skin. Acantholysis is induced by autoantibodies against intercellular adhesion molecules. There are several types (Table 6.5), out of which pemphigus vulgaris (PV) is the most common. The average age of onset is 40 to 60 years. The lesions are thin-walled, delicate blisters that usually rapidly rupture and erode (Figure 6.3). They occur anywhere on the skin surface and very frequently occur within the mouth and throat, where they cause much discomfort and disability. The disorder is persistent, although fluctuating in intensity. Before adequate treatment became available, it was usually fatal. Pemphigus foliaceus is another variant where blistering occurs in the superficial layers of the epidermis. Clinically, blisters are seen rarely and erosions with crusting are seen mainly over the scalp, face, and seborrheic areas. It can sometimes become generalized and the patient may go into erythroderma. Though a chronic disease, its course is more benign than pemphigus vulgaris.

Laboratory findings

In more than 90% of patients, there is a detectable circulating antibody directed to the intercellular adhesion molecules. The titre of the antibody reflects the severity of the disease. The presence of the antibody and its titre are determined by indirect immunofluorescence methods. Biopsy reveals the intraepidermal split, with rounded up epidermal cells, known as acantholytic cells. The cells over the basement membrane lose intercellular adhesion and appear as a 'row of tombstones'. Direct immunofluorescence examination of the perilesional involved skin is the gold standard and will show the presence of antibody of the IgG class in a fishnet pattern and the complement component C3 between epidermal cells.

TABLE 6.5

Intraepidermal blistering diseases

Disease	Cutaneous distribution	Mucosal involvement	Clinical features	Special features
Pemphigus vulgaris	Face, scalp, trunk	May be severe	Flaccid bullae, erosions	Rare association with thymoma, may be drug-induced
Pemphigus vegetans	Flexures	Less severe	Vegetating lesions in flexures	Cerebriform tongue
Pemphigus foliaceus	Scalp, seborrheic areas	None	Erosions with crusting, blisters seen rarely	May go into erythroderma
Endemic pemphigus foliaceus	Upper body	None	Flaccid blisters, erosions	Endemic to South America, may progress into erythroderma
Intercelluar IgA Dermatosis	Flexures, scalp, proximal limbs	none	Flaccid pustules, Circinate appearance	IgA monoclonal gammopathy
Paraneoplastic Pemphigus	Significant palmoplantar involvement, generalized lesions may be there	Severe	Polymorphic lesions-bullae, erosions, 'target lesions', lichenoid lesions	Lymphoproliferative disease,

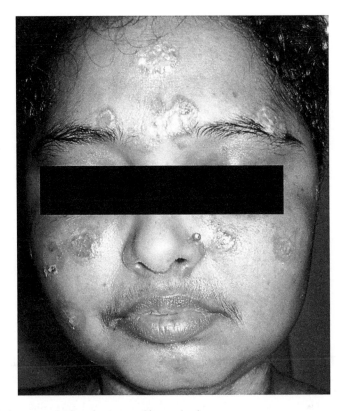

FIGURE 6.3   Eroded areas on the face due to pemphigus vulgaris.

Treatment

The patients should be treated as though they had burns and, if severely affected, need inpatient care. High doses of systemic steroids are the mainstay of therapy as they provide rapid improvement in the disease. Immunosuppressive therapy with azathioprine or mycophenolate mofetil should be started simultaneously to reduce the steroid dose gradually. In resistant cases, other therapeutic modalities should be used, which include cyclophosphamide, rituximab, intravenous immunoglobulins, plasmapheresis, and immunoadsorption.

7

Skin disorders in AIDS, immunodeficiency, and venereal disease

Indrashis Podder
Rashmi Sarkar

Introduction

Acquired immune deficiency syndrome (AIDS) is a symptom complex caused by a lymphotropic retrovirus, now known as the human immunodeficiency virus (HIV). The virus is acquired either by sexual intercourse (homosexual or heterosexual) or from the accidental introduction of material contaminated by HIV into systemic circulation. Although unprotected sexual intercourse remains the major route of transmission of this deadly condition, intravenous drug abuse, and contaminated blood transfusion facilitate its spread.

Epidemiology

Today, this disorder has reached epidemic proportions, with approximately 36.7 million people living with HIV/AIDS at the end of 2015 worldwide. Amongst them, 1.8 million were found to be children (<15 years), most of them acquiring the infection from their HIV-positive mothers during pregnancy, childbirth, or breastfeeding. The vast majority of these people live in low- and middle-income countries, with sub-Saharan Africa being the worst affected region, accounting for almost 70% of these cases (25.6 million).

Pathogenesis

The virus incapacitates the T-helper lymphocytes, thus preventing the proper functioning of the cell-mediated immune response. It uses the CD4 antigen as its receptor and employs the T-cell's genomic apparatus to replicate, destroying the cell as it does so. It can also infect reticuloendothelial cells (including Langerhans cells) and B-lymphocytes.

After gaining access, the virus usually stays latent and the infected individual remains free of symptoms for a long period, but the virus may cause a systemic illness in a relatively short time after infection and before or at the time of seroconversion. This illness is characterized by pyrexia, malaise, and a rash resembling infectious mononucleosis. The median period for progression from HIV infection to AIDS is 9–10 years but is very variable.

Usually, there are no symptoms for several years, even after an antibody response develops until the virus is 'activated' by an intercurrent infection such as herpes simplex. AIDS is characterized by

TABLE 7.1

Dermatological manifestations of HIV/AIDS

Infectious conditions	Non-infectious conditions
• Fungal infections (characteristic deep fungal infections viz. histoplasmosis, blastomycosis, dermatophytosis, etc.)	• Cutaneous malignancy (Kaposi sarcoma, non-melanoma skin cancers, etc.)
• Viral infections (warts, molluscum contagiosum, etc.)	• Seborrhoeic dermatitis (more severe and more common)
• Bacterial infections (exaggerated manifestations of tuberculosis, syphilis, bacillary angiomatosis, etc.)	• Psoriasis (increased incidence of psoriatic arthritis)
• Parasitic infestation (crusted/Norwegian scabies, acanthamoebiasis)	• Reiter's syndrome
	• Generalized pruritus
	• Ichthyosis/xerosis
	• Drug reactions (more severe than in normal patients; SJS, TEN)
	• Acne conglobata
	• Mucosal changes (increased occurrence of oral aphthae)
	• Hair changes (thin lustreless hair, different varieties of alopecia, long eyelashes)
	• Nail changes (characteristic finding is proximal subungal onychomycosis)
	• IRIS (immune reconstitution inflammatory syndrome)

depressed delayed hypersensitivity, and a reduction in the number of circulating T-helper cells is a constant finding. Indeed, the progress of the disease can be monitored by checking the lymphocyte count and estimating the viral RNA load. Skin disorders are prominent in AIDS, and patients often present with a skin complaint.

Some important dermatological manifestations of HIV/AIDS are given in Table 7.1.

Infectious conditions

When the disease is activated, the patient becomes subject to opportunistic infections as well as to an increased incidence and severity of usually mild and commonplace infections, such as viral warts and oral thrush, as a result of profound immunosuppression.

The introduction of highly active antiretroviral therapy (HAART) has greatly reduced the development of these complications in patients with HIV infection. However, these complications may become severe or life-threatening in the absence of proper and adequate treatment.

Fungal infections

Dermatophyte infections, including nail infection, become extensive and are difficult to clear. Recurrent candidiasis is often a major problem, especially in the mouth and oropharynx with varied clinical presentations (erosive, membranous, vegetative, and angular cheilitis). Even systemic spread of *Candida* infection, especially oesophageal involvement (an AIDS-defining criterion), is not uncommon and often a terminal event. Occasionally, it may result in disseminated disease or sepsis, which is characterized by the occurrence of proximal muscle tenderness along with maculopapular rash. Proximal subungual onychomycosis is the characteristic pattern of fungal nail infection in these patients. *Pityrosporum ovale* may cause extensive pityriasis versicolor, thus resulting in troublesome and persistent truncal folliculitis (Figure 7.1) in some patients and severe seborrhoeic dermatitis in others. Various 'deep fungal' infections like histoplasmosis, blastomycosis, cryptococcosis have gained prominence, particularly in hot and humid parts of the world. Organisms that do not usually infect humans may sometimes cause problems – such as the *Penicillium* species. Invasive deep fungal infections have been reported to be one of the major causes of mortality in HIV/AIDS patients, accounting to almost 50% of all AIDS-related deaths globally.

Viral infections

Viral warts may become very extensive and troublesome. Molluscum contagiosum lesions may be larger than usual and present in very large numbers, often on the face and eyelid. Inflamed lesions are common.

Recurrent herpes simplex infection may be a particular problem, with extensive bilateral and persistent skin involvement often resulting in scarring. Severe, chronic, and progressive orolabial, genital, or anorectal ulcers may occur. Even an unsuspecting lesion of chronic herpetic whitlow may be the first manifestation of HIV/AIDS.

Herpes zoster is similarly a troublesome infection in AIDS and maybe the initial manifestation. It may not resemble 'ordinary' herpes zoster, typically resulting in echthymatous, verrucous, and necrotic lesions, causing considerable pain and tissue destruction, as well as spreading outside the dermatomes in which it began (non-contiguous dermatomes). A characteristic pattern called disseminated zoster often occurs in these patients (more than 2 non-contiguous, scattered lesions outside the affected dermatome). Epstein-Barr virus (EBV) causes a characteristic condition in these patients called oral hairy leukoplakia (OHL), which serves as a marker for HIV/AIDS.

Bacterial infections

Severe and extensive staphylococcal infections (pyoderma) are common (Figure 7.2). Tuberculosis and syphilis are both major problems for individuals with AIDS. Both disorders progress rapidly and are

FIGURE 7.1   Folliculitis due to Pityrosporum ovale infection in a patient with human immunodeficiency virus infection (from Marks and Motley, 18th edition).

responsible for extensive and severe disease in AIDS patients. Extrapulmonary disease is quite common in late HIV disease. It has been reported that these patients are 30 times more likely to develop active TB, compared to the general population. Cutaneous TB also occurs more frequently in these patients. The most common form is military tuberculosis in contrast to scrofuloderma being the most common form in non-reactive patients. Infections with mycobacterial species that do not generally infect humans may also be seen in these patients. Bacillary angiomatosis, a characteristic feature of HIV/AIDS, occurs due to infection with a bacterial microorganism similar to the bacillus-causing 'cat-scratch' disease. It causes Kaposi's sarcoma-like lesions and a widespread eruption of red papules. Another infection characteristic of HIV/AIDS is pneumonia due to *Pnemocystis jiroveci*. Recently, trials are going on the long-term use of co-trimoxazole to prevent serious bacterial infections in HIV-infected children. A group of researchers are also exploring the role of vaginal microbiota in HIV transmission and infection. Syphilis can also present with some unusual manifestations in immunosuppressed AIDS patients like multiple, painful and giant chancres, increased chance of lues maligna (secondary syphilis with vasculitis and systemic involvement) and more rapid progression to tertiary syphilis. There might be limited antibody response to treponemal antigens or false-negative non-treponemal tests, making the serologic diagnosis of syphilis unreliable in these patients.

Parasitic infestations

Scabies seems to spread very quickly and cause extensive and severe skin involvement in patients with AIDS, leading to the formation of hyperkeratotic lesions called 'crusted or Norwegian' scabies. Erythroderma may occur and itching may be almost non-existent. Other rare parasitic

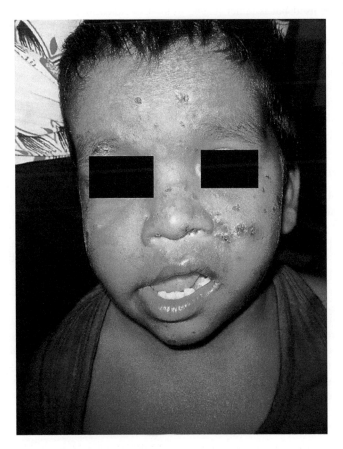

FIGURE 7.2 Severe, extensive pyoderma in an HIV-positive child (courtesy of Dr. Nidhi Gupta, Medical College, Kolkata, India).

infections may also occur with increased frequency in these patients viz. acanthamoebiasis, onchocerciasis, etc.

Skin cancers

Depressed delayed hypersensitivity also results in failure of 'immune surveillance' and the development and rapid progression of many forms of skin cancer. Viral infection may also be at work in the development of the disorder known as Kaposi's sarcoma, which mainly accompanies AIDS contracted from homosexual contact. A herpes-type virus is suspected of being responsible for this (HHV-8). Mauve, red, purple, or brown macules, nodules, or plaques may ulcerate and may spread to involve the viscera. Kaposi's sarcoma is a frequent cause of death in patients with AIDS. Other common skin cancers seen in HIV-positive patients include superficial basal cell carcinomas (BCCs) of the trunk, SCCs in sun-exposed areas, genital HPV-induced SCC, and extranodal B- and T-cell lymphomas.

Other skin manifestations

Pruritus and dryness of skin (xerosis)

The skin of patients with AIDS may become dry and ichthyotic, making AIDS one of the causes of 'acquired ichthyosis', which, in turn, is one of the causes of persistent pruritus. Pruritus occurs in almost 30% of AIDS patients and is considered to be one of its markers. However, pruritus is not usually caused by the disease itself but is rather related to the associated inflammatory dermatoses. The most common type of lesions are papular, pruritic eruptionpapules, collectively called 'papular pruritic eruption,' which can be either follicular (temperate regions) or non-follicular (tropical and subtropical regions). Eosinophilic folliculitis (EF) is the most common type of follicular pruritic eruption, clinically characterized by the development of urticarial papules on the upper trunk, face, neck, and scalp; while the histologic hallmark is eosinophilic infiltration around the upper part of hair follicles. Non-follicular pruritic eruptions are mostly insect-bite reactions, followed by scabies, prurigo nodularis, atopic dermatitis, seborrheic dermatitis, and transient acantholytic dermatosis (Grover's disease). These lesions are treated using topical corticosteroids, phototherapy (UVB or PUVA), and antihistamines.

Seborrhoeic dermatitis

Seborrhoeic dermatitis is one of the common causes of chronic, itchy scaly eruption in these patients. Its incidence is much more than in seronegative patients, affecting also 85% of all seropositive patients at some point of their disease. It is quite often the presenting feature of HIV (Figure 7.3). Often this condition becomes extensive in patients with AIDS, presumably due to massive overgrowth of *Pityrosporum ovale* other causative microorganisms, occasionally resulting in erythroderma.

Psoriasis

Pre-existing psoriasis may develop an 'explosive phase', or psoriasis may develop *de novo* as an aggressive, rapidly spreading eruption. Severe psoriatic variants like psoriatic arthritis, pustular psoriasis, and erythrodermic psoriasis are more common in HIV-infected patients. Several explanations have been proposed lately for this "psoriasis HIV-1 paradox" including HIV-1induced destruction of regulatory CD^4 + T cells, an increase in the number of memory CD^8 + T cells late in disease, or HIV-1 proteins acting as superantigens.

Reiter's syndrome

Patients often present with migratory arthritis along with keratotic limpet-like scales. Circinate balanitis and plantar fasciitis are common, but urethritis and uveitis are often absent.

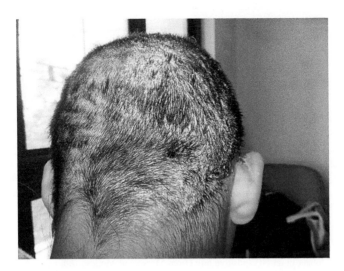

FIGURE 7.3 Extensive seborrhoeic dermatitis in an AIDS patient (courtesy of Dr. Nidhi Gupta, Medical College, Kolkata, India).

Drug reactions

Cutaneous adverse drug reactions (CADRs) occur more frequently in patients suffering from HIV/AIDS; ranging from morbilliform eruptions to erythroderma and even Stevens–Johnson syndrome. Commonly implicated drugs include sulphonamides (cotrimoxazole), nevirapine, abacavir, rifampicin, and carbamazepine.

Acne conglobata

This is a severe and extensive form of acne responding well to oral retinoids or HAART (Figure 7.4).

Mucosal lesions

Mucosal lesions like aphthae occur more frequently in these patients.

Hair changes

Lustreless hair, thin hair, various types of alopecia, discoloration, premature greying, and long eyelashes have been described.

Nail changes

Some of the important nail changes reported to occur more frequently in seropositive patients are leukonychia, pigmentation, half and half nail, clubbing, yellow nail syndrome, paronychia, and proximal subungual onychomycosis (PSO). PSO is a marker of HIV infection.

IRIS (Immune reconstitution inflammatory syndrome)

IRIS refers to a paradoxical worsening of a known condition or the appearance of a new condition in HIV positive patients after initiation of antiretroviral therapy occurring as a result of restored immunity. Mycobacterial infections have been reported to be the commonest triggering factor for IRIS, apart from viral (herpetic, HPV, hepatitis group, etc.), fungal (cryptococcal, histoplasma), parasitic (Strongyloides

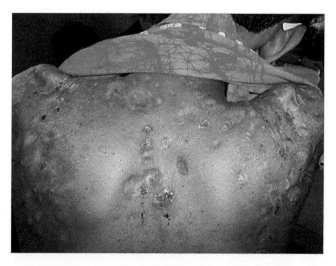

FIGURE 7.4   Acne conglobata in an HIV-positive boy (from Marks and Motley, 18th edition).

infestation), and other non-infectious conditions like Guillain–Barre syndrome, autoimmune thyroiditis, non-Hodgkin's lymphoma, and myopathy. HAART must be continued along with symptomatic treatment in all cases apart from a few life-threatening cases which may require discontinuation of HAART along with systemic corticosteroids.

Treatment of skin manifestations of AIDS

Treatment of the cutaneous manifestations include treatment of the disease proper (AIDS) and symptomatic treatment of the cutaneous condition (infections, pruritus, etc.)

Treatment of the disease proper (HIV/AIDS)

Several drugs have shown efficacy in treating HIV infection; some of the important antiretroviral drugs are tabulated in Table 7.2.

The first effective treatment for AIDS was zidovudine (AZT, azidothymidine), a reverse transcriptase inhibitor, given at 500–1500 mg per day in four to five divided doses. The drug slows down the progress of the HIV infection but comes nowhere near eliminating the viral infection. Unfortunately, it causes nausea, malaise, headache, and rash as well as many other side effects. Several other classes of antiretroviral drugs are now available. Other nucleoside analogue reverse transcriptase inhibitors include lamivudine, nevirapine, stavudine, delavirdine, and efavirenz. Other classes of drugs in use include protease inhibitors and non-nucleoside reverse transcriptase inhibitors. Optimal regimens now usually consist of at least three drugs from two classes of antiretroviral agents. The newer antiviral drugs include enfuviritide (fusion inhibitor), maraviroc (blocks the entry of virus into cell by blocking the CD4 protein), and the integrase inhibitors (raltegravir, dolutegravir). Although promising, trials are going on to assess the efficacy of these drugs.

Symptomatic treatment of cutaneous conditions

Ganciclovir and foscarnet are indicated for cytomegalovirus complications. Aciclovir is used for herpes simplex and herpes zoster. Various antibiotics and other antimicrobials are used as indicated for bacterial infections. Fluconazole, itraconazole, and ketoconazole are particularly useful for serious and life-threatening *Candida* infections. Recombinant interferon-alpha 2B and other interferons have been used with some success in Kaposi's sarcoma. The new retinoid bexarotene (Targretin®) is used topically to

TABLE 7.2

Important antiretroviral drugs

Category/Family of drugs	Principal mechanism of action	Names of drugs
Nucleoside reverse transcriptase inhibitors (NRTI)	After phosphorylation, gets incorporated into the growing viral DNA to cause premature chain termination	Zidovudine, Didanosine, Zalcitabine, Stavudine, Lamivudine, Abacavir, Emtricitabine
Non-nucleoside reverse transcriptase inhibitors (NNRTI)	Binds directly to the viral (HIV) reverse transcriptase enzyme and blocks its function	Nevirapine, Delavirdine, Efavirenz
Nucleotide reverse transcriptase inhibitors	Prevents the entry of viral DNA into the host cell nucleus	Tenofovir
Protease inhibitors	Inhibit protease enzymes resulting in the formation of immature, defective viral particles	Indinavir, Ritonavir, Saquinavir, Nelfinavir, Amprenavir, Atazanavir, Tipranavir, etc.
Fusion inhibitor	Blocks the fusion of viral membrane with the host cell membrane	Enfuvirtide
Entry inhibitor	Blocks receptors on the host cell (CD4)	Maraviroc
Integrase inhibitors	Blocks the integration of viral DNA into host cell DNA	Raltegravir, Dolutegravir, Elvitegravir

induce regression in individual lesions. Other cutaneous manifestations also require symptomatic treatment like topical corticosteroids (psoriasis), antipruritics (generalized pruritus), and emollients (xerosis and ichthyosis).

Drug-induced immunodeficiency

Patients who undergo organ transplantation and those suffering from chronic disorders like auto-immune disorders such as systemic lupus erythematosus, rheumatoid arthritis, and some eczematous diseases, including severe recalcitrant atopic dermatitis, receive immunosuppressive drugs like corticosteroids and azathioprine, ciclosporin, or tacrolimus for varying lengths of time. The cutaneous side effects from the immunosuppression are not usually as prominent as in AIDS patients but depend on the extent and length of the immunosuppression. They include severe and extensive bacterial and other opportunistic infections.

Patients with renal allografts have most problems, perhaps because they are treated continuously for longer periods than most of the other groups. They are prone to the development of numerous warty lesions on the hands and face. These are either viral warts or solar keratoses, or lesions in which it is really quite difficult to determine their nature. It may be that many viral warts directly transform into premalignant lesions (Figure 7.5).

It should be noted that photochemotherapy with ultraviolet radiation of the 'A' type (PUVA) treatment also causes depression in delayed hypersensitivity due to depletion of antigen-presenting cells of the skin (Langerhans cells), and this probably results in the delayed development of skin cancer in few patients with psoriasis treated with PUVA.

Other causes of acquired immunodeficiency

Lymphoreticular proliferative diseases such as Hodgkin's disease, leukemias, and sarcoidosis also result in depressed delayed hypersensitivity. Hypovitaminosis A, chronic malnutrition, and chronic alcoholism also result in depressed immune defences, although the depressed immunity in these instances is contributory to causing disease rather than being directly causative.

Congenital immunodeficiencies

Some congenital/primary immunodeficiency disorders present with eczematous dermatitis as the cutaneous manifestation. Some of such prominent disorders are listed in Table 7.3.

Dermatological aspects of venereal disease

Several skin infections, although not exclusively 'venereal', are nonetheless spread by venereal contact. Such disorders include genital warts, herpes simplex (type II virus), molluscum contagiosum, scabies, and pubic lice.

Reiter's syndrome

This disorder occurs as a sequel to non-specific urethritis in men and, less commonly, to bowel infection, and probably results from infection with a *Mycoplasma* organism. There is usually accompanying migratory arthritis with spondylitis and occasionally conjunctivitis. Thick, red psoriasiform skin lesions develop on the soles and elsewhere on the feet. These are often severe, persistent, aggressive, and pustular (keratoderma blenorrhagica). Inflamed red scaling patches may also develop on the glans penis (circinate balanitis). There is a curious and unexplained preponderance of patients with the human leucocyte antigen (HLA) B27 haplotype. Although arthritis in a characteristic involvement is the most common presentation, urethritis and conjunctivitis may or may not be present; thus the classical triad of arthritis, urethritis, and conjunctivitis is extremely rare in occurrence.

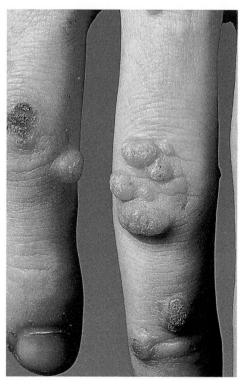

FIGURE 7.5   Warty lesions on the hands in a patient after 8 years on azathioprine and prednisolone following renal allograft; the lesions are either viral warts or solar keratoses, or somewhere in between (from Marks and Motley, 18th edition).

Gonorrhoea

This venereal disease, which predominantly affects urethral epithelium, is caused by a delicate intracellular Gram-positive diplococcus – the gonococcus. The skin is only affected during gonococcaemia, when small purpuric and pustular vasculitic lesions suddenly appear in the course of a pyrexial illness (Figure 7.6). These are similar to the purpuric pustular lesions that develop in meningococcaemia and subacute bacterial endocarditis.

Chancroid (soft sore)

This venereal infection is caused by the Gram-negative bacillus *Haemophilus ducreyi*. One to 5 days post-infection, a soft sloughy ulcer appears on the areas of contact on the penis or vulva. Other sites may be affected, and inguinal adenitis occurs in 50% of patients, usually unilateral in distribution. Both the genital ulcer and lymphadenopathy are painful, a characteristic feature of this condition.

Differential diagnosis includes syphilitic chancre, herpetic ulceration, granuloma inguinale, and traumatic ulcers. The treatment of choice is Azithromycin (1 gm orally in a single dose) or Injection Ceftriaxone 250 mg i.m. in a single dose or Ciprofloxacin (500 mg twice daily for 3 days) or Erythromycin (500 mg 6-hourly for 14 days).

TABLE 7.3

Important immunodeficiency disorders

Disorders	Features
1. Infantile/X-linked agammaglobulinaemia	X-linked recessive disorder; absence of plasma cells in the marrow making patients more susceptible to severe pyoderma and numerous warts.
2. Severe combined immunodeficiency (SCID)	Sex-linked recessive or autosomal recessive inheritance, complete deficiency of both cell-mediated and humoral immunity due to depression of circulating lymphocytes, increased susceptibility to all infections leading to death between the ages of 1 and 2 years.
3. Ataxia telangiectasia	Autosomal recessive disorder characterized by cerebellar degeneration, telangiectasia on exposed skin developing progressively, lymphopenia and depressed circulating levels of IgA antibody.
4. Hyper-IgE syndrome (HIES)/Job syndrome/Buckley syndrome	Autosomal dominant disorder, mutation in STAT3 gene; recurrent cutaneous and sinopulmonary infections, dermatitis from birth or early childhood, coarse facial features, and very high levels of immunoglobulin E (IgE).
5. Wiskott–Aldrich syndrome	X-linked recessive inheritance, mutation in WAS gene, life-threatening primary immunodeficiency associated with a bleeding tendency, eczema, and recurrent pyogenic infection.

Syphilis

Syphilis has recently generated renewed interest because of the rising incidence of AIDS; the syphilitic chancre serves as a portal of entry for the HIV virus as well as the more dramatic presentation of syphilis in AIDS patients. The disease is caused by the delicate spirochaetal microorganism *Treponema pallidum*, which is transmitted by contact between mucosal surfaces.

Clinical features

Characteristically, the incubation period is 9–90 days and the first sign is the appearance of the chancre at the site of inoculation, usually on the glans penis, prepuce or, less often, on the shaft of the penis in men and on the vulva in women. In homosexuals, the chancre may appear around or in the anus. The chancre is of variable size (0.5–3 cm in diameter) and has a sloughy and markedly indurated base. Untreated, it heals after 3–8 weeks.

This primary stage of the disease is followed by a brief quiescent phase of from 2 months to up to 3 years before the secondary stage occurs. In secondary syphilis, there are signs of a usually mild systemic upset with slight fever, headache, mild arthralgia, and generalized lymphadenopathy. In addition, there are skin manifestations, which include an early widespread pink macular rash, involving the palms and soles (Figure 7.7) and a later papular or lichenoid eruption. Thickened, broad-based warty areas (condylomata) appear perianally and in other moist flexural sites (Figure 7.8). Ulcers appear on the oral mucosa (snail-track ulcers).

After resolution of the secondary stage, there is a latent period without signs or symptoms, lasting for 5–50 years. The tertiary stage takes protean forms and includes cardiovascular disease with aneurysm formation (particularly aortic aneurysm), central nervous disorder, either as tabes dorsalis or general paralysis of the insane, and ulcerative or gummatous lesions that may occur on the skin or on mucosal surfaces.

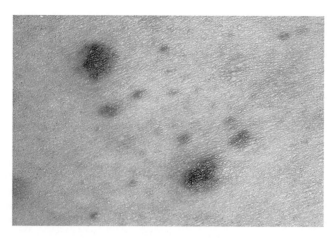

FIGURE 7.6   Vasculitis (from Marks and Motley, 18th edition).

Diagnosis

Diagnosis is made by identification of the spirochaete from wet preparations of the chancre or moist secondary-stage lesions (dark ground illumination microscopy) and by serological tests detecting either lipoidal substance liberated by infected tissues (non-treponemal tests) or the presence of antibodies to the microorganism (treponemal tests).

The older Wassermann reaction (WR) has been replaced by the Venereal Disease Reference Laboratory (VDRL) test, a flocculation test, which, although not specific, is quite sensitive and becomes

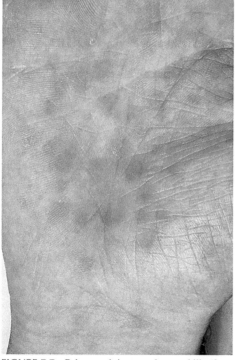

FIGURE 7.7   Palmar rash in secondary syphilis (from Marks and Motley, 18th edition).

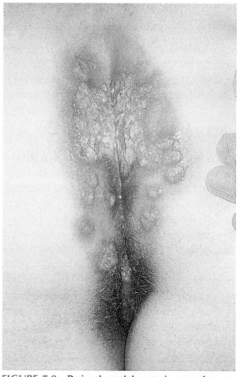

FIGURE 7.8   Perianal condylomata in secondary syphilis (from Marks and Motley, 18th edition).

positive early in the disease. It can also be used to monitor therapy as it becomes negative around 6 months following adequate therapy. The WR and the VDRL tests (and other similar tests) depend on lipoidal antigens. The *T. pallidum* haemagglutination assay (TPHA) is currently the most widely used specific test and depends on antibodies to the microorganism.

Treatment

The treatment of syphilis includes one dose of Benzathene penicillin (240000 IU) intramuscular for early stages or 3 weekly 240000 IU intramuscular doses for late latent/unknown duration disease. Recently, comparable efficacy has been reported with oral Doxycycline 100 mg twice daily for 14 days for early stages and 100 mg twice daily for 28 days for late latent/unknown duration stages (Antonio MB, Cuba GT, Vasconcelos RP, Alves AP, da Silva BO, Avelino-Silva VI. Natural experiment of syphilis treatment with doxycycline or benzathine penicillin in HIV-infected patients. *Aids*. 2019; 33:77–81). A proportion of patients develop a fever and possibly a rash after starting treatment (Jarisch–Herxheimer reaction). More serious reactions can also occur. However, in penicillin-sensitive patients, the drug of choice is erythromycin.

8

Eczema (dermatitis)

Sumit Sethi

The term 'eczema' includes several disorders (Table 8.1) in which inflammation is focused on the epidermis. Typically, epidermal cells become swollen and accumulate oedema fluid between them (spongiosis), leading to the formation of vesicles in acute cases. Odema, vasodilation along with perivascular mononuclear infiltrate, is seen in the dermis.

Some types of eczema stem from yet uncharacterized constitutional factors ('endogenous' or constitutional eczema), whereas others are the result of an external injury (exogenous). The clinical picture varies according to the nature of the provocation, the acuity of the process, the susceptibility of the individual, and the site of involvement.

Atopic dermatitis

Definition

This is a very common, chronic relapsing inflammatory skin condition characterized by extreme itching. The eczematous lesions typically affect the face and extensors in infants, while flexural surfaces are involved in children, adolescents, and young adults. It is often associated with a personal or family history of other atopic disorders, such as asthma and allergic rhinoconjunctivitis.

Clinical features

Signs and symptoms

Atopic dermatitis (AD) is a highly pruritic inflammatory skin disease characterized by a chronic or chronically relapsing course that begins during infancy (early onset) but occasionally may present in adulthood (late-onset). Dry lackluster skin, intense pruritus, and cutaneous hyperreactivity are cardinal features of AD. Pruritus may be present intermittently throughout the day but is usually worse in the evening and night. The itchiness is made worse by changes in temperature, by rough clothing (such as woollens), and by other minor environmental alterations. The incessant scratching gives the fingernails a 'polished' appearance and results in eczematous lesions, prurigo papules, and lichenification. Early/ acute skin lesions appear as intensely pruritic papules and vesicles on erythematous base, associated with excoriations, vesicles, and serous exudate (Figure 8.1). Erythematous, excoriated, scaling papules characterize subacute dermatitis (Figure 8.2). Chronic AD is characterized by thickened hyperpigmented plaques of skin with accentuated skin markings (lichenification) and pruritic papules (Figure 8.3). The distribution pattern of eczema varies according to the patient's age. During infancy, the lesions are more acute and primarily involve the face, scalp, and extensor surfaces of the extremities. The diaper area is usually spared. Older children, and those with long-standing skin disease, develop a chronic form of AD, with lichenification and distribution of the rash to the flexural folds of the extremities. AD often decreases in severity as the patient grows older, leaving an adult with skin that is prone to itching and inflammation when exposed to exogenous irritants. Chronic hand eczema may be the presenting manifestation of many adults with AD.

TABLE 8.1

Common types of eczema

Type	Synonyms	Frequency/Age group	Cause
Atopic dermatitis	Neurodermatitis Besnier's prurigo Infantile eczema	Very common, mostly occurs in infants and the very young	Unknown, but appears to be immunologically mediated
Seborrhoeic dermatitis	Infectious eczematoid dermatitis	Very common in all age groups	Probably microbial with overgrowth of normal skin flora being responsible
Discoid eczema	Nummular eczema	Uncommon, mainly in middle-aged individuals	Unknown
Lichen simplex chronicus	Circumscribed neurodermatitis	Quite common, mainly in young and middle-aged adults	Initially appears to be a localized itch causing an 'itch–scratch cycle'
Eczema craquelée	Asteatotic eczema	Uncommon, restricted to the elderly	Low humidity and vigorous washing
Venous eczema	Stasis dermatitis Gravitational eczema	Common in the age group that has gravitational syndrome	Multiple; a common variety is allergic contact dermatitis to medicament
Allergic contact dermatitis		Common in all adult age groups except the very old	Delayed hypersensitivity to a specific agent
Primary irritant contact dermatitis	Occupational dermatitis Housewives' eczema	Very common in all adult age groups except the very elderly	Both mechanical and chemical trauma
Photosensitivity eczema		Not uncommon, mainly in adults	Both phototoxic and photoallergic types occur

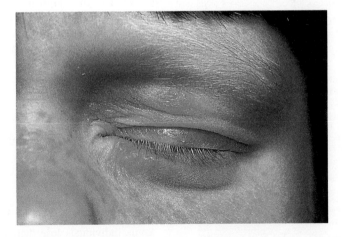

FIGURE 8.1   Inflamed, thickened eyelids and some loss of eyebrows and eyelashes due to perpetual eye rubbing in atopic dermatitis (from Marks and Motley, 18th edition, with permission).

In many patients, there is a widespread fine scaling of the skin, described as 'dryness' or xerosis; it is sometimes incorrectly diagnosed as ichthyosis, but is really the result of the eczematous process itself. Another feature sometimes incorrectly ascribed to ichthyosis is the presence of increased prominence of the skin markings on the palms Figure 8.4) – the so-called hyperlinear palms. The cheeks are often pale,

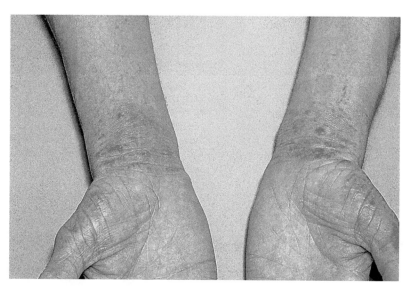

FIGURE 8.2 Excoriations of the wrists in atopic dermatitis (from Marks and Motley, 18th edition, with permission).

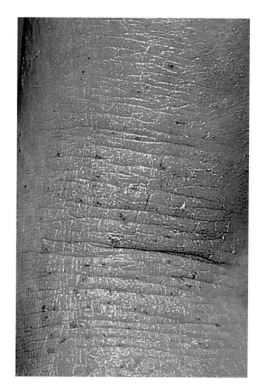

FIGURE 8.3 Exaggeration of skin surface marking (lichenification) due to scratching (from Marks and Motley, 18th edition, with permission).

with crease lines just below the eyes (known as Dennie Morgan folds) due to continual rubbing, making the facial appearance quite characteristic (Figure 8.5). In addition, the eyebrows tend to be sparse. Running a blunt instrument (such as a key) over affected skin produces a white line in about 70% of patients, known as 'white dermatographism'. This is the reverse of the normal triple response and disappears when the condition improves. This paradoxical blanching is similar to that seen after intracutaneous injection of methacholine in atopic dermatitis patients.

Clinical variants

In patients with black skin, there are often numerous small follicular papules in affected areas. In lichenified areas in black-skinned patients, there may be irregular pigmentation, with hyperpigmentation at some sites and loss of pigment at others.

Some individuals lose their childhood eczema only to develop chronic palmar eczema in later years with scaling, hyperkeratosis, and cracking. This is also believed to be a manifestation of atopic disease.

Associated disorders

Atopic dermatitis, asthma, and hay fever seem to share pathogenetic mechanisms in which aberrant immune processes play an important part. These three 'atopic' disorders cluster in families and the tendency to one or

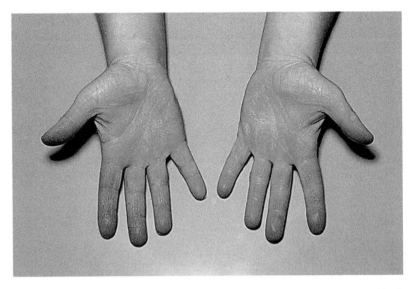

FIGURE 8.4   Prominent skin surface markings of the palms (hyperlinear palms) in atopic dermatitis (from Marks and Motley, 18th edition, with permission).

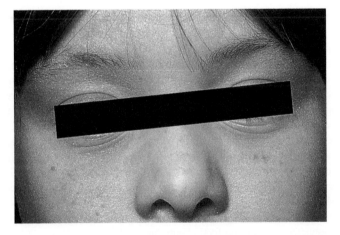

FIGURE 8.5   Prominent crease beneath the eyes in a child with atopic dermatitis – Denny Morgan fold (from Marks and Motley, 18th edition, with permission).

the other or all is inherited in an as-of-yet uncharacterized way. Chronic urticaria and alopecia areata occur more often in atopic dermatitis patients. The skin of patients with atopic dermatitis is more vulnerable to both chemical and mechanical trauma and has an unfortunate tendency to develop irritant dermatitis. Many of these associated problems may be due to a general defect in the barrier function of atopic skin.

Occupational and chronic hand eczema are much more common in patients with atopic dermatitis.

Complications

Patients with atopic dermatitis are frequently troubled by skin infections. Pustules and impetiginized areas represent bacterial infection (mostly staphylococcal) and are the most common expression of this propensity. They are easily treated but tend to recur. Cellulitis may also develop, giving rise to fever and systemic upset. Viral warts and molluscum contagiosum are also more frequent and more extensive than in non-eczematous subjects.

Herpes simplex sometimes causes a severe and extensive rash in atopic dermatitis patients, who may develop fever and severe systemic upset, but recover after 10–14 days.

Epidemiology and natural history

Atopic dermatitis occurs in families, but the mode of inheritance has been difficult to work out.

AD is very common and has 15–20% prevalence in some developed countries. It typically begins during infancy; 50% of patients present it by 1 year of life and an additional 30% between the ages of 1 and 5 years. Between 50–80% of patients with AD develop allergic rhinitis or asthma later in childhood. Many of these patients outgrow their AD as they develop respiratory allergy.

Laboratory findings and aetiopathogenesis

Skin biopsy of an acute eczematous lesion reveals spongiosis, epidermal thickening, parakeratosis and an inflammatory cell infiltrate (mostly lymphocytes), oedema, and vasodilatation in the dermis.

Elevation of serum IgE antibodies is seen in approximately 70–80% of AD patients. These are 're-aginic', precipitating antibodies to various environmental allergens, including foods and inhaled materials, which become fixed to mast cells. Atopic patients often have multiple positive reactions to various foods, house dust mite allergen, and pollens.

The susceptibility to skin infection, association with other disorders with immunopathogenetic component, and elevated IgE level, suggest an abnormality of the immune system in the pathogenesis of atopic dermatitis. Part of the problem may be an imbalance in the relative proportions of two sub-populations of T-helper lymphocytes – TH1 and TH2. The TH1 subset typically secretes gamma in-terferon and is important in turning off the secretion of immunoglobulins by B-lymphocytes. TH2 cells predominantly secrete interleukin-4 (IL-4) and are thought to be dominant in atopic dermatitis.

A marked decrease in skin barrier function is observed in AD patients due to the downregulation of cornified envelope genes (filaggrin and loricrin), reduced ceramide levels in epidermis, enhanced transepidermal water loss, and increased levels of endogenous proteolytic enzymes. Frequent use of alkaline soap and detergents raise the pH of skin, increasing the activity of endogenous protease enzymes, leading to further decrease of epidermal barrier function. Exogenous proteases from *Staphylococcus aureus* (*S. aureus*) and house dust mites also take a toll on the epidermal barrier. Deficiency of few endogenous protease inhibitors in atopic skin worsens the situation. The defective epidermal barrier leads to increased allergen absorption and microbial colonization of the skin. Epicutaneous sensitization to these environmental allergens, chemicals, and antigens results in inflammatory responses and a high level of immunologic memory, thus predisposing these children to the development of respiratory allergy and food allergy later in life.

Management

Several points need to be kept firmly in mind.

The disease is persistent but unpredictably active and subject to recurrent flares, making it important to develop a good relationship with patients and their immediate relatives over what may be many years.

The disorder causes discomfort and disability because of the intense and persistent itching, resulting in anxiety and depression in those affected by it. The sleep disturbance associated with intense pruritus affects the entire family.

The use of bland, greasy emollients gives symptomatic relief and provides protection from further antigenic insults.

Infection plays an important role in the aggravation of the disease and antimicrobial therapy, both local and systemic, may help to rapidly terminate an exacerbation. This is particularly true in cases of *Staphylococcus aureus* infections, to which there appears to be a specific susceptibility in atopic patients.

Topical corticosteroids

Topical corticosteroids are the most useful topical agents for the treatment of atopic dermatitis. However, these drugs are only suppressive and may need to be given over long periods to maintain a reasonable quality of life. Toxic side effects include skin atrophy, striae distensae, and pituitary–adrenal axis suppression, with the possibility of adrenal collapse and masked infection. Sudden withdrawal of corticosteroids can lead to a severe 'rebound' aggravation of eczema, and, thus, it is prudent to use the least potent corticosteroid preparation that is effective. Acquired tolerance or tachyphylaxis is another problem associated with the use of topical corticosteroids, which makes them less effective with continued use. However, changing to another preparation of similar potency will help regain control.

Steroid formulations specifically tested for safety and approved by the US Federal Drug Administration (FDA) for use in younger children include desonide hydrogel and nonethanolic foam, fluticasone 0.05% cream, and fluocinolone acetonide oil. Mometasone cream and ointment are approved for children aged 2 years and older. Ointments are preferred over creams, lotions, and gels as vehicles for steroids, as they do not contain preservatives and tend to have a better emollient effect.

Non-steroidal topical immunosuppressive agents – like tacrolimus (Protopic® 0.03% and 0.1%) and pimecrolimus (Elidel® 1.0%) – are alternatives to topical steroids and particularly useful for the treatment of areas such as the face and intertriginous regions. Tacrolimus ointment 0.03% has been approved for intermittent treatment of moderate to severe AD in children aged 2 years and older, with tacrolimus ointment 0.1% approved for use in adults; pimecrolimus cream 1% is approved for the treatment of patients aged 2 years and older with mild-to-moderate AD. These agents are effective, but expensive, and should only be used when the corticosteroids are contraindicated or prolonged application is required.

Topical phosphodiesterase inhibitors

Crisaborole is a topical PDE4 inhibitor indicated for the treatment of mild to moderate atopic dermatitis in adult and pediatric patients 3 months of age and older. It can be used on the face and skinfolds but may sting when applied. It is most useful as maintenance therapy for mild to moderate eczema.

Moisturizers

Moisturizers have hydrating effects on the skin in eczema because of their occlusive and emollient properties. Many moisturizers also contain 'humectants', which attract and retain water. They reduce scaling and improve skin texture and appearance. They improve the elasticity of skin, reduce fissuring, and decrease the pruritus and inflammation.

All moisturizers seem to have the same degree of efficacy, provided they are sufficiently greasy and occlude the skin surface. The most important issues are how frequently they are applied and patient compliance. They should ideally be applied within 3 minutes of a warm soaking bath to retain moisture. Hydration of skin improves its barrier function and decreases transepidermal water loss.

Tar preparations

Coal tar has anti-inflammmatory and anti-pruritic properties. The generic preparations (e.g. tar ointment or tar and salicylic acid ointment BP) are not popular because of the smell and messiness associated with their use. Modern proprietary preparations are more acceptable (e.g. Exorex® cream). They are not to be used on inflamed skin and are best employed for chronic lichenified type of eczema. Side effects include folliculitis, irritation, and photosensitivity.

Systemic agents

Patients with severe recalcitrant disease do not respond to topical measures. For this group, options include NBUVB (narrowband UVB), systemic steroids, cyclosporine, 'biologicals', and other immunosuppressants (methotrexate and azathioprine).

Some patients improve after sun exposure, and in 50%–75% of severely affected patients, phototherapy of some type may be of assistance, but has to be balanced against the long-term hazards of skin ageing and cutaneous malignancy. In a hot and humid climate, sunlight may trigger sweating and pruritus, thereby being deleterious to atopic patients. Systemic steroids suppress eczema, but have long-term side effects, including osteoporosis, skin fragility, susceptibility to infection, and pituitary–adrenal axis suppression, which probably outweigh the short-term benefits. They are appropriate to manage short-term exacerbation and should be gradually tapered followed by an intensive regimen of skincare to prevent rebound phenomenon.

Cyclosporine is a fungal metabolite peptide with immunosuppressive effects, which is helpful for patients with severe, generalized atopic dermatitis at a dose of 3–5 mg/kg body weight per day. Nephrotoxicity and hypertension are side effects of cyclosporine and therapy requires regular blood pressure and kidney function test-monitoring.

Alitretinoin

This is an oral retinoid drug that has been shown to be helpful in the treatment of chronic hand eczema. The recommended dose is 30 mg daily for a 12–24-week period. The drug has many of the retinoid group toxicities, including teratogenicity.

Dupilumab

This is an IL-4 alpha receptor inhibitor that blocks the function of IL-4 and IL-13. It is a targeted therapy approved by the FDA for the treatment of moderate-to-severe atopic dermatitis in patients aged 12 years and older whose disease is not adequately controlled with topical prescription treatments. It is injected every 2 weeks after a loading dose and decreases pruritus and Eczema Area and Severity Index (EASI) scores. The most common significant side-effects are injection site reactions, eye and eyelid inflammation, and cold sores.

Antimicrobial agents

Patients with atopic dermatitis are particularly prone to skin infection, which contributes to the flare-up of dermatitis. Infection with staphylococci and possibly other bacteria cause pustules, impetiginized lesions, and cellulitis. Bacterial swabs from suspected infected lesions should be taken before starting treatment with either topical or systemic antibacterial agents. Diluted bleach baths may reduce the bacterial load and decrease skin infections. The infected area can be soaked or bathed in 1 in 8000 potassium permanganate solution or aluminium subacetate solution. Topical mupirocin may be used, but other antibiotics should be avoided because of the risk of inducing microbial resistance and allergic contact dermatitis. If the infection is severe, systemic antibiotics should be given.

Seborrhoeic dermatitis

Definition

This is a common, chronic, superficial inflammatory disorder that characteristically affects regions with high sebum production and the flexural areas of the body. Both infantile (Figure 8.6) and adult forms exist. It is believed to be due to the overgrowth of lipophilic yeast *Malessezia*, sebaceous activity, immunologic abnormality, and patient susceptibility.

Clinical features

Signs and symptoms

Sharply demarcated patches or thin plaques varying in color from pink-yellow to dull red to red-brown appear at predisposed sites rich in the sebaceous gland, like the scalp, face, ears, presternal region – and

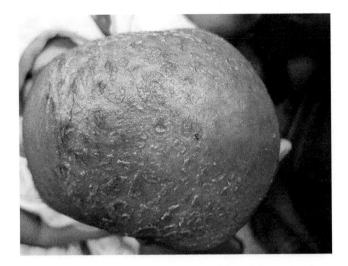

FIGURE 8.6   Cradle cap.

body folds. Depending on the acuteness and severity, scaling may be bran-like in dandruff (pityriasis sicca) to flaky "greasy" scaling in frank seborrhoeic dermatitis or exudative and crusted in severe involvement. Scaling and erythema of the eyelid margins (marginal blepharitis) may also occur. Seborrhoeic folliculitis is marked by numerous small monomorphic itchy papules and papulopustules originating in the hair follicles of scalp and beard. The usually commensal yeast-like microorganism *Malassezia ovalis* (*Pityrosporum ovale*) seems to have taken on an aggressive role, causing the inflammatory lesions.

Other sites involved

The condition may erupt suddenly to cause exudative lesions in the major body flexures. This is especially likely to occur in the summer months in overweight elderly individuals. In the elderly, seborrhoeic dermatitis may spread rapidly to become generalized. This 'erythrodermic' picture is quite disabling, but fortunately quite uncommon.

The disorder causes mild itching and discomfort as compared to other eczematous disorders. It can give rise to severe soreness and discomfort when it is exudative and affects the major flexures. Round or annular scaling patches, which develop over the central chest and the central upper back, are particularly common in the middle-aged and the elderly, as are erythematous areas in the groins, especially in overweight people.

Differential diagnosis

In the groin area, it is important to distinguish from flexural psoriasis and ringworm infection (tinea cruris; Table 8.2). Ringworm is usually asymmetrical and does not reach up into the groin apices. There is usually a raised, slightly scaly advancing edge to ringworm and a tendency to clear centrally. Mycological testing is simple and prevents misdiagnosis. Psoriatic lesions have more pronounced erythema with silvery-white scales that peel in layers. Characteristic psoriasis lesions elsewhere and nail involvement may differentiate from seborrheic dermatitis.

Aetiopathogenesis

The current view is that seborrheic dermatitis is an inflammatory response to the overgrowth of yeast-like microorganism, *Malassezia ovalis* (*Pityrosporon ovale*). This is a 'normal' denizen of human hair

TABLE 8.2

Differential diagnosis of rashes in the groin

Diagnosis	Clinical features	Tests
Ringworm	Often not symmetrical, very itchy, rapidly spreading	Microscopy and culture of scales
Seborrhoeic dermatitis/ intertrigo	Tends to be symmetrical and to involve apices of groins; other areas may be affected	None available
Clothing dermatitis	May resemble seborrhoeic dermatitis; likely to affect other areas	Patch testing
Flexural psoriasis	Psoriasis elsewhere tends to be symmetrical surface scaling	None available

follicles. In the human immunodeficiency virus (HIV) disease, Parkinson's and stroke patients, the *M. furfur* population increases and causes dermatitis.

Natural history and epidemiology

The condition is common at all ages and in both sexes. Severe and widespread seborrhoeic dermatitis is a particular problem for elderly men, but the milder forms are no more common in the elderly than in younger age groups. In the newborn, yellow or brown scaly lesions with adherent epithelial debris are known as 'cradle cap'. There is no racial predilection for the disorder and it appears to affect all social groups and occupations. Left untreated, the condition waxes and wanes over many years.

Treatment

The major aim of treatment in seborrhoeic dermatitis is the removal of the precipitating microbial cause and the suppression of the eczematous response. Topical preparations containing both corticosteroids or an imidazole, such as miconazole, econazole, or clotrimazole may be all that is required for patients with limited glabrous disease. Topical antifungal agents or topical calcineurin inhibitors are preferred on facial and intertriginous skin.

Exudative intertriginous areas in the major body fold respond rapidly to bed-rest, which avoids further friction between opposing skin surfaces, and weak, non-irritating antimicrobial solutions for bathing and wet dressings.

Discoid eczema (nummular eczema)

Definition

Discoid eczema is a common eczematous disorder of unknown cause, characterized by the appearance of erythematous, round, scaly patches on the arms, legs, and, less frequently, the trunk.

Clinical features

Signs and symptoms

Slightly raised, pink–red, well-defined, scaly discs, varying in diameter from 1 to 4 cm, appear on the extensor arms and lower legs and dorsum of hands (Figure 8.7). The disorder is quite itchy and is often associated with dry skin on arms and legs.

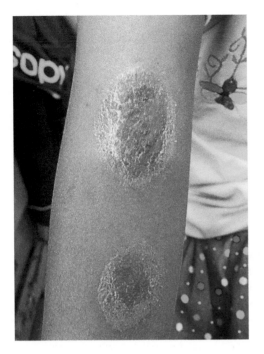

FIGURE 8.7 Discoid eczema.

Natural history and epidemiology

Discoid eczema is most common in middle-aged and elderly people and presents as an intensely itchy outbreak of three or four discoid lesions on the leg. The condition responds to potent topical steroid therapy. Regular use of emollients is important to prevent recurrence.

Differential diagnosis

The condition has to be distinguished from psoriasis, in which the margins are more distinct; from ringworm, which usually spreads peripherally and has a raised margin; and from Bowen's disease, which is mostly restricted to the light-exposed areas and is usually manifested as one or two solitary red, scaling patches (Table 8.3) that gradually increase in size.

Treatment

Potent topical steroid ointments with regular emollients and emollient cleansers are required.

Eczema craquelée (asteatotic eczema)

Definition

Eczema craquelée is an eczematous disorder that occurs on the extensor aspects of the limbs of elderly individuals and is characterized by very dry skin and a 'crazy pavement' appearance.

Clinical features

Signs and symptoms

The most common affected sites are the shins, the fronts and sides of the thighs, extensor aspects of the upper arms and forearms, and the upper and mid-back. The involved skin is pink, roughened, and superficially fissured, giving a 'cracked' appearance (Figure 8.8). The areas affected are more sore than itchy.

Natural history and epidemiology

The disorder is restricted to the elderly and is more common in winters, when there is low ambient relative humidity. Vigorous prolonged hot baths and use of harsh soaps aggravate the condition.

TABLE 8.3

Differential diagnosis of round, red, scaling patches

Dianosis	Features
Psoriasis	Well-defined, thickened, scaly plaques, usually multiple
Discoid eczema	Only a moderately well-defined edge; slightly scaly, pink patches, limited in number
Ringworm	May be annular with central clearing; microscopy and culture of scales will reveal fungal mycelium
Bowen's disease	Often slightly irregular in shape; edge is well-defined; biopsy is decisive

Treatment

The condition responds to the frequent use of emollients and, if necessary, corticosteroid ointment. Taking short tepid showers, using acid pH synthetic detergent soaps, and application of emollient after bathing prevent recurrence.

Lichen simplex chronicus (circumscribed neurodermatitis)

Definition

Lichen simplex chronicus is an intensely pruritic rash, sharply localized to one or a few sites. Affected areas are characterized by hyperpigmentation, thickening, and exaggeration of the skin surface markings.

Clinical features

The medial aspect of the ankle, the back and sides of neck, scalp, the elbows, and adjoining extensor aspects of the forearms, the wrists, and the genitalia are among the areas of skin that are prone to develop patches of this disorder. The individual lesions vary greatly in size but are mostly 2.5–7.5 cm in diameter. Characteristically, the lesions are raised hyperpigmented scaling plaques with a well-defined, if somewhat irregular, margin. They are intensely itchy, often bearing excoriations, and the perpetual rubbing and scratching causes skin hypertrophy with exaggeration of the skin surface markings (Figure 8.9). In extreme cases, large nodules form, and the condition is known as prurigo nodularis (Figure 8.10).

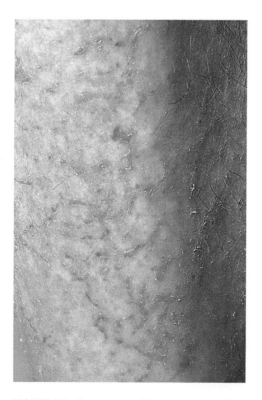

FIGURE 8.8   Eczema craquelée; note the 'crazed appearance' (from Marks and Motley, 18th edition, with permission).

Natural history and epidemiology

The disorder is quite common in middle-aged individuals regardless of sex or race. It is a very stubborn disorder, which is very resistant to treatment and recurrences are frequent. Prurigo nodularis is similarly persistent.

Differential diagnosis

Hypertrophic lichen planus may be difficult to distinguish, although this disorder tends to be more mauve or pigmented and be less regularly lichenified than lichen simplex chronicus. Biopsy may be needed to distinguish these disorders with certainty. Lichen simplex chronicus may also resemble a patch of psoriasis or a patch of Bowen's disease.

Pathology and pathogenesis

Histologically, there may be striking epidermal hypertrophy, which, in extreme cases, may resemble epitheliomatous change (pseudoepitheliomatous hyperplasia). More usually, the hypertrophy is quite regular and may resemble psoriasis (psoriasiform). The persistent scratching causes an increased rate of epidermal cell production and accounts for the hypertrophy; there is always marked hyperkeratosis and some parakeratosis.

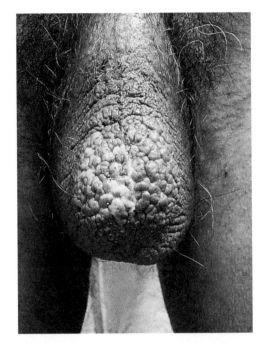

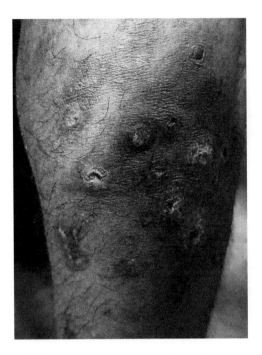

FIGURE 8.9 Lichen simplex chronicus affecting scrotum; note the hyperpigmentation and exaggerated skin surface markings.

FIGURE 8.10 Prurigo papules with excoriations involving the knee.

Treatment

The condition tends to persist and recur regardless of the treatment prescribed. High-potency topical corticosteroids, intralesional corticosteroids, or preparations of coal tar are sometimes helpful. Medium potency steroid impregnated tape can be particularly helpful. It is applied to affected skin overnight for several weeks until the lesions remit.

Contact dermatitis

Contact dermatitis may be caused by direct toxic action of a substance on the skin, the so-called primary irritant dermatitis, or by a substance inducing a delayed hypersensitivity reaction, allergic contact dermatitis. Both are common and cause considerable loss of work and disability.

Primary irritant dermatitis

Definition

Primary irritant dermatitis is a non-specific inflammatory rash that results from direct contact with toxic 'irritating' materials. The degree and the severity of damage are dependent on both the concentration of the toxic material, duration of contact as well as the condition of the skin at the time of contact.

Clinical features

Scaly, red, and fissured areas appear on the irritated skin (Figures 8.11 and 8.12). The hands are the most frequently affected. The palmar skin is often affected, but the areas between the fingers and elsewhere on the hands may also be involved. The condition may become exudative and very inflamed if the

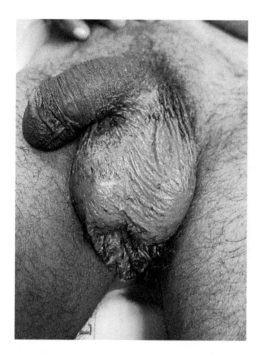

substances contacted are very toxic. This form of contact dermatitis causes considerable soreness and irritation. The fissures make movement very difficult and effectively disable the victims.

Differential diagnosis

The condition must be distinguished from allergic contact dermatitis by a carefully taken history and patch testing. Psoriasis of the palms may resemble contact dermatitis, but the areas affected are better marginated and nearer to the wrist and are usually accompanied by signs of psoriasis elsewhere. Ringworm usually affects one palm only and is marked by diffuse erythema and silvery scaling. If there is any doubt, scales should be examined for fungal mycelium under the microscope.

Natural history and epidemiology

An 'irritant' substance will injure anyone's skin if there is sufficient contact. The duration of the contact is as important as is its intimacy.

FIGURE 8.11 Primary irritant contact dermatitis to chloroxylenol containing antiseptic on scrotum.

Occlusion enhances the penetration of irritants and so worsens dermatitis. The simultaneous application of more than one irritant will often compound an irritant reaction synergistically. However, some individuals are more prone to develop primary irritant contact dermatitis – especially atopic subjects.

The disorder is seen particularly often in manual workers (occupational dermatitis) and housewives (housewives' dermatitis). Builders, mechanics, hairdressers, cooks, and laundry workers are some of the

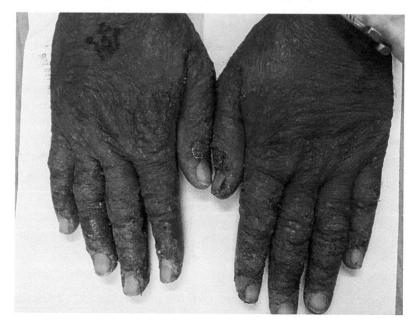

FIGURE 8.12 Primary irritant contact dermatitis affecting the back of the hand.

groups that are frequently affected. The condition causes considerable economic loss due to loss of work. Contact with alkalis, organic solvents, detergent substances, cement, and particulate waste is often responsible.

Prevention and management

The identification of potential irritant substances, use of non-toxic substances as substitutes for more irritating traditional agents, prevention of skin contact, use of protective gloves, use of emollients and worker education are all important in prevention. When present, the cause must be identified and further contact should be prevented. When the condition is severe, rest from manual work is required.

Moisturizers are an important component of treatment. They prevent contact with irritants by forming a barrier and minimize fissuring. Moderately potent to potent corticosteroids should help reduce the inflammation and accelerate healing.

Allergic contact dermatitis

Definition

Allergic contact dermatitis is an eczematous rash that develops after contact with an agent to which delayed (cellular) hypersensitivity has developed.

Clinical features

The rash develops at the sites of skin contact with the 'allergen' but occasionally spreads outside these limits for unknown reasons. The severity and area of involvement vary enormously depending on the 'dose' of allergen to which the patient has been exposed and the susceptibility of the individual. When very acute, the reaction develops within a few hours of contacting the responsible substance; e.g. with 'poison ivy', which is common in the USA. Itching is noticed as a sign after exposure first and then the area involved becomes red, swollen, and vesicular. Later, the area becomes scaly and fissured.

An enormous number of substances are capable of causing allergic contact dermatitis. Nickel dermatitis is one of the most common examples – about 5% of women (or more) in the UK are said to be sensitive to nickel. Affected individuals cannot wear stainless-steel jewellery because of the nickel content in the steel (Figure 8.13) and develop a rash beneath steel studs, clips, and buckles.

Other examples include allergy to chemicals in rubber, e.g. mercaptobenzthiazole (MBT) and thiouram. Allergies to lanolin (in sheep-wool fat and in many ointments and creams) and to perfumes can cause dermatitis after the wearing of cosmetics. Modern-day 'lanolin' is much less of a problem because the potent allergenic components of natural wool have been removed during purification. Lanolin, ethylenediamine, Vioform, neomycin fragrances, and local anaesthetics are amongst the many substances that may cause dermatitis after using in a cream or an ointment (dermatitis medicamentosa). Dyes (such as the black hair dye paraphenylenediamine) can also be the cause of allergic contact dermatitis (Figure 8.14). Some materials are notorious for causing sensitivity and are not often used topically because of this, e.g. penicillin and sulfonamides.

Natural history and epidemiology

Allergic contact dermatitis is quite common but not as common as primary irritant dermatitis. It is rare in children and uncommon in the elderly. It is seen in all racial groups, although less so in black-skinned individuals. Once allergic dermatitis has developed, the sensitivity persists throughout life.

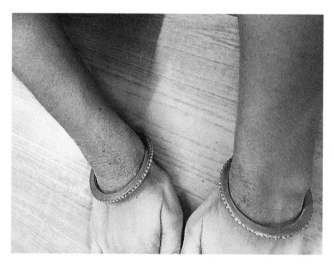

FIGURE 8.13   Allergic contact dermatitis to nickel in metal bangles.

Diagnosis of allergic contact hypersensitivity

Accurate history taking and careful clinical examination to identify all involved areas are very important. The definitive technique for diagnosing allergic contact hypersensitivity is patch testing. In this test, possible allergens are placed in occlusive contact with the skin for 48-hour periods, and the area is inspected 48–72 hours after removal of the patch. A positive test is revealed by the development of an eczematous patch with erythema, swelling, and vesicles at the site of application. In practice, low concentrations of allergen are applied to avoid false-positive primary irritant reactions.

In most cases, a battery of the commonest allergens causing allergic contact dermatitis in that community is applied in appropriate concentrations (Table 8.4).

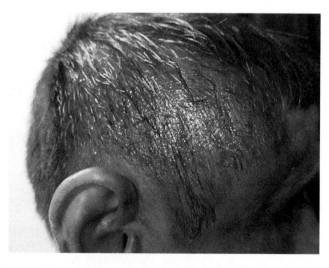

FIGURE 8.14   Allergic contact dermatitis due to paraphenylenediamine hair dye.

Pathology and pathogenesis

The sensitizing chemical (antigen) crosses the stratum corneum barrier and is picked up by the Langerhans cells in the epidermis. The antigen is then 'processed' by the Langerhans cell and passed on to T-lymphocytes in the peripheral lymph nodes. Here, some of the T-lymphocytes develop a specific 'memory' for the particular antigen and their population expands. This process of sensitization takes some 10–14 days in humans. After this period, when the particular antigen contacts the skin once again, the primed T-lymphocytes with the 'memory' for this chemical antigen rush to the contacted site and liberate cytokines and mediators that injure the epidermis and cause the eczematous reaction.

Treatment

It is vital to identify the sensitizing material and prevent further contact with it. Eczema will subside rapidly in most cases after removal from the antigen. The use of weak or moderately potent topical corticosteroids and emollients will speed the resolution of the eczematous patches.

Venous eczema (gravitational eczema; stasis dermatitis)

Definition

Venous eczema occurs on the lower legs and is the result of chronic venous hypertension.

TABLE 8.4

Common antigens and concentrations used in patch testing and concentrations

Antigen	Percent
Balsam of Peru	25
Benzocaine	5
Chlorocresol	1
Chloroxylenol	1
Cobalt chloride	1
Colophony	1
Dowicil 200	1
Epoxy resin	1
Ethylene diamine	1
Formalin	1
Kanthon CG	0.67
Mercaptobenzthiazole	2
Mercapto-mix	2
Neomycin	20
Nickel sulfate	5
Parabens	15
Paraphenylene diamine base	1
Perfume-mix	8
Potassium dichromate	0.5
Primin	0.01
Thiuram-mix	1
Wool alcohols	30

Clinical features

Itchy, pink scaling areas develop on a background of the changes of chronic venous hypertension. The affected areas are often around venous ulcers, but the margins of the eczematous process are poorly defined. Occasionally, the process spreads to the contralateral leg and even to the thighs and arms.

In most cases, venous eczema is actually an allergic contact hypersensitivity to one of the substances used to treat the venous ulcer. Such substances include lanolin, neomycin, ethylenediamine, and rubber additives (in the dressings and bandages). Allergy to topical steroids may also develop.

Treatment

The presence of allergic contact hypersensitivity must be identified and the patient should be advised to avoid using the agent responsible. The simplest of topical applications should be used – white soft paraffin is suitable as an emollient and 1% hydrocortisone ointment is suitable as an anti-inflammatory agent.

9

Psoriasis and lichen planus

Shruti Barde

Introduction

Psoriasis is a multisystem inflammatory syndrome that affects people of all ages globally. It is more usually seen in adults than in children, with two peaks of presentation in the age groups 16–22 years and 57–60 years. There is no gender difference in the morbidity profile of psoriasis, although females reportedly develop it earlier than males. Geographically, its prevalence increases farther away from the equator. Prevalence rates are between 0.09% and 11.4% globally, whereas in developed nations, the rates are between 1.5% and 5%. Studies also show differences in prevalence based on ethnic origin, with the rates being higher in Caucasians compared to those in Africans, Hispanics, and people of other ethnic origins. Due to its chronicity, recurrent, and disfiguring nature, and multisystem involvement, psoriasis has a deep psychological impact on the patients and their Quality of Life (QoL).

Presentation

Psoriasis presents itself with well-defined, raised, pinkish, scaly patches predominantly on the extensor aspects of the body like elbows and knees, lower back, and scalp, mostly symmetrical in distribution (Figure 9.1). Scalp involvement does not cause alopecia (Figure 9.2). Lesions are mildly pruritic or non-pruritic. The scales are due to the dead cell build-up, giving it a shiny silvery-white appearance (Figure 9.3). The lesions vary considerably in shape and size, and mucosal involvement is almost never seen. When lesions cover the joints, fissuring may be seen. Facial skin is usually not affected, except the scalp margins, retro auricular folds, and sometimes the nasal folds.

Auspitz's sign

Pinpoint bleeding is seen after removing psoriatic scales by glass slide, due to breach in the suprapapillary epithelium. The bleeding occurs when the glistening white Bulkeley's membrane is scraped off from the lesions, exposing the dilated suprapapillary blood vessels. This is a quick test useful for diagnosis in the OPD.

Woronoff's ring

A clear halo surrounding a psoriatic plaque due to vasoconstriction.

Nails

Pitted, discolored, and deformed nail plates can be seen in psoriatic patients, often due to nail plate separation from the nail bed (onycholysis). Nail changes are seen in about 50% of the patients with psoriasis, sometimes after as long as a decade of onset of the cutaneous lesions (Figure 9.4).

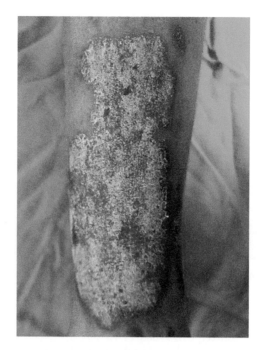

FIGURE 9.1   Typical red, scaling plaques of psoriasis on the leg.

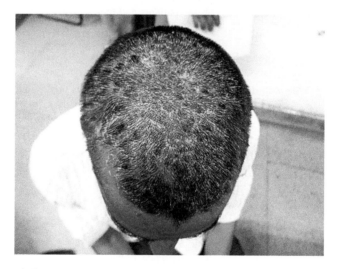

FIGURE 9.2   Scalp psoriasis.

Koebner's phenomenon/Isomorphic response

This involves the appearance of new psoriatic patches at the site of cutaneous trauma (scratching, burns, cuts, etc.) and scars (Figure 9.5). The lesions appear about a week or two after the injury. This can also be seen in other conditions such as vitiligo and lichen planus. Pseudokoebnerization is seen in warts and molluscum contagiosum due to autoinoculation. The lesions appear about a week or two after the injury.

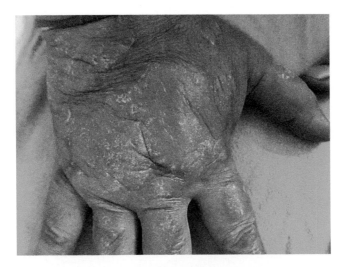

FIGURE 9.3 Psoriasis on the dorsum of hand – a site of predilection.

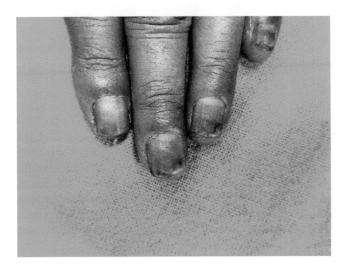

FIGURE 9.4 Nail psoriasis with discoloration, subungual hyperkeratosis, and oil spot/salmon patch.

Genetics

The chance of children being affected varies according to family history. With one positive parent history, chances are 14%, which goes up to about 41% with both parents being clinically affected. A range of "susceptibility genes" in the MHC (major histocompatibility complex) determine the incidence and severity of psoriasis in a person. HLA-C (mainly HLA Cw6) is the main gene associated with the disease. HLA-B27 is a marker for sacroiliitis associated with psoriasis.

Pathogenesis

The two main pathological processes involved in dermal lesions are epidermal proliferation and dermal inflammation. One very obvious abnormality in psoriasis is the hyperplastic epidermis with increased

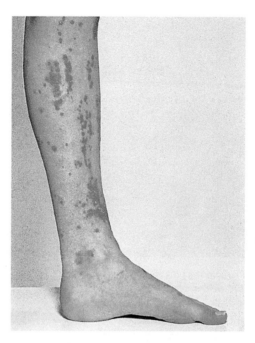

FIGURE 9.5   Psoriasis appearing at sites of injury (from scratching) – the isomorphic response (from Marks and Motley,18th edition, with permission).

mitotic activity, and initial therapeutic interventions were directed at the control of epidermal cell production in this disease. Attention has now diverted to dermal inflammation and immune-suppression to control the disease since increased mitotic activity and epidermal thickness were found to be secondary phenomena.

In histologic sections, epidermal findings include parakeratosis (epidermal nuclei are retained in the inefficient horny layer), hyperkeratosis, and marked exaggeration of the rete pattern. Collection of polymorphs in the parakeratotic stratum corneum results in the formation of Munro's microabscesses, which is the most important diagnostic sign to clinch the diagnosis. Epidermal cell turnover is faster and is about 3–4 days instead of about 28–30 days. Inflammation results from lymphocyte infiltration and an increased number of tortuous capillaries in the dermis.

Morphological classification of psoriasis

Plaque psoriasis

This is the most common type of psoriasis, has an onset in the second or third decade of life, can involve other systems (metabolic syndrome), and can be resistant to treatment (Figure 9.6). Small plaque psoriasis (plaques < 2 mm) occurs at any age and responds well to treatment such as phototherapy.

Guttate psoriasis

This type of psoriasis is seen in children and young adults usually after acute streptococcal infections of throat. It presents with small lesions of 2 mm–1 cm distributed uniformly throughout the body, but mainly on the trunk, arms, and legs (Figure 9.7). Palms and sole involvement is rare. An elevated antistreptolysin O, streptozyme or anti-DNase B titer is found in nearly half of the patients, indicating a recent streptococcal infection. Resolution occurs within 2–3 months.

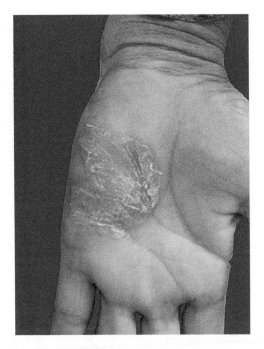

FIGURE 9.6   Well-defined erythematous, scaly patch on the palm due to psoriasis.

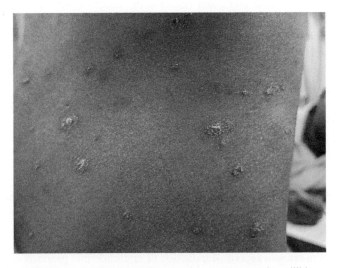

FIGURE 9.7   Multiple small papules of guttate psoriasis seen after a streptococcal tonsillitis.

Flexural/Inverse psoriasis

As the name suggests, this type of psoriasis is seen on the flexural aspects on the body, namely groin, gluteal clefts, axilla, and inframammary folds (Figure 9.8). This presentation is common in overweight or obese people with psoriasis. The lesions often are shiny and without appreciable scales due to these areas being humid. Failure of anti-fungals and antibiotics in suspected candidal or bacterial infections should arouse suspicion. Another common differential is seborrhoeic dermatitis and both conditions can coexist simultaneously.

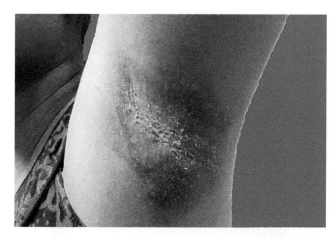

FIGURE 9.8   Flexural psoriasis.

Uncommon types of psoriasis

- **Elephantine type:** As the name suggests, the skin becomes very thick and scaly. It is usually seen on back, hips, or thighs.
- **Rupioid type:** Here the lesions resemble the oyster shells and have a conical thick crust. They appear waxy and yellowish and could resemble the lesions of secondary syphilis or keratotic scabies. Biopsy is needed to confirm.
- **Lichenified type:** Due to repeated scratching and rubbing the area, the skin becomes thicker and darker in these lesions.
- **Koebnerized type:** Lesions can develop on the areas that have suffered cutaneous trauma due to scratching or itching and on previous scars.
- **Photosensitive type:** UV Light is helpful in most but in some, it could worsen the condition, causing an increased inflammatory response.

Erythrodermic psoriasis

In erythrodermic psoriasis, the characteristic plaque-like lesions disappear and progress to generalized, diffuse skin involvement. The skin becomes red and scaly throughout the body. It is a very severe subtype of psoriasis that could be fatal; hence, close monitoring is advised. Some provoking factors include blatant use of topical and oral corticosteroids and the use of irritant agents such as dithranol and tar. There are also reports of induction of erythrodermic psoriasis due to bupropion and intereferon alpha and ribavarin. Due to excessive inflammation in the skin, there is a lot of heat loss and water loss resulting in dehydration. Because of shunting the blood to the skin, there is hyperdynamic circulation which could result in cardiac failure and loss of protein, electrolytes, and metabolites via the shed scales.

Drug aggravated and drug-induced psoriasis

Some drugs (Table 9.1) can aggravate existing psoriasis, precipitate psoriasis, cause recurrence in patients, and even lead to the development of treatment-resistant psoriasis; beta-blockers, in particular, are known to cause psoriasiform eruptions.

TABLE 9.1

Drugs associated with psoriasis

ACE inhibitors/AT II antagonists

Antimalarials

Beta-blockers

Calcium channel blockers

Carbamazapine

Corticosteroids

Imiquimod

Interferon-alpha/interferon-gamma

Lithium

Metformin/gemfibrozil

NSAIDs

Sodium valproate

Pustular psoriasis

This is classified further into three classes: palmoplantar pustulosis, generalized pustulosis, and others.

Palmoplantar pustulosis

Patients with palmoplantar pustulosis develop yellowish-white, sterile pustules on the central parts of the palms and soles (Figure 9.9). Older lesions after 1–2 weeks take on a brownish appearance and are later shed on a scale at the surface (Figure 9.10). The affected area can become generally inflamed, scaly, and fissured and, although relatively small areas of skin are affected, the condition can be very disabling.

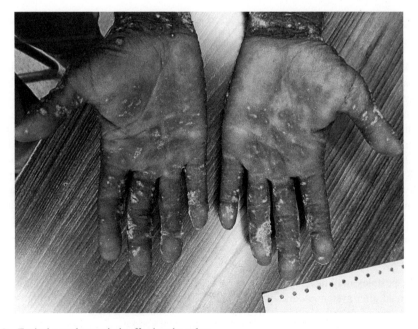

FIGURE 9.9   Typical pustular psoriasis affecting the palms.

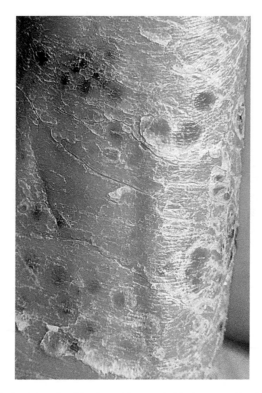

FIGURE 9.10   Pustular psoriasis of the sole of the foot with several older brown scaling lesions that were pustules (from Marks and Motley,18th edition, with permission).

The disorder is common in smokers and resistant to treatment.

Generalized pustular psoriasis

This is also known eponymously as Von Zumbusch's disease and is one of the most potentially serious disorders dealt with by dermatologists. In its classic form, attacks occur suddenly and are characterized by severe systemic upset, swinging pyrexia, arthralgia, and a high polymorphonuclear leucocytosis accompanying the skin disorder.

The skin first becomes erythrodermic and then develops sheets of sterile pustules 2–4 mm in diameter over the trunk and limbs. Sometimes, the pustules become confluent so that 'lakes of pus' develop just beneath the skin surface. Various provoking agents include infections, hypocalcemia, irritating topical treatment (Koebner phenomenon), and sudden withdrawal of oral corticosteroids. These patients are very unwell and require hospitalization. They can usually be brought into remission by modern treatments but are subject to recurrent attacks.

Other forms of pustular psoriasis

Occasionally, pustules may develop locally after strong topical corticosteroids have been used or become widespread after systemic corticosteroids have been administered and then abruptly withdrawn. Other rare variants of pustular psoriasis include:

TABLE 9.2

Types of psoriasis arthritis

Presentation	Involvement
Asymmetric	Distal interphalangeal, metacarpophalangeal joints
Rheumatoid arthritis	Symmetrical polyarthritis
Axial	Resembling ankylosing spondylitis (+/− peripheral joints)
Arthritis mutilans	Joint destruction

- Acrodermatitis continua, in which there is a recalcitrant pustular erosive disorder on the fingers and toes around the ends of the fingers and the nails and occasionally elsewhere.
- Pustular psoriasis in pregnancy is known as impetigo herpetiformis.

Associations

It has been seen that psoriasis results in systemic inflammation which results in the following:

- Arthritis: the various types of presentation are given in Table 9.2. Psoriatic arthritis can range from mild inflammation to a severe mutilating form known as arthritis mutilans (Figure 9.11). The rheumatoid factor is absent in this arthritis and it is accompanied with tendon, ligament, and joint capsule inflammations (enthesitis) and dactylitis.
- Inflammatory bowel disease
- Cardiovascular disease: psoriasis has been known to cause an increase in CRP levels and BMI, resulting in hyperlipidemia and increased waist circumference which increases the risk of an adverse cardiovascular event.
- Depression

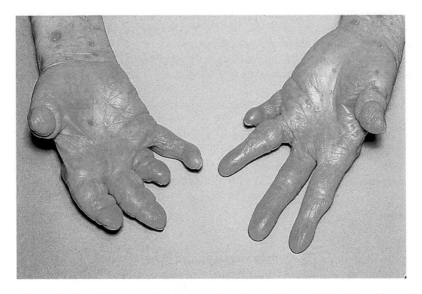

FIGURE 9.11   The results of psoriatic arthropathy (arthritis mutilans) (from Marks and Motley, 18th edition, with permission).

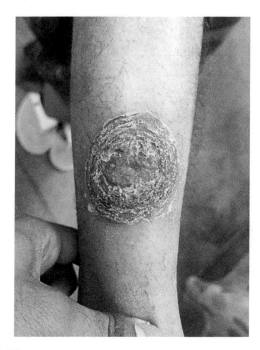

FIGURE 9.12   Psoriasiform plaque in the leg in reactive arthritis.

Differential diagnosis

Scaly rash in plaque psoriasis can be confused with conditions like *seborrhoeic dermatitis, discoid eczema, lichen simplex chronicus, Bowen's disease, ringworm infection, psoriasiform napkin dermatitis* etc. (Figure 9.12). In seborrhoeic dermatitis, the rash is rather diffuse unlike the distinct plaques of psoriasis. In Lichen simplex, the history of intense itching results in excessive rubbing and lichenified skin which is often dark and pigmented. Ringworm infection can be confused with flexural psoriasis but the KOH treated scrapings can provide the distinction.

Mycosis fungoides – a T-cell lymphoma of skin – often evolves through a phase in which there are many red psoriasiform lesions on the trunk, but these differ from psoriasis by being more varied in thickness and more irregular in shape and persistent.

On the legs, raised, round, red, scaling psoriasiform patches often turn out to be patches of *Bowen's disease* in the elderly or discoid eczema. Lichen simplex chronicus around the ankles may also be difficult to distinguish.

Pityriasis rubra pilaris is an uncommon disorder of no known cause, which may mimic psoriasis in some cases. It is characterized by large red scaling areas on the face and trunk often with an orangish tinge and prominent follicular orifices containing keratinous debris. Psoriasis of the palms may be difficult to distinguish from eczema but typically has a sharper border.

Superficial basal cell carcinoma lesions are sometimes several centimetres in diameter and quite psoriasiform in appearance, but have a fine raised, 'hair-like', 'pearly' margin.

Treatment

Inflammatory reactions in psoriasis affect many systems in the body, the symptoms of which may arise at random points in the course of the diseases. It has been reported that the cases of psoriasis are often undertreated and physicians often do not have a long-term and customized perspective in tailoring treatments. Many factors need to be considered before deciding on treatment options for

TABLE 9.3

Factors to be considered before treatment

1	Age
2	Occupation
3	Psychosocial disability
4	Extent of disease
5	Financial backing
6	Pregnancy
7	Treatment history
8	Need for monotherapy
9	Other comorbidities
10	Patient preferences

psoriasis (Table 9.3). Treatment of psoriasis includes topical and systemic treatment options (Table 9.4).

Correct and long-term treatment planning, initiating oral treatments at the right time and referral to the dermatologist at the correct time are imperative.

Topical therapy

Topical treatments for skin lesions aim at decreasing the rate of mitosis and keratolysis of the thickened stratum corneum, thus improving the appearance of lesions. However, in severe disease, topicals are not the first-line treatments and systemic treatments are preferably started with topicals.

Patients with just a few small plaques do well with an emollient such as white soft paraffin, by itself or with 3–6% salicylic acid twice daily. Salicylic acid, combined with topical steroids, has a higher efficacy.

With more lesions and symptoms, more active topical treatment is needed. Tar-containing preparations are less popular because of stinging, unpleasant smell, and staining of clothes. Tar has anti-inflammatory and cytostatic activity and certainly has a mild anti-psoriatic effect. Proprietary tar preparations have some advantages over the British National Formulary formulations with regard to aesthetic qualities. Tar shampoos for scalp involvement are still popular.

Analogues of vitamin D3 are effective topical treatments; calcipotriol used once or twice daily results in an improvement in some 60% patients after 6 weeks of treatment. Used alongside medium-potency corticosteroids, the efficacy is increased and the skin irritation decreased. Apart from skin irritation, there is the concern that a sufficient amount of these D3 analogues will be absorbed to cause hypercalcaemia. Fortunately, this has not proved to be a frequent problem thus far. Other vitamin D analogues being tried for topical therapy include maxacalcitol and tacalcitol. Calcipotriol with steroid combinations has been shown to be better than either of them used alone.

Anthralin (dithranol) is a potent reducing agent that has marked therapeutic activity in psoriasis. It is generally used in ascending concentrations, starting at 0.1% or 0.05% and rising to 5.0%. Dithranol often irritates and burns the skin and care must be taken to match the concentration used to the individual patient's tolerance. It also causes a distinctive brown–purple staining of clothes (Figure 9.13), towels, and skin. Apart from the irritation and staining, dithranol has no serious side effects.

The role of topical corticosteroids in the treatment of psoriasis is limited owing to their side effect profile and rebound flare-up of the disease after stopping them. Life-threatening generalized pustular psoriasis can result after sudden withdrawal. They are useful for patients with flexural lesions for which other irritant preparations are not suitable. For the same reason, weak topical corticosteroids are also suitable for lesions on the genitalia and the face where potent topical corticosteroids cannot be used.

TABLE 9.4

Treatment options for psoriasis

Grade	BSA	Treatment	Side effects and monitoring requirements	Assessment	Other support
Mild	<10%	Topical therapies	Corticosteroids: Atrophy, striae, telangiectasia, tachyphylaxis, hypopigmentation	PASI score calculated before and after 6–24 weeks for assessment	• Psychological support • Rehabilitative support • Nursing care • Climatotherapy • Day care treatment: modified Goeckerman
			Anthralin: Irritation, staining dermatitis	Improvement assessed as follows:	
			Tar: Irritant dermatitis	PASI score	
			Tazarotene: Retinoid dermatitis	>= 75%: GOOD response	
			Calcipotriene: Slight irritation, staining	50–75%: PARTIAL response	
			Emollients: Liquid paraffin and other hydrating moisturizers		
Moderate	10–30%	Systemic	Methotrexate: KFT, LFT, CBC, platelet counts to be monitored monthly		
			Retinoids (Acitretin): LFT, Cholesterol monthly, pregnancy tests if indicated		
			Cyclosporine A: KFT, BP, LFT, Uric acid every 2–4 weeks (short-term use preferred)		
Moderate	10–30%	Systemic	Others: Mycophenolate Mofetil, Hydroxyurea, Sulfasalazine, Cellcept etc.	<50%: FAILED treatment. Other assessment tools are DQLI (Dermatology Quality Life Index), PGA, SKINDEX-16	
		Phototherapy	PUVA: Nausea after ingestion of psoralen, burns (start after 24hours of exposure), development of lentigenes, malignant melanoma, eye irritation, and dryness.	In case of incomplete response or compliance issues, consider combination treatments or use of Biologicals.	
			NBUVB		
			BBUVB		
			Lasers: Excimer (308 nm): Burns		

(Continued on next page)

TABLE 9.4 (*Continued*)

Grade	BSA	Treatment	Side effects and monitoring requirements	Assessment	Other support
Severe	>30%	Biologics	Given below	If ADL affected, consider more potent treatment.	
		Systemic +/− Phototherapy	As above		
		Biologics Alefacept	CD4 levels monitored weekly Platelet counts monitored weekly		
		Etanercept	LFT		
		Infliximab	Latent screening, KFT, PPD, LFT TB		
		Adalimumab	Latent screening, KFT, PPD, LFT TB		
Severe: Erythrodermic psoriasis/Pustular psoriasis		Systemic	Acitretin (most common), methotrexate, cyclosporine A, anti-TNF agents, systemic steriods (occasionally)		

Note: BSA: body surface area; PASI: Psoriasis Area and Severity Index; KFT: kidney function tests; LFT: liver function tests; CBC: complete blood counts; BP: blood pressure; PUVA: psoralen + ultraviolet A; NBUVB: narrow-band ultraviolet B; BBUVB: broad-band ultraviolet B; ADL: activities of daily living.

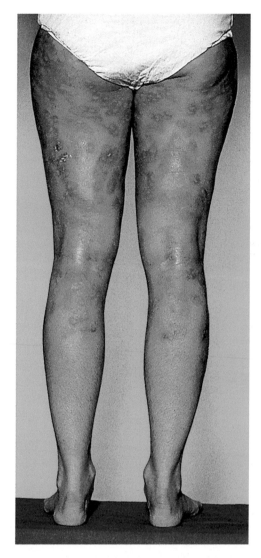

FIGURE 9.13 Brownish-purple staining on the skin due to dithranol (from Marks and Motley, 18th edition, with permission).

Systemic steroids can be used ONLY in the following indications:

- Generalized pustular psoriasis of pregnancy/erythroderma: this is the ONLY definitive indication for using oral steroids.
- Persistent and uncontrolled erythrodermic psoriasis causing metabolic complications.
- Generalized pustular psoriasis if other drugs are contraindicated or not effective.
- Severe polyarthritis that could lead to irreversible joint damage.

Another, quite different, treatment is a topical retinoid analogue called tazarotene (0.05% or 0.1%). This is quite an effective agent, showing 65% improvement in 6 weeks. When used alongside medium-potency topical corticosteroids, its efficiency is increased and the irritation experienced by around 15% of users is decreased.

Both the vitamin D3 analogues and tazarotene may improve psoriasis by modulating gene activity and redirecting differentiation and by reducing the epidermal proliferation. When more than 10% of the body surface area is involved, topical treatment becomes very difficult. The same is true of erythrodermic psoriasis and generalized pustular psoriasis, which require systemic treatment.

TABLE 9.5

The use of methotrexate in psoriasis

Indications
- Severe psoriasis involving >20% BSA
- Resistant psoriasis (resistant to topicals, retinoids, PUVA)
- Erythroderma
- Pustular psoriasis
- Psoriatic arthritis

Contraindications
- Compromised liver functions (cirrhosis, acute hepatitis, etc.)
- Compromised renal function
- Pregnancy or nursing
- Decreased blood counts (anaemia, leukopenia, thrombocytopenia)

Methotrexate

This antimetabolite is a competitive antagonist of tetrahydrofolate reductase, blocking the formation of thymidine and thus DNA. It is thought that this anti-proliferative activity may be important in reducing epidermal and lymphocyte proliferation. It is also quite toxic, producing hepatotoxicity in patients who stay on the drug for long periods. The drug also suppresses haematopoiesis and may cause gastro-intestinal upset. Hence, it is used in moderate to severe cases of erythrodemic or pustular psoriasis, where psoriasis involves >20% BSA, is resistant to topicals therapies, or in debilitating psoriatic arthritis. The indications and contraindications for using methotrexate in psoriasis are listed in Table 9.5.

It is given once weekly in doses of 5–25 mg orally, subcutaneously, or intramuscularly. To minimize the possibility of serious side effects, patients must be monitored frequently (preferably monthly) by blood counts and blood biochemistry.

It is recommended that a liver biopsy be performed both before treatment begins and after a cumulated dose of 1.5 gm in patients at high risk of methotrexate toxicity and after a 3.5 gm cumulative dose in low-risk individuals. Many clinicians believe that information concerning incipient hepatic toxicity can be obtained by measuring blood levels of procollagen peptides. Ultrasound scanning has also been used to assess hepatic damage non-invasively. Methotrexate is also a teratogen, and fertile women should use contraceptive measures. It is mainly suitable for those who would otherwise be disabled by the disease, and for some elderly patients with severe psoriasis.

Retinoids are analogues of retinol (vitamin A). They exert important actions on cell division and maturation, and acitretin is of particular value in psoriasis. The drug benefits patients with all types of severe psoriasis after 3–4 weeks of administration but is most effective when used in combination with some form of ultraviolet treatment. Its major drawback is that it is markedly teratogenic and can only be given to fertile women if they use contraception and are prepared to continue using efficient and reliable contraceptive measures for 3 years after stopping treatment. Other significant toxicities include hyperlipidaemia and a possibility of hyperostosis and extraosseous calcification. In addition, it does have some hepatotoxicity in a few patients. These 'significant' toxicities are not common; but minor mucosal side effects occur in all patients, including drying of the lips and the buccal, nasal, and conjunctival mucosae. Minor generalized pruritus and slight hair loss also occur. Oral retinoids should only be prescribed by dermatologists, i.e. those who are familiar with their actions and effects.

Cyclosporin

Cyclosporin is an immunosuppressive agent and appears to work by inhibiting the synthesis of cytokines by T-lymphocytes. It is also dramatically effective in psoriasis when given in doses of 3–5 mg/kg per day. Its toxic side effects include severe renal damage, hypertension, hyperlipidemia, and hypertrichosis.

Its place in the treatment of disabling and severe psoriasis is assured, but great care and constant monitoring are required.

Treatment with ultraviolet radiation

A form of UVR treatment known as PUVA (photochemotherapy with ultraviolet radiation of the A [long-wave] type) is used in psoriasis. The UVA is supplied by special fluorescent lamps that emit at wavelengths of 300–400 nm, housed in cabinets or special frames over beds.

A photosensitizing psoralen drug is given orally 2 hours before exposure or topically shortly before irradiation. The main psoralen used is 8-methoxy psoralen, but 5-methoxy psoralen and trimethoxy psoralen are also sometimes used. The dose of 8-methoxy psoralen is 0.6 mg/kg.

Alternatively, the patient bathes in water containing a psoralen and is then exposed to UVR a few minutes later. Ordinary 'sun lamps' emitting UVB (290–320 nm) can also be used to treat psoriasis. The dangers of burning may be greater and the dangers of skin cancer are similar to PUVA.

Narrowband UVB light (311 nm) is increasingly the phototherapy treatment of choice, especially in extensive involvement of more than 30% surface area. It is given 3 times a week. Both PUVA and UVB can be combined with topical dithranol, calcipotriol, and tazarotene or oral acitretin. These combinations reduce the cumulative dose and side effects of these therapies.

The dose of UVA is calculated (in joules) from the output of the lamps and the time of exposure. The dose required for clearance is approximately 50–100 J/cm^2, and care is taken to keep the dose as low as possible and certainly below a total cumulated dose of 1500 J/cm^2 to reduce the possibility of long-term side effects, which are as follows:

- Increased incidence of squamous cell carcinoma of the skin – up to 10 or 12 times that in a control group of patients with psoriasis after 10 years. Carcinoma of the external genitalia in men is a particular problem. There is an increased incidence of basal cell carcinoma and melanoma in PUVA-treated psoriatic patients as well.
- Increased solar elastotic degenerative change, with the appearance of ageing and alteration of skin elasticity.
- Cataracts can develop and all patients who receive PUVA must wear effective UVA protective goggles or sunglasses during exposure and for 24 hours afterwards.

In the short term, nausea is often experienced and, if too long an exposure is given, burning can occur. Patients who are 'sensitive to the sun' or who coincidently have a disorder that can be aggravated by UVA exposure, such as lupus erythematosus or porphyria cutanea tarda, should not be treated by any form of UVR.

Biological treatments

It appears that tumor necrosis factor (TNF)-alpha is an important cytokine component in the pathogenesis of psoriasis, and since 2004, agents have been available that block the action of this factor. They are all quite effective and can be given IM, SC, or IV. Since they do not disturb the Cyt.P450 system, there are no drug interactions seen when they are administered along with other systemic therapies such as methotrexate, etc. The agents concerned are of three types: 'humanized' monoclonalantibodies to TNF-alpha (such as adalimumab or infliximab); recombinant human cytokines; and fusion proteins.

Biologicals are usually considered in patients having 5–10% BSA involvement with a Psoriasis Area and Severity Index (PASI) score of 10–12. Prior to the start of treatment it is essential to do baseline counts and rule out any chronic infections such as tuberculosis (TB). The treatment cycles are generally

12–14 weeks and results are evaluated on PASI score, Dermatology Quality of Life Index (DQOLI), and lesion improvement. Although short-term use of biologicals does not show any renal or hepatic side effects, the long-term safety profile, especially with respect to immunosuppression is not well documented and will need further studies.

Lasers in psoriasis

Xenon chloride excimer laser (308 nm) is the laser of choice for treating the dermal lesions in psoriasis. Laser provides a targeted phototherapy and this treatment can be initiated in children as well as adults. The energy given (J/cm^2) depends upon the lesion's thickness and the response achieved. The target chromophore is cellular DNA. Laser causes death of the T cells and regulates epidermal proliferation. The advantage of laser over other phototherapies is that it is more site-specific, reduces UV exposure to normal skin, thereby reducing side effects, and hence allows a higher dosage of energy per session.

Importance of attention for psychological health

Psoriasis is known to be associated with depression. This is not only because of the extent of the disease and its disabling nature, but also because of the stigma attached to it, which prevents patients from taking the treatment in the first place. Social morbidity leading to employment worsen the burden. QoL is affected, especially in those having lesions on exposed body parts, particularly scalp and face. WHO has raised concerns due to the increasing incidence and prevalence of psoriasis over the years and is urging health organizations to increase awareness about the same. Physicians are also encouraged to refer patients for group therapy or psychotherapy sessions.

Pityriasis rubra pilaris

Definition

Pityriasis rubra pilaris (PRP) is an uncommon papulosquamous skin disorder of unknown etiology, presenting with follicular keratosis, erythema, and palmoplantar hyperkeratosis.

Clinical features and histology

PRP is divided into six clinical subtypes: adult type (classical and atypical), juvenile type (classical, circumscribed, and atypical) and HIV-virus associated. Adult type is the most common. Usually, the disease begins on the face and scalp after trauma or bacterial infection and progresses in the cephalo-caudal direction. It is associated with pinkness and scaling, and spreads within a few days or a week to involve the rest of the body. There is a characteristic orange hue to the redness, and on the thickened palms there is a characteristic yellowish discoloration (Figure 9.14). Scattered among the red, scaling rash are islands of spared white skin on the hands and thighs, and sometimes elsewhere there is a typical follicular accentuation due to the presence of hyperkeratotic spines. Typical lesions called nutmeg papules are seen on the dorsum of hands on the knuckles. The juvenile type of pityriasis rubra pilaris, although similar in many ways to the adult form, tends to be much more stubborn and resistant to treatment.

The histological appearance is distinctive in that, although there is considerable epidermal thickening, the accentuation of the dermal papillae and the undulations of the dermo-epidermal junction are much less marked than in psoriasis.

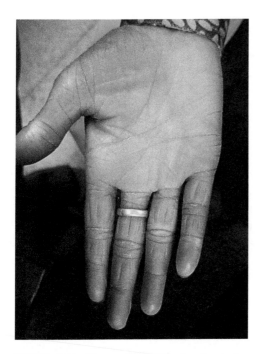

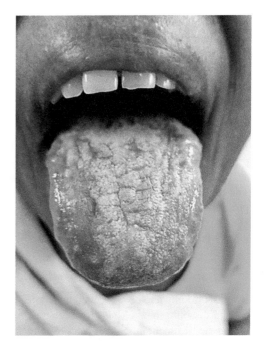

FIGURE 9.14 Waxy palmar thickening due to hyperkeratosis in pityriasis rubra pilaris (PRP Sandle).

FIGURE 9.15 Lichen planus papules affecting the tongue.

Treatment

Treatment is challenging; however, patients respond well to TNF inhibitors, oral retinoids (acitretin and isotretinoin), and anti-IL 12/23 because of their anti-proliferative anti-inflammatory and immune modifying properties. Recently, alitretinoin has been tried with very good results. Treatment with methotrexate or cyclosporine has also been advocated.

Lichen planus

Lichen planus (Greek *leichen*, 'tree moss'; Latin *planus*, 'flat') is an inflammatory disease affecting skin, mucosa (Figure 9.15), scalp, and nails. The term 'lichenoid' refers to the histologic description of inflammatory infiltrate and basal cell liquefaction and used to characterize the pathology of diseases resembling lichen planus. This is the only papulosquamous disorder that presents itself without scales.

Epidemiology

Lichen planus occurs between the third and the fifth decades of life without any specific gender or race predilection.

Aetiology

The exact aetiology of LP is unknown; however, it results from an immune response to the basal layer of epidermis. The following are associated with the onset of this autoimmune disorder:

- Drugs: diuretics (thiazides, spirolactone, furosemide), gold, anitmalarials, β–blockers, penicillamine, phenothiazines, ACE-inhibitors, quinidine
- Infections: hepatitis C infection and post viral chronic active hepatitis
- Immunological disorders: primary biliary cirrhosis, autoimmune chronic active hepatitis

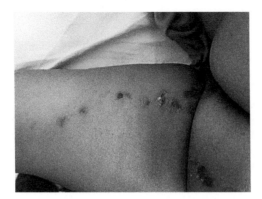

FIGURE 9.16 Red–mauve papules of lichen planus in linear distribution. Some of these have a faint white network pattern on the surface (Wickham's striae).

Lesions

A classical cutaneous lesion of lichen planus (LP) is a **p**ruritic **p**olygonal, **p**urple, flat-topped **p**apule or **p**laque often having a whitish lace pattern on it (Wickham's striae, Figure 9.16). Lichen planus tends to involve the flexor aspects of extremities, wrists, arms, and legs in a bilaterally symmetric distribution. Koebner's phenomenon is seen in LP too (Figure 9.17). Nails, mucosa, and scalp should always be examined. Nail involvement is seen in 10% of the cases and presents as thinning, longitudinal ridging, pterygium formation (Figure 9.18), distal splitting, onycholysis, and anonychia (in long-standing cases) of the nail plate.

Lichen planus is one of the primary causes of scarring alopecia on the scalp. Lesions heal with a pigmented patch, which persists for some weeks.

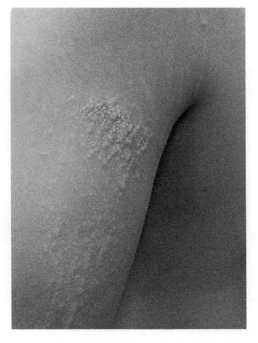

FIGURE 9.17 Many papules of lichen planus affecting the arm, showing Koebner phenomenon.

Variants

Hypertrophic lichen planus (Figure 9.19) is commonly present on extremities with thickened, hyperpigmented, extremely pruritic plaques while in Annular lichen planus lesions individual papules fuse to give a ring-type configuration. This presents mostly in blacks and commonly involves genitalia. Lichen nitidus is a variant of lichen planus in which many tiny, pale, flat-topped papules develop in clusters. Bullous lichen planus is a very rare variant in which blistering occurs due to bullae forming sub-epidermally in some lesions. Lichen planopilaris involves the hair follicles resulting in scarring alopecia and affected sites look like horny spines with perifollicular scaling and pigmentation. Atophic lichen planus presents with bluish to erythematous papules and plaques with central superficial atrophy. Ulcerative type is a progression of bullous lichen planus and results in extensive scarring of feet. Nail and mucosal involvement is common.

Histopathology

The exact prevalence of lichen planus is unknown but it is a rather common disease in Asian countries. T-cell mediated proinflammatory and counterregulatory mechanisms against an unknown antigen in epidermis, function in the pathogenesis of lichen planus. Ultimately there is damage to the basal cells, leading to their hydropic degeneration.

- A band of lymphocytes and histiocytes is seen subepidermally. Among the inflammatory cell infiltrate are clumps of melanin pigment as a result of damage to the epidermis.
- Damage to the basal epidermal cells causes a 'sawtooth' profile, vacuolar degenerative change, and scattered eosinophilic cytoid bodies representing dead epidermal cells. A cleft formed due to epidermal separation is called a Max Joseph histological cleft.
- Variable epidermal thickening with increase in thickness of the granular cell layer and hyperkeratosis is seen.

Immunofluorescence studies show a dense, ragged band of fibrin at the dermoepidermal junction and clumps of IgM deposit. The basic process is thought of as an immunological attack on the basal layer; the presence of inflammatory cells and the other epidermal alterations is believed to be a secondary event.

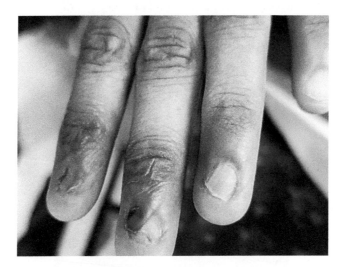

FIGURE 9.18   Pterygium of the nail in lichen planus.

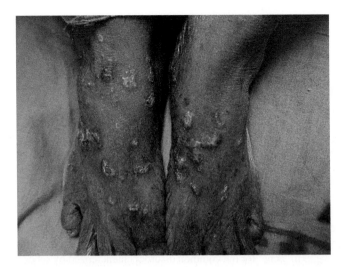

FIGURE 9.19   Hypertrophic lichen planus.

TABLE 9.6

Treatment overview for lichen planus

Lesion	Treatment of choice
1 Localized LP	Topical corticosteroids, Tacrolimus ointment
2 Extensive LP	Oral corticosteroids/PUVA/acitretin
3 LP of nail and scalp	Oral corticosteroids
4 Mucosal LP	Oral corticosteroids/cyclosporine/acitretin

The disease mostly remits spontaneously, so that most patients require very little treatment. Despite severe pruritis, LP patients are not seen to scratch as much, since scratching induces pain. This is called Brocq's phenomenon. When patients are severely affected with a generalized eruption, systemic corticosteroids are sometimes helpful, as are the oral retinoids such as acitretin for the more recalcitrant patients. Treatment options depend on the type of LP and its severity (Table 9.6).

10

Acne, rosacea, and similar disorders

Pooja Agarwal

The disorders described in this chapter are common, inflammatory, characterized clinically by papules, and occur on the face pre-eminently. Traditionally disorders of this kind were given the term 'acne' as a prefix. However, we now no longer subscribe to the view that they are related in any significant way, and it is better to reserve the term 'acne' for the common disorder characterized by seborrhoea and comedones.

Acne

Acne is one of the most common skin disorders. It has been estimated that the prevalence of acne ranges from 35% to 90% in adolescents. There are some differences in the prevalence in different ethnic types – it is uncommon, for example, among the Inuit. It is mostly a disorder of puberty but can occur at any age.

Definition

Acne (acne vulgaris) is a disorder in which hair follicles develop, obstructing horny plugs (comedones). Later, inflammation may develop around the obstructed follicles, which can lead to surrounding tissue inflammation also and scar formation.

Clinical features

The earliest feature of the disorder is an increased rate of sebum secretion at puberty, making the skin look greasy (seborrhoea). Comedones usually accompany the greasiness. They often occur over the sides of the nose and the forehead but can occur anywhere. Comedones are follicular plugs composed of follicular debris, desquamated corneocytes, and compacted sebum. They have pigmented tips from the melanin pigment deposited by the follicular epithelium at this level (Figure 10.1).

Inflamed, erythematous papules develop from blocked follicles. These are a shade of bright red, often irregular in shape, and quite tender to the touch and may be set quite deep within the skin (Figure 10.2). Sometimes, they develop pus at their tips (pustular acne), but these may also arise independently (Figure 10.3). In a few patients, some of the papules become quite large and persist for long periods – they are then referred to as nodules.

In severely affected patients, the nodules liquefy centrally so that fluctuant cysts are formed. In reality, the lesions are pseudocysts, as they have no epithelial lining. These lesions are seen in the most severely affected patients, and they cause the worst scarring. This type of severe acne is known as cystic or nodulocystic acne and can be very disabling and disfiguring (Figure 10.4).

When the large nodules and cysts eventually subside, they leave in their wake firm, fibrotic, nodular scars, which sometimes become hypertrophic or even keloidal. The scars are often quite irregular and tend to form 'bridges' (Figure 10.5). Even the smaller inflamed papules can cause scars, and these tend to be pock-like (Figure 10.6) or are triangular indentations ('ice-pick scars', Figure 10.7). Other types of scars that can be seen in acne are rolling scars – which are broad depressions with sloping edges (Figure 10.8) – and boxcar scars – which are broad depressions with sharply defined edges (Figure 10.9).

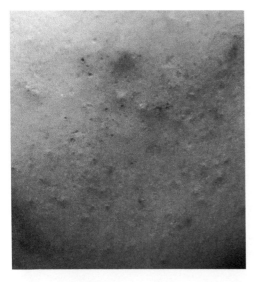

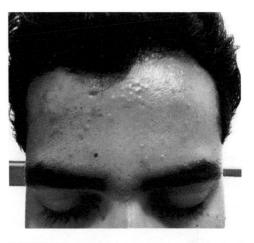

FIGURE 10.2 Multiple acne papules over the forehead.

FIGURE 10.1 Multiple open and closed comedones; note the blackened tips from melanin.

There is a very rare and severe type of cystic acne known as acne fulminans, in which the acne lesions quite suddenly become very inflamed. At the same time, the affected individual is unwell and develops fever and arthralgia. Laboratory investigation often reveals a polymorphonuclear leucocytosis and odd osteolytic lesions in the bony skeleton. The cause of this disorder is not clear, although it has been

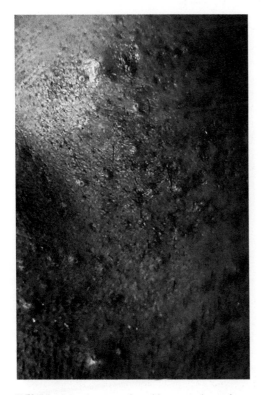

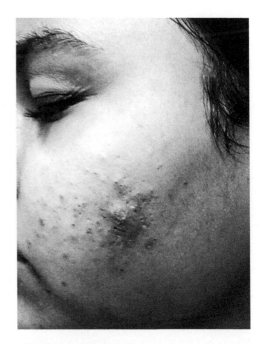

FIGURE 10.3 Acne papules with scattered pustules.

FIGURE 10.4 Cystic acne over cheek; note the surrounding inflammation.

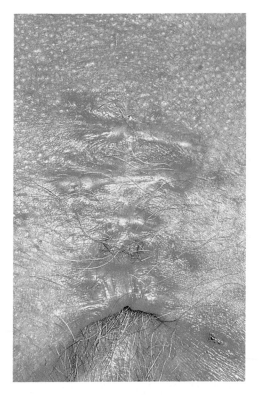

FIGURE 10.5   Hypertrophic scarring in a bridging pattern (from Marks and Motley, 18th edition).

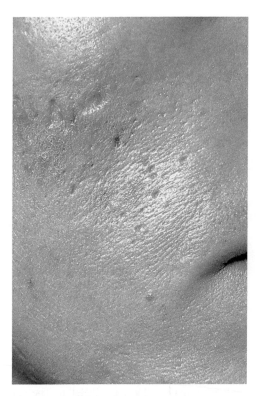

FIGURE 10.6   Pock scarring of acne (from Marks and Motley, 18th edition).

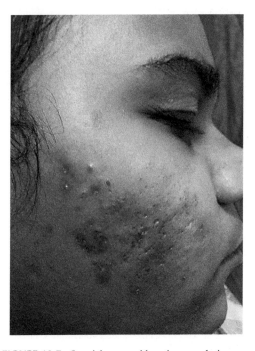

FIGURE 10.7   Ice pick scars with active acne lesions.

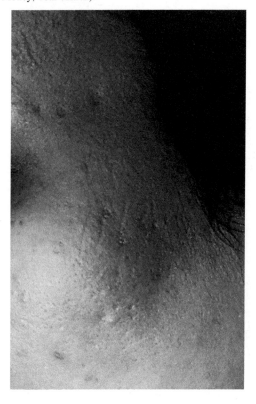

FIGURE 10.8   Multiple rolling scars.

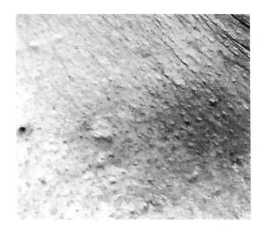

FIGURE 10.9 Boxcar scars.

suggested that it is due to the presence of a vasculitis that is somehow precipitated as a result of the underlying acne. Rarely, Gram-negative folliculitis can develop in acne patients where topical antimicrobials are inadvertently used (Figures 10.10 and 10.11).

Sites affected

Any hair-bearing skin can develop acne, but the areas on the front and back of the trunk and the face are much more vulnerable than others. These acne-prone areas tend to have hair follicles with small terminal hairs and larger sebaceous glands (sebaceous follicles). The face and, particularly, the skin of the cheeks, lower jaw, chin, nose, and forehead are usually affected. The scalp is usually not involved. In patients with severe acne, it is quite common for other areas to be affected, including the outer aspects of the upper arms, the buttocks, and thighs.

Clinical course

For most of those affected, the disorder is annoying, troublesome, and persistent, with wave after wave of new lesions. Although the natural tendency is for resolution, it is difficult to know in any individual patient when the condition will improve. The majority lose their acne by the age of 25 years, but some tend to have the occasional lesion for much longer. In some women, there is a pronounced premenstrual flare of their acne some 7–10 days before the menses begin and right through their reproductive life.

Occasionally, acne may make an unwelcome appearance (sometimes for the first time) in the fifth or sixth decades.

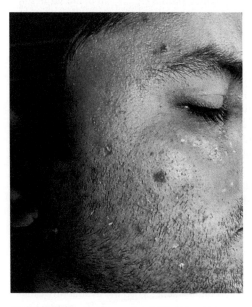

FIGURE 10.10 Gram-negative folliculitis with severe erythema.

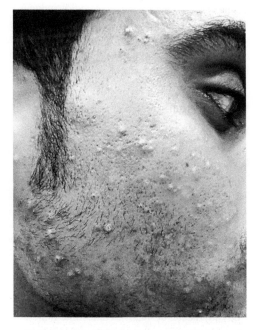

FIGURE 10.11 Gram-negative folliculitis with acne lesions.

People with acne in hot, humid climates often become disabled by its suddenly worsening, with large areas of skin covered by inflamed and exuding acne lesions. This is termed as tropical acne.

Epidemiology

About 35–90% of the population develops a degree of clinically evident acne at some point during adolescence and early adult life, but perhaps only 10–20% seek medical attention for the problem. This proportion varies in different parts of the world, depending on the racial background, affluence, and the sophistication of medical services. The variations in incidence in different ethnic groups have not been well-characterized, although it does appear that Eskimos and Japanese experience less acne than do Western Caucasians.

Onset is usually at puberty or a little later, although many patients do not appear troubled until the age of 16 or 17 years. Men appear to be affected earlier and more severely than women. However, in post-adolescent ages, females are affected predominantly. Older age groups are not immune, and it certainly is not rare to develop acne in the sixth, seventh, or even eighth decade of life.

Special types of acne

Acne conglobata

It is a severe form of acne, which most commonly affects young males. Back, chest, and buttocks are the most severely affected sites. Large nodular-cystic lesions with draining sinuses and resultant severe scarring occur. In contrast to acne fulminans, systemic symptoms are absent in acne conglobata.

Acne induced by drugs

Androgens provide the main normal 'drive' to the sebaceous glands. It is the increased secretion of these hormones that is responsible for the increased sebum secretion at puberty.

The systemic use of glucocorticoids induces troublesome acne (Figure 10.12). The acne that results is curiously monomorphic in that sheets of acne lesions appear (unlike ordinary acne) all at the same stage of development. Interestingly, corticosteroid creams can, uncommonly, also cause acne spots at the site of application. Paradoxically, corticosteroids are sometimes required for their anti-inflammatory actions in the treatment of severe acne and are given for a short duration.

Occupational acne/Chloracne

Workers who come into contact with lubricating and cutting oils develop an acne-like eruption at the sites of contact, consisting of small papules, pustules, and comedones. This is often observed on the fronts of the thighs and forearms, where oil-soaked overalls come in contact with the skin. A similar 'acneiform folliculitis' sometimes arises at sites of application of tar-containing ointments during the treatment of skin diseases (Figure 10.13).

Chloracne is an extremely severe form of industrial acne caused due to exposure to complex chlorinated naphthalenic compounds and dioxin. Typically, numerous large cystic-type lesions occur in this form of industrial-acne-causing massive cosmetic disability.

Acne cosmetica

Some cosmetics contain comedo-inducing (comedogenic) agents, such as cocoa butter, iso-propylmyristate, derivatives and some mineral oils, which can induce acne. With the availability of less comedogenic cosmetics, its prevalence has lessened. Use of thick, oil-based hair products contributes to acne development on the forehead, which is termed as pomade acne.

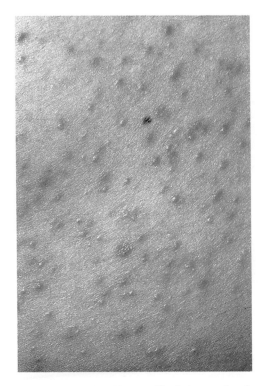

FIGURE 10.12 Steroid acne. The lesions tend to be more uniform in appearance than in 'ordinary' acne (from Marks and Motley, 18th edition).

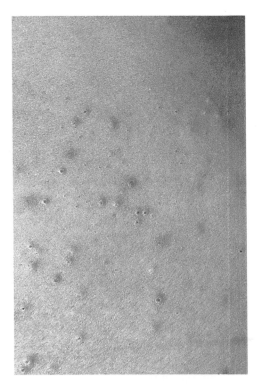

FIGURE 10.13 Comedones and inflamed follicular papules from tar application (from Marks and Motley, 18th edition).

Excoriated acne

This disorder is most often seen in young women. Small acne spots around the chin, forehead, and on the jawline are picked, squeezed, and otherwise altered by manual interference. The resulting papules are crusted and often more inflamed than routine acne spots. Often, the patients have little true acne and the main cosmetic problem is the result of the labour of their fingers! Mostly, this is a minor problem, which can be improved by counselling, but there are some more seriously affected patients in whom the problem is persistent.

Other rare variants of acne

1. Acne mechanica: it is the result of blocked pilosebaceous ducts as a result of repeated friction, such as by backpack straps, etc.
2. Neonatal and infantile acne: a benign self-resolving condition occurring in

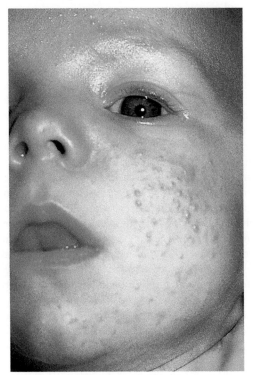

FIGURE 10.14 Infantile acne (from Marks and Motley, 18th edition).

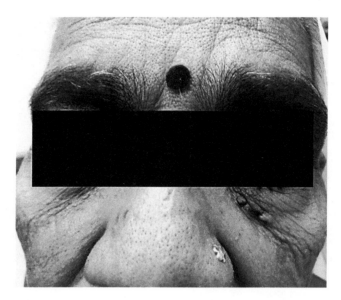

FIGURE 10.15 Senile comedones.

children under the influence of maternal androgens (Figure 10.14)

3. Senile comedones: comedones seen in old age, usually in periorbital area due to laxity of skin (Figure 10.15)
4. SAPHO syndrome: synovitis, acne, pustulosis, hyperostosis, and osteitis
5. PAPA syndrome: sterile pyogenic arthritis, pyoderma gangrenosum, and acne
6. SAHA syndrome: seborrhea, acne, hirsutism, and alopecia

Pathology, aetiology, and pathogenesis

Histologically, the essential features are those of a folliculitis with considerable inflammation. The exact histological picture depends on the stage reached at the time of biopsy. Usually, it is possible to make out the remnants of a ruptured follicle. In the earliest stages, a follicular plug of the horn (comedone) can be identified. Later, fragments of horn appear to have provoked a violent mixed inflammatory reaction with many polymorphs and, in places, a granulomatous reaction with many giant cells and histiocytes (Figure 10.16). In older lesions, fibrous tissue is deposited, indicating scar formation.

The sequence of events leading to acne development is not yet fully understood. However, it is agreed upon that sebum production, follicular hyperkeratinization, growth of *Propionibacterium acnes,* and inflammation are the key events involved in the pathogenesis. Acne first appears at puberty, at which time there is a sudden increase in the level of circulating androgens. Sebaceous glands are predominantly 'androgen-driven,' and thus sebum production increases at puberty. However, the composition of sebum lipids is more influential for acne development than the amount of sebum produced. Alterations in sebum lipid composition (increased levels of desaturated free fatty acids and decreased levels of linoleic acid) are seen to be associated with follicular hypercornification through modulation of the immune system. Lipid peroxidation products also have a proinflammatory effect.

Follicular obstruction plays an important role in the development of acne lesions. Micro comedones are the earliest lesions, and inflammation has been seen at the microcomedone level also. Previously it was thought that abnormal follicular keratinization occurred first, but studies have recently demonstrated expression of IL-1α and other cytokines preceding abnormal keratinization. These local cytokines along with the alteration of serum lipid composition, sensitivity to androgens, and *P. acnes* overgrowth cause epithelial hyperproliferation.

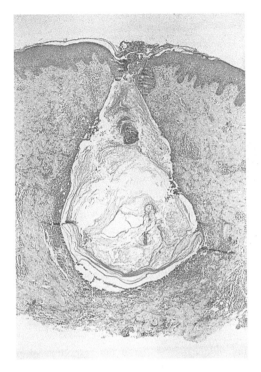

FIGURE 10.16 Pathology of inflamed acne papules showing a ruptured follicle and a dense inflammatory cell infiltrate composed predominantly of polymorphs (from Marks and Motley, 18th edition).

P. acnes is a Gram-positive bacilli thriving in the anaerobic environment provided by sebum lipids and the pilosebaceous apparatus. Earlier thought to be nonpathogenic, P. acnes-driven inflammatory responses lead to acne. Enzymes secreted by *P. acnes* promote the follicular wall degradation and follicle rupture. These also digest the sebum lipids into fatty acids, which have a pro-inflammatory action by stimulating the antimicrobial peptides (defensins, cathelicidin, and granulysin). *P. acnes* also directly engages the Toll-like receptors located on keratinocytes and inflammatory cells and leads to the recruitment of neutrophils and macrophages to the follicle. *P. acnes* also promotes follicular hyperkeratinization by inducing integrin and filaggrin and biofilm production. An acceptable hypothesis is that the important inflammatory lesions of acne are the result of follicular leakage and eventually rupture.

The role of diet in acne pathogenesis still remains controversial. Stress, on the other hand, appears to have a slight correlation with acne development.

Treatment

Perhaps no other dermatological ailment demands as much attention as teenager's acne. Although not physically disabling, the psychological impact of acne can be striking, leading to low self-esteem and depression. The appropriate course of acne treatment requires a detailed assessment of clinical type and severity of acne, previous treatments, aggravating factors, and the presence of post-inflammatory changes.

Basic principles

Medical therapies for acne target the four key factors involved in acne pathogenesis.

- Follicular hyperproliferation and abnormal desquamation, encouraging the shedding of the follicular horny plugs to free the obstruction (comedolytic agents)
- Increased sebum production – reducing the rate of sebum production, either directly by acting on the sebaceous glands (sebotrophic agents) or indirectly by inhibiting the effects of androgens on the sebaceous glands (anti-androgens)
- *Propionibacterium acnes* proliferation – reducing the bacterial population of the hair follicles to cut down the hydrolysis of lipids (antimicrobial agents)
- Inflammation – reducing the damaging effects of acne inflammation on the skin with anti-inflammatory agents

General measures

Patients with acne are often depressed and may need sympathetic counselling and support. There is no evidence that particular foodstuffs have any deleterious effect or that washing vigorously will help remove lesions. These and other myths should be dispelled and replaced with a straightforward explanation of the nature of the disorder, its natural history, and treatment, with firm reassurance that they will improve.

Topical treatment

Currently, the most popular form of topical preparation is a gel, cream, or alcohol-based lotion.

1. Topical retinoids
   These enhance desquamation and facilitate the removal of comedones (comedolytic). They are useful for the treatment of both inflammatory and non-inflammatory acne and preferably should be used as the first-line management. Tretinoin and its *cis*-isomer – isotretinoin (systemic) – both are used successfully for the treatment of acne. Adapalene and tazarotene are the newer retinoids.
   The side effects from the use of retinoid preparations include some pinkness and slight scaling of the skin surface, especially in fair, sensitive-skinned individuals. For the most part, this 'dryness' of the treated area is tolerable and decreases after continued usage. It is the same with both tretinoin and isotretinoin. All the topical retinoids cause increased sensitivity to the sun – due to the thinning of the stratum corneum. Though tazarotene is considered as the most effective, it is also the most irritating topical retinoid, while adapalene is the best-tolerated one.
   In addition to the treatment of active acne, retinoids also fasten the resolution of post-inflammatory hyperpigmentation. They are also used as maintenance therapy in the patients.
2. Topical antimicrobials
   Clindamycin (1%) preparations are quite effective for mild and moderate types of acne. Bacterial resistance to clindamycin frequently develops when used as monotherapy. Topical dapsone (5% and 7.5% gel) is a novel and effective treatment for acne vulgaris. The greatest improvement is seen in inflammatory lesions. Nadifloxacin, a potent synthetic bactericidal fluoroquinolone, is also reported as having potent action against *P. acne.*

Other antimicrobial compounds

Benzoyl peroxide (2.5–10.0%) is quite effective and is used as a cream, gel, or lotion. Its prime action is as an antibacterial agent but it also has some comedolytic action. It is quite irritating and causes some pinkness, scaling, and soreness. Combination of other antibiotics with benzoyl peroxide reduces the chances of development of antibiotic resistance.

3. Other topical preparations
   a. Azelaic acid: it is a natural dicarboxylic acid with comedolytic, antimicrobial, and mild anti-inflammatory action. Due to its inhibitory effect on tyrosinase, it is also useful in improving post-acne pigmentation. It is available as a 15% gel and 20% cream.
   b. Salicylic acid: in patients who are not able to tolerate topical retinoids, topical salicylic acid (0.5–2%) gel can be used as an alternative comedolytic agent.

Systemic treatment

Antibiotics: they are mainly indicated in patients with moderate and severe inflammatory acne and acne resistant to topical treatment.

Tetracyclines

Systemic tetracyclines have been the sheet anchor of treatment for moderate and severe acne for many years. Patients with many papular inflammatory lesions involving several sites are suitable for systemic tetracyclines. In the past, tetracycline was the primary agent used, but with the advent of newer tetracyclines, its use has been reduced greatly. The newer minocycline and doxycycline are given in smaller doses (50 mg or 100 mg) once or twice per day, and their absorption does not seem to be affected by food. Extended-release formulation of minocycline given once a day is now an additional option available for the treatment of acne.

Side effects of the tetracyclines are few and not usually serious. Gastrointestinal discomfort and diarrhoea occasionally occur. Photosensitivity was mainly a problem with older, now no longer used, analogues. Fixed drug eruption and, rarely, other acute drug rashes develop. Minocycline can cause a dark-brown pigmentation of the skin or acne scars or acral areas on the exposed parts of the skin after long-continued use in a small number of patients. Minocycline may also provoke a rare reaction similar to drug-induced lupus erythematosus with hepatitis, arthritis, and pneumonitis.

Tetracyclines must not be given to pregnant women, as they are teratogenic, and must not be given to children and adolescents, as they cause a bone and tooth dystrophy, in which these structures become deformed and discolored.

Macrolides

Erythromycin, earlier considered as one of the main agents for treating acne, is now being used less because of development of antibiotic resistance. The efficacy of erythromycin in acne is similar to that of the tetracyclines, and its use is now recommended only in patients with contraindication to tetracycline and its derivatives. Azithromycin, another macrolide antibiotic, has proved efficacious in the treatment of acne.

Other antibiotics and antimicrobials

Clindamycin, quinolones, dapsone, and sulfonamides are other drugs that have been used systemically for acne. None is more effective than the tetracyclines, but they may be suitable for patients who are either intolerant or who no longer respond to the tetracyclines or erythromycin. Side effects are more common and sometimes of a serious nature (e.g. blood dyscrasias).

Isotretinoin (13-*cis*-retinoic acid)

The large majority of patients with acne will respond to topical or some combination of topical and systemic drugs. However, some severely affected patients may not, and for them there is another drug that can offer relief. This agent is the *cis*-isomer of tretinoin – isotretinoin. It reduces sebum secretion by shrinking the sebaceous glands and may also alter keratinization of the mouth of the hair follicle and have an anti-inflammatory action.

In order to reduce treatment-induced flares, it is typically started at 0.5 mg/kd/day during the first month, and then slowly increased to 1 mg/kg/day. The total treatment goal is to achieve 120 to 150 mg/kg cumulative dose, which is usually reached in four to six months.

The response after a few weeks is to inhibit new lesions in more than 80% of patients. Patients with many large cystic lesions affecting the trunk, as well as the head and neck region, take longer to respond and may need more than one 4-month course. Isotretinoin is the only acne medication that can alter the natural course of acne permanently.

Unfortunately, side effects are frequent. They range from common drying and cracking of the lips, to the very serious, which include teratogenicity, hepatotoxicity, bone toxicity, and a blood lipid-elevating effect. The teratogenic effects are very worrisome, as the acne age group is almost identical to the reproductive age group. The effects on the fetus include facial, cardiac, renal, and neural defects and are most likely to arise if the drug is taken during the first trimester. Some 30–50% of

TABLE 10.1

Treatments for acne

Topical		Oral	
Antimicrobial	Comedolytic	Antimicrobial	Sebum suppressive
Benzoyl peroxide	Tretinoin	Tetracycline	Isotretinoin
Erythromycin	Adapalene	Minocycline	Cyproterone
Clindamycin	Tazarotene	Doxycycline	Ethinylestradiol
Azelaic acid		Erythromycin	Spironolactone
Dapsone			
Nadifloxacin			

pregnancies during which the drug was taken have been affected. Because of this, it is strongly recommended that if it is planned to prescribe isotretinoin for women who can conceive, effective contraceptive measures must also be planned and used during and for 1 month after stopping the drug.

Hepatotoxicity is rare, although a small rise in liver enzymes is common. A rise in triglycerides and cholesterol, such that the ratio of very-low-density lipoproteins to high-density lipoproteins is increased, regularly occurs, and overall there is a 30% rise in lipid levels. This is not likely to be a problem for most patients with acne, but maybe for older patients. The same is true of bone toxicity. A variety of bone anomalies have been described, including disseminated interstitial skeletal hyperostosis and osteoporosis, but these are not likely to be a problem for acne subjects. The drug has also been accused of causing severe depression, leading to suicide in some cases. The evidence for this is not strong, as patients with severe acne are often depressed before starting treatment.

Hormonal therapy

Hormonal treatments include inhibitors of androgen production, either from the ovary (oral contraceptives) or adrenal gland (low-dose corticosteroids), anti-androgens blocking the androgen receptors effect on the sebaceous gland.

Oral contraceptives containing a combination of progestin and oestrogen are used in women with resistant acne. The commonly used progestins are cyproterone acetate and drospirenone. They are not suitable for men because of the feminizing properties. Acne improvement is seen after some 6–8 weeks of use, but is not as effective as isotretinoin. It is associated with a number of minor side effects, essentially those associated with taking oral contraceptives.

Spironolactone, a potassium-sparing diuretic, has also been found to have anti-androgenic effects and has occasionally been used as a treatment for acne.

Treatment of acne is summarized in Table 10.1.

Rosacea

Definition

Rosacea is a chronic inflammatory disorder of the skin of the facial convexities, characterized by persistent erythema and telangiectasia punctuated by acute episodes of flushing, papules, and pustules.

Classification

There are four subtypes of rosacea: erythematotelangiectatic (facial redness and visible blood vessels), papulopustular (acne), rhinophymatous (thickening of the skin on the nose), and ocular rosacea (the eye area). Patients may present with features suggestive of one or multiple subtypes.

Epidemiology

Rosacea is quite a common disorder, but its exact prevalence is not known and varies in different communities. The disorder is essentially one of fair-skinned Caucasians. It seems particularly common in Celtic peoples and in individuals from northwest Europe. It is only occasionally seen in darker-skinned and Asian skin types and is rare in black-skinned individuals. It occurs primarily in adults over the age of 30. Women are more frequently affected, except in the case of rhinophymatous rosacea, where males are predominantly affected.

Aetiology and pathogenesis

The cause of rosacea remains uncertain. Various contributing factors have been proposed, which include abnormalities in the immune system, ultraviolet damage, various microorganisms, and vascular dysfunction.

a. Immune response – dysfunction of the innate immunity may contribute to the development of vascular abnormalities and chronic inflammation in rosacea. This is proposed to occur through the production of cathelicidin peptides, which have inflammatory and vasoactive properties.

b. Microorganisms – the role of the mite *Demodex folliculorum*, a normal commensal of the hair follicle, is quite unclear. Although it is found in vastly increased numbers in rosacea, this increase may result from the underlying disorder in which there is follicular distortion and dilatation. The mite is a normal inhabitant of adult facial hair follicles, but it does not seem to do any harm. Similarly, gastrointestinal colonization by the microorganism *Helicobacter pylori* has been suspected (but not confirmed) of having a role in the aetiopathogenesis.

c. Ultraviolet damage – ultraviolet radiations through stimulation of reactive oxygen species and angiogenic peptides are believed to contribute to rosacea development. The disorganization of the upper dermal collagen, the excess of solar elastotic degenerative change, and the predominance in fair-skinned types all point to the importance of solar damage to the upper dermis.

d. Vascular dysfunction – vascular hyperactivity is seen in patients with rosacea.

Clinical features

Sites affected

The cheeks, forehead, nose, and chin are the most frequently affected areas, making a typical cruciate pattern of skin involvement (Figure 10.17). The flexures and periocular areas are conspicuously spared. Occasionally, the front of the neck and the bald area of the scalp in men are also affected. Sometimes only one or two areas of the face are affected, and this makes diagnosis quite difficult.

The lesions

The most characteristic physical sign is that of persistent erythema, often accompanied by marked telangiectasia. The disorder may not progress beyond this 'erythemato-telangiectatic' state but, even if it does not, the bright red face causes considerable social discomfort and often marked depression. Such patients also complain of frequent flushing at the most trivial stimuli.

Superimposed on this persistent background of erythema are episodes of swelling and papules (Figure 10.18). The papules are dull red, dome-shaped, and non-tender, in contrast to acne, in which they tend to be irregular and tender. Pustules also occur, but are less frequent than in acne; blackheads, cysts, and scars do not occur in rosacea.

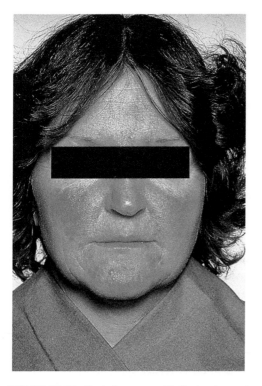

FIGURE 10.17 Typical rosacea with the involvement of the cheeks, forehead, and chin. Note the sparing of the periocular area and flexural sites (from Marks and Motley, 18th edition).

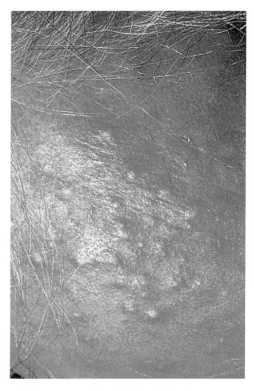

FIGURE 10.18 Papules of facial skin in rosacea (from Marks and Motley, 18th edition).

Natural history

Rosacea tends to be a persistent disease and the tendency for patients to develop episodes of acute rosacea remains for many years after appropriate treatment has calmed down an attack. However, the disease becomes less common in the seventh decade and seems quite rare in the elderly.

Pathology

A characteristic constellation of features seen in histological sections makes skin biopsy a useful test when the clinical diagnosis is uncertain. A feature common to all rosacea skin samples is the presence of dermal disorganization, solar damage, and oedema and telangiectasia in the upper dermis. When there are inflammatory papules, the blood vessels are encircled by lymphocytes and histiocytes, among which giant cell systems are sometimes found. In a small proportion of biopsies, the granulomatous aspect is striking and may even resemble a tuberculous granuloma. In rhinophyma, apart from abnormalities in the fibrous dermis and inflammation, there is also marked sebaceous gland hyperplasia.

Differential diagnosis

Any red rash of the face may be confused with rosacea. Papular rashes of the face seem to cause most problems. The most common differential diagnoses are summarized in Table 10.2.

TABLE 10.2

Differential diagnosis of rosacea

Disorder	Positive discriminants
Skin disorders	
Acne	Scars, seborrhoea, cysts, back and chest involvement
Seborrhoeic dermatitis	Greasy scaling, involvement of nasolabial, retroauricular areas
Perioral dermatitis	Micropapules, perioral and paranasal involvement
Systemic disorders	
Systemic lupus erythematosus	Rash on light-exposed areas, arthropathy, positive antinuclear factor, haematological findings
Dermatomyositis	Mauve–lilac rash around the eyes, with swelling, rash on backs of fingers, muscle tenderness, pain, and weakness, positive laboratory findings
Carcinoid syndrome	Marked telangiectasia, flushing attacks, hepatomegaly
Polycythaemia rubra vera	General facial redness and suffusion, possibly hepatosplenomegaly
Superior vena caval obstruction	Facial suffusion, distended neck veins

Complications

Rhinophyma

This occurs mainly in elderly men, although it occasionally occurs in women too. The nose becomes irregularly enlarged and 'craggy', with accentuation of the pilosebaceous orifices. The nose also develops a dull-red discoloration with prominent telangiectatic vessels (Figure 10.19). Popular names for this include 'whisky-drinkers nose' and 'grog blossom'. Rarely, the chin, the earlobes, and the forehead are similarly affected.

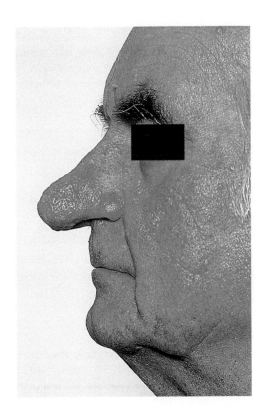

FIGURE 10.19 Rhinophyma with prominent telangiectasia (from Marks and Motley 18E).

Lymphoedema

Persistent lymphoedema is another unpleasant, though uncommon, complication of rosacea seen predominantly in men. The swollen areas are usually a shade of dull red and may persist when the other manifestations of rosacea have remitted.

Ocular complications

About 30–50% of patients with acute papular rosacea have a blepharoconjunctivitis. This is usually mild, but some patients complain bitterly of soreness and grittiness of the eyes. Some of this may be the result of keratoconjunctivitis sicca, which appears to be quite common in rosacea. Styes and chalazion are also more common in rosacea. Keratitis is a rare, painful complication occurring in men, in which a vascular pannus moves across the cornea, producing severe visual defects and, ultimately, blindness.

General management

Patients with rosacea are often very sensitive about their appearance and may be depressed. They should be strongly reassured and managed sympathetically. Regular use of sunscreens, mild facial cleansers, emollients, and avoidance of aggravating factors are advised in every subtype.

Treatment

Treatment depends on the subtype of rosacea

Erythemato-telangiectatic rosacea: Topical alpha receptor agonists like brimonidine (0.5%) have shown the strongest efficacy in controlling facial erythema in rosacea. Another alpha receptor agonist, oxymetazoline, has also shown good results. Topical tacrolimus has been shown to cause improvement in a small number of cases. In patients not responding to topical treatment, low-dose β-blocking medications, e.g. propranolol should be considered. Laser therapy (using pulse dye laser, intense pulsed light) can also be used to eliminate the malar telangiectatic vessels. In recalcitrant lesions, botulinum toxins have been found to be helpful to reduce facial flushing.

Papulopustular rosacea: Most patients with active inflammatory lesions can be managed with topical therapies. Metronidazole (0.75%) gel or cream, azelaic acid (15%) gel, ivermectin(1%) cream and sulfacetamide (10%) with sulphur 5% preparations are the commonly used agents. Topical retinoids and benzoyl peroxide-clindamycin combinations have also been found useful. Systemic therapy is typically used in patients with unsatisfactory response to topical therapy. Tetracycline, doxycycline, and minocycline are the first-line antibiotics for papulopustular rosacea. In patients who cannot tolerate tetracyclines, alternative antibiotics include macrolides (erythromycin) and oral metroronidazole. Low-dose isotretinoin can be considered in resistant cases.

Rhinophymatous rosacea: Early cases with inflammation benefit with topical therapies. Chemical peels and low dose isotretinoin are useful to reduce seborrhoea. In severe cases, debulking with carbon dioxide laser, or surgical remodelling are indicated.

Ocular rosacea: Daily lid hygiene in form of lid massage and warm compression, along with the use of lubricant eye drops is recommended. Topical antibiotics like metronidazole may improve mild lid inflammation. Topical cyclosporine is also seen to minimize inflammation. For moderate to severe ocular rosacea, oral tetracyclines or macrolides, or metronidazole are often needed.

Perioral dermatitis

Definition

Perioral dermatitis is a common inflammatory disorder of the skin around the mouth, characterized by the occurrence of micropapules and pustules.

Epidemiology

Perioral dermatitis is most common in young women aged 15–25 years, being quite uncommon in men and in older women.

Pathogenesis

The pathways leading to the development of perioral dermatitis are unclear. Topical corticosteroid use is commonly reported with perioral dermatitis. The classic history is of a popular facial eruption which initially improves with corticosteroid use and then worsens or recurs upon continued use. Several other factors have also been proposed as contributors to its development e.g. fluoridated toothpaste, cosmetic products, *Candida albicans,* and oral contraceptive therapy.

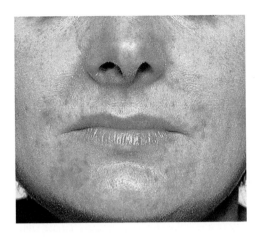

FIGURE 10.20 Perioral dermatitis. There are many tiny papules around the mouth (from Marks and Motley, 18th edition).

Clinical features

Many minute, slightly pink scaly papules and pustules develop around the mouth, sparing the area immediately next to the vermillion of the lips (Figure 10.20). Lesions sometimes involve the nasolabial grooves and, in severely affected patients, also affect the skin at the sides of the nose. There is no background of erythema, distinguishing the condition from rosacea.

Treatment

No definitive treatment has been recommended for perioral dermatitis. Tapering followed by discontinuation of topical corticosteroids is advised. Use of a milder corticosteroid cream is recommended to avoid flare of disease. Topical calcineurin inhibitors, e.g. pimecrolimus (1%), topical erythromycin, and topical metronidazole 1% have been used in mild-to-moderate cases. In severe cases, oral tetracyclines or low dose isotretinoin may be indicated.

11

Wound healing and ulcers

Shekhar Neema

Principles of wound healing

Wound healing is fundamental to the survival of an organism. Injury to tissue initiates a complex cellular and biochemical activity, which results in wound healing. Wound healing is divided into three distinct, but overlapping, phases: (a) hemostasis and inflammation; (b) proliferation; (c) the remodelling phase (Figure 11.1).

Wounds that do not progress through normal stages of wound healing become chronic and result in poor anatomical and functional outcomes. Non-healing wounds are a major cause of morbidity and have an enormous impact on healthcare expenditures.

Factors affecting wound healing

There are various local as well as systemic factors that affect the process of wound healing. Oxygenation and nutrition are important for the wound healing process. The presence of infection or of a foreign body in the wound results in impaired wound healing. Advanced age, obesity, stress, diseases such as diabetes, chronic renal disease, chronic liver disease, smoking, medications such as glucocorticoids, and chemotherapeutic agents negatively impact wound healing.

Venous ulcers

The common causes of leg ulcers are listed in Table 11.1.

Epidemiology

Venous leg ulcers account for 70% of chronic leg ulcers. The prevalence of venous leg ulcers increases with increasing age and is more common in men more than 60 years of age and in women.

Pathogenesis

The venous system in lower extremity comprises superficial, communicating, and deep veins. It contains bicuspid valves, which ensure the unidirectional flow of blood towards the heart. In a standing position, the pressure in the venous system is equal to the hydrostatic pressure in the legs (80 mm Hg). During muscle contraction, calf muscles exert pressure on deep veins, and blood is pushed upwards. Normal valve functioning maintains a unidirectional flow of blood and prevents transmission of high venous pressure to the superficial venous system. After the deep venous system empties, the pressure reduces and blood flows from the superficial venous system to the deep venous system through its

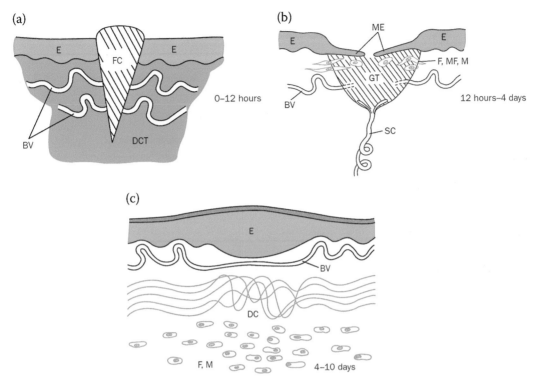

FIGURE 11.1 The sequence of events after incisional wounding of the skin. (a) 0 to 12 hours. Initially, the small blood vessels constrict and then platelets plug the endothelial gaps. The extravasated blood clots form a temporary plug for the wound. White cells accumulate at the interface between the damaged and the normal tissue. (b) 12 hours to 4 days. After about 18–24 hours, epidermal cells actively move on to the surface of the defect. Epidermal cells at the sides of the wound divide some hours later to make up for the loss. Epidermis also sprouts from the cut ends of the sweat coils and hair follicles. After 2–4 days, new capillaries start to sprout and vascularize the granulation tissue in the wound cavity. Damaged connective tissue is destroyed and removed by macrophages, and new collagen is secreted by fibroblasts. Myofibroblasts are fibroblastic cells that develop the power to contract and are responsible for wound contraction. (c) 4 to 10 days. Between 4 and 10 days after wounding, the wound cavity becomes covered with the new epidermis, whose stratum corneum does not possess normal barrier efficiency until the end of this period. The granulation tissue is replaced by a new dermis whose collagenous fibres are not yet orientated. In the later stages, remodelling takes place so that the orientation of the dermal collagenous bundles to the original lines of stress occurs. Scar formation occurs when there has been significant damage to the dermis. The epidermis ultimately develops a normal profile and the vasculature is also restored to normal contractility. E = epidermis; DCT = dermal connective tissue; BV = blood vessel; FC = fibrin clot; ME = migrating epidermis; F = fibroblasts; MF = myofibroblasts; M = macrophages; GT = granulation tissue; SC = sweat coil; DC = dermal collagen. (From Marks and Motley, 18th edition, with permission.)

communicating system. In cases where there is any obstruction in the deep venous system, valve dysfunction or reflux, it will result in ambulatory venous hypertension.

The exact pathomechanism for venous ulceration is not known. Various theories have been proposed, one being the fibrin cuff theory, which postulates that increased intraluminal pressure in capillaries causes leakage of fibrinogen and formation of fibrin cuff, thereby impairing oxygen and nutrition diffusion to tissues. Another theory proposes that trapped white cells release proteolytic enzymes, which promote ulceration. Extravasation of red blood cells results in the deposition of a hemosiderin pigment in macrophages, resulting in a brownish pigment of the skin (Figure 11.2).

Clinical features

The patient complaints of heaviness or a dull ache in the lower legs, which is increased after prolonged standing and relieved after rest or leg elevation. Pitting ankle oedema is usually the earliest sign. Dilated

TABLE 11.1

Common causes of leg ulcers

Vascular	Venous, arterial, mixed
	Vasculitis – polyarteritis nodosa, rheumatoid arthritis, Wegener's granulomatosis
	Livedoid vasculopathy
Neuropathic	Diabetes, syringomyelia, leprosy, peripheral neuropathy
Decubitus ulcer	Elderly, bedbound, spinal cord injury
Hematologic	Sickle cell disease, polycythemia rubra vera, thalassemia, cryoglobulinemia
Infection	Mycobacterium tuberculosis, atypical mycobacteria, leishmaniasis, fungal – blastomycosis, cryptococcosis, coccidioidomycosis, histoplasmosis, sporotrichosis
Neoplastic	Marjolin's ulcer, squamous cell carcinoma, basal cell carcinoma, melanoma, Kaposi sarcoma
Metabolic	Diabetes mellitus, alpha-1 antitrypsin deficiency, prolidase deficiency
Misc	Pyoderma gangrenosum, trauma, factitious, cold injury, radiation, burns, panniculitis, medications – hydroxyurea

tortuous veins can be visualized best with the patient in the standing position. In prolonged disease, the skin develops a brownish discoloration and becomes thick and hard, which is known as lipodermatosclerosis. A venous ulcer is usually solitary, develops on the lower one-third of leg and is superficial (Figure 11.3).

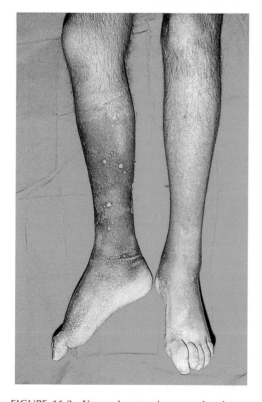

FIGURE 11.2 Venous hypertension; note the pigmentation and appearance of the skin, suggesting that it is bound down to the underlying tissues (from Marks and Motley, 18th edition, with permission).

Complications

Infection: The ulcer may get infected.

Eczema: Allergic contact dermatitis is commonly seen in patients with a venous ulcer. It results from various medications applied for the treatment of ulcer (e.g. neomycin, sisomycin).

Malignant change: Malignant transformation can occur in any chronic wound; however, such transformation in venous ulcer is extremely rare.

Bleeding

Lipodermatosclerosis – hyperpigmentation and induration of the skin.

Treatment

Treatment is aimed at wound care and improving venous drainage.

Wound care

- Clean the wound with normal saline.
- Wound debridement, if required, may be surgical, autolytic or mechanical.
- The infected ulcer should be treated with appropriate antibiotics based on swab culture and sensitivity.

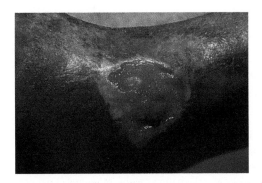

FIGURE 11.3   Typical venous ulcer.

- A dressing that maintains a moist wound bed should be used; topical antimicrobial should be avoided.

Improving venous drainage

- Compression therapy increases the leg ulcer healing rate. It also reduces the risk of recurrence. Multicomponent compression bandages are more effective than single-component bandages. The presence of arterial insufficiency is a contraindication for compression therapy.

- Sclerotherapy, superficial endoscopic perforator surgery, endovenous ablation, or saphenofemoral junction ligation can be performed for the treatment of reflux.

Supportive therapy consists of weight reduction; exercise to improve the calf muscle pump; pentoxifylline, flavonoid, doxycycline, or zinc help in ulcer healing; split-thickness skin grafting can be used for ulcers with a healthy wound bed; or stanozolol or danazol for lipodermatosclerosis.

Ischemic ulceration

Ischemic ulcers are also a common clinical problem; however, they occur more commonly as mixed ulcers in combination with a venous ulcer or a diabetic ulcer.

Pathogenesis

Arterial insufficiency can be acute or chronic. Acute limb ischemia results from an embolic phenomenon and results in gangrene and acute ulceration. Progressive atherosclerosis is the commonest aetiology resulting in chronic ischemia. It affects large vessels. Other diseases that can cause ischemic ulceration are thromboangiitis obliterans, vasculitis, livedoid vasculopathy, and cryoglobulinemia.

Clinical features

Arterial ulcers usually occur in a patient older than 45 years, who have risk factors for atherosclerosis such as diabetes mellitus, smoking, hypertension, hyperlipidemia, or obesity and a sedentary lifestyle. Patients present with intermittent claudication. Arterial ulcers are extremely painful and the pain worsens on leg elevation and improves on dependency.

Ulcers are punched out, have a sharply demarcated border and are present over sites of pressure or trauma. They may be associated with diminished peripheral pulses and a prolonged capillary filling time.

Treatment

Treatment in arterial ulcers is aimed at the treatment of the underlying atherosclerosis. It is of utmost importance to cease smoking and control diabetes, blood pressure, or dyslipidemia and reduce weight. A gradual increase in the walking distance improves the blood supply to ischemic extremities. Wound care includes moist wound dressing, sharp debridement, and systemic antibiotics for infection. An interventional vascular procedure like percutaneous transluminal angioplasty or bypass surgery can be performed for stenotic vessels. Aspirin is effective for the secondary prevention of coronary artery disease and cerebrovascular disease.

Decubitus ulcers

This is better known as the pressure ulcer. It is defined as an area of unrelieved pressure over a defined area, usually over a bony prominence, resulting in ischemia and tissue necrosis.

Pathophysiology

Pressure ulcers result from constant pressure, which impairs local blood flow to soft tissue for an extended period. The arterial capillary closing pressure is 32 mm Hg, and the venous capillary closing pressure is 8–12 mm Hg. The external pressure exerted should be more than 32 mm Hg, and for an extended time, so as to impair inflow and the resultant ischemia. Ischemia results in pain and patients shift position; however, in the unconscious or immobile patient, this protection is lost and a pressure ulcer is produced. Poor nutritional status, incontinence, or maceration increase the vulnerability of tissue to develop pressure ulcers.

Clinical features

Pressure ulcer occurs on pressure points in patients who are unconscious, unable to move or bed-bound due to some reason. The National Pressure Ulcer Advisory Panel (NPUAP) has classified pressure ulcer into four stages.

STAGE 1: Intact skin with signs of impending ulceration; this presents as non-blanchable erythema
STAGE 2: Partial-thickness skin loss; this presents as a shallow ulcer with a pink wound bed
STAGE 3: Full-thickness skin loss with extension into the subcutaneous tissue
STAGE 4: Full-thickness tissue loss with extension into muscle, bone, tendon, or joint capsule

Treatment

It is of utmost importance to prevent pressure sore in an immobile, unconscious patient by good nursing care. Changing position regularly, proper bed positioning, protection of vulnerable bony prominences, removal of skin secretions and nutritional support are some of the interventions to prevent the formation of pressure ulcers.

The treatment of pressure ulcers depends on the stage of an ulcer. Stages 1 and 2 can be treated conservatively by moist wound dressing, while stages 3 and 4 require surgical intervention such as flap reconstruction. Antibiotics are used if the wound is infected.

Neuropathic ulcers

Neuropathic ulcers result from repeated inadvertent injury to an anaesthetic or hyperesthetic area of skin, subsequent to nerve injury. Nerve injury can result from various causes such as metabolic, infections, or toxic causes. The most common causes are diabetes mellitus and leprosy.

Clinical features

Ulcers usually occur in long-standing cases of uncontrolled diabetes mellitus or lepromatous leprosy. Neuropathic ulcers usually occur on the soles of the feet as punched out, deeply penetrating, painless ulcers (Figure 11.4).

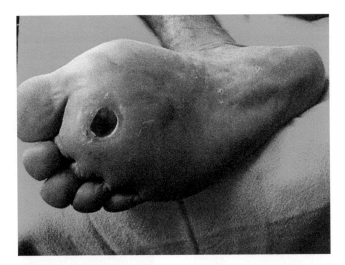

FIGURE 11.4   Neuropathic ulcer in a patient of leprosy.

Treatment

The treatment of neuropathic ulcers requires offloading of the affected limb, wound care by appropriate dressing to maintain moist wound environment, antibiotic for wound infection, optimal control of blood glucose in cases of diabetes, and multi-drug therapy in cases of leprosy.

Less common causes of ulceration

Pyoderma gangrenosum

This is a rare disease of uncertain etiology, associated with an underlying systemic condition in almost 50% cases. Diagnosis is made by excluding other causes of ulceration.

Aetiopathogenesis

Commonly associated diseases are inflammatory bowel disease, rheumatoid arthritis, leukemia, and monoclonal gammopathy. Dysregulation of the immune system – especially neutrophil chemotaxis – occurs, which results in ulceration and the pathergy phenomenon.

Clinical features

A patient presents with red papules or pustules, which ulcerate and then increase in size. It is associated with pain, arthralgia, and malaise. Ulcers have a violaceous border and undermined edges (Figure 11.5).

Treatment

Treatments include systemic therapies such as corticosteroids, cyclosporine, mycophenolate mofetil, azathioprine, or dapsone. Topical therapies include gentle wound care, topical tacrolimus and pimecrolimus. Surgical debridement should be avoided as the pathergy phenomenon can lead to enlargement of the wound.

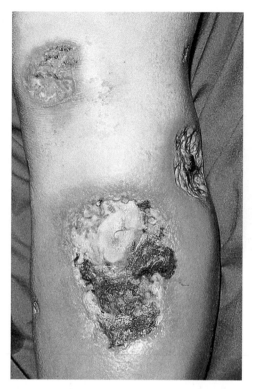

FIGURE 11.5 Multiple ulcers of the leg in pyoderma gangrenosum that developed over a 3-day period (from Marks and Motley, 18th edition, with permission).

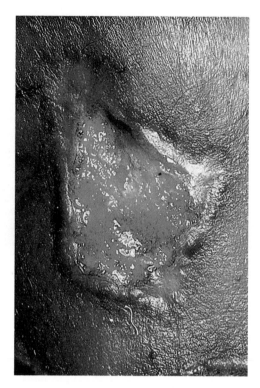

FIGURE 11.6 Vasculitic ulcer (from Marks and Motley, 18th edition, with permission).

Vasculitic ulcer

Ulceration may occur when small or medium vessels become thrombosed due to inflammation of the vessel wall. Vasculitic ulcers are wedge-shaped, have irregular borders and are usually bilateral (Figure 11.6). Inflammation of the vessel wall may occur due to primary vasculitis like polyarteritis nodosa or Wegener's granulomatosis or vasculitis secondary to other illnesses, such as rheumatoid

TABLE 11.2

Diagnosis of ulcers based on clinical examination

1.	Venous ulcer	Location – ulcer in the lower third of the calf and 1 inch below malleolus (Gaiter area), sloping edges.
		Surrounding skin – telangiectasia, varicose vein, eczema, lipodermatosclerosis, oedema
2.	Arterial ulcer	Location – distal regions, bony prominences
		Vertical edges
		Surrounding skin – poor capillary refill time, diminished peripheral pulses
		Pain increases on elevating limb
3.	Neuropathic ulcer	Location – sole of feet (heel or base of great toe), punched out edges
		Surrounding skin – hypoaesthetic or anesthetic, deformity might be present
4.	Vasculitic ulcer	Presence of livedo reticularis and thigh ulcers in polyarteritis nodosa, stellate ulcers in livedoid vasculopathy
5.	Miscellaneous	Rolled out edges in basal cell carcinoma
		Violaceous border and undermined edges in pyoderma gangrenosum

TABLE 11.3

Investigations in a patient with a leg ulcer.

Sr No	Clinical suspicion	First-line investigation
1.	Venous ulcer	**Imaging**
		• Duplex ultrasonography to diagnose venous reflux and rule out deep venous thrombosis • Contrast venography
2.	Arterial ulcer	Ankle – brachial index
		Imaging
		• Arterial duplex ultrasonography • Magnetic resonance angiography • CT angiography • Conventional angiography
3.	Neuropathic ulcer	Nerve conduction studies Electromyography
4.	Pyoderma gangrenosum or malignant ulcer	Biopsy from the edge of the ulceration
5.	Vasculitic ulcer	Serology – ANA, ANCA, APLA
6.	Miscellaneous investigations	• Wound swab and culture – should be done in all cases where the infection is suspected • Biopsy from the edge of the ulcer can be done in cases where the exact cause is not known • Complete blood count, blood sugar fasting and postprandial • Coagulation studies including protein C, protein S, Factor V leiden, Antithrombin III levels in cases where vasculopathy is suspected • Special test for sickle cell anaemia

arthritis, scleroderma, or systemic lupus erythematosus. The treatment of vasculitic ulcer is by wound care and treatment of underlying vasculitis, usually by immunosuppressive therapy such as corticosteroids.

Malignant disease

In rare cases, basal cell carcinoma or squamous cell carcinoma can present as a non-healing ulcer. Kaposi sarcoma in immunosuppressed individuals can also present as leg ulcers. Squamous cell carcinoma can develop in a burn wound, radiation injury, lichen planus hypertrophicus, or other chronic dermatoses.

Infective causes

Tuberculosis, leishmaniasis, tertiary syphilis, or deep fungal infection can result in leg ulcers.

Diagnosis and assessment of leg ulcers

Diagnosis of leg ulcer is very important before a specific therapy is planned. Diagnosis depends on the appearance of the ulcer and physical examination (Table 11.2) and special investigation (Table 11.3).

12

Benign tumors

Rashmi Sarkar
Isha Narang

Many different cell and tissue types in the skin are responsible for the enormous number of tumors that may arise from it (Figure 12.1). Some important benign tumors of dermatological relevance (Figure 12.2) are discussed in this chapter. Treatment of benign tumors is summarized in Table 12.1.

Adipocytic tumors

Lipoma

Lipomata are common, solitary, or sometimes multiple, slowly growing benign tumors of fat, mostly found in the subcutaneous tissue. Histologically, they consist of mature fat cells.

Clinical features

They are soft, skin-colored subcutaneous nodules and have poorly defined edges. They may be enormous in size or only 1–2 cm in diameter and can occur anywhere (Figure 12.3). Multiple lipomas can be found in association with Proteus syndrome, Cowden's disease, and Bannayan's syndrome.

Lipomatosis is diffuse infiltration with non-encapsulated adipose tissue. It is found in conditions like multiple symmetrical lipomatosis, Dercum's disease, etc.

Fibrohistiocytic tumors

Dermatofibroma (fibrous histiocytoma, histiocytoma, sclerosing haemangioma)

It is a benign dermal or subcutaneous tumor. Its line of differentiation is uncertain, and it is also not certain whether the dermatofibroma is a benign neoplasm or some form of a localized chronic inflammatory disorder. The lesions have no serious clinical significance but are sometimes mistaken for melanomas.

These lesions are classified as fibrohistiocytic tumors due to their histopathology. It consists of many spindle-shaped and banana-shaped mononuclear cells in a whorled pattern, which may be fibroblast-derived, and there is a variable amount of new collagenous dermal connective tissue. There are also many histiocytic cells present, which often contain lipid or iron pigment, both of which may derive from the large number of small blood vessels also contained in the lesion. The presence of Touton giant cells loaded with hemosiderin is thought to be pathognomonic of dermatofibroma.

Clinical features

They are firm or hard intracutaneous nodules. They are usually found on the limbs as solitary lesions, but sometimes two or three or even more are found in the same patient. Generally, they are brownish in color (from the haemosiderin pigment) and have a rough or warty surface because these dermal nodules have the

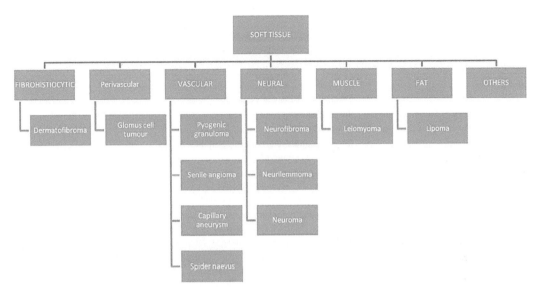

FIGURE 12.1   Classification of soft-tissue tumors.

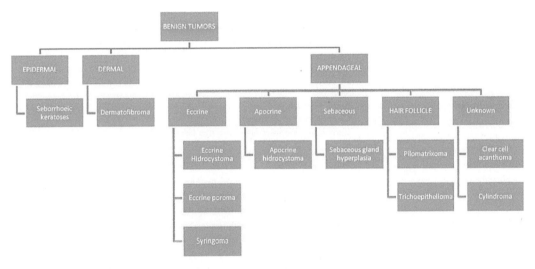

FIGURE 12.2   Classification of benign tumors.

propensity to thicken up the epidermis immediately above them. On squeezing the overlying epidermis, the 'dimple sign or Fitzpatrick sign' is seen, due to tethering of the overlying epidermis to the underlying lesion (Figure 12.4). Multiple dermatofibromas are associated with systemic lupus erythematosus, chronic myeloid leukemia, HIV, and patients on immunosuppressive therapy.

Pericytic (Perivascular) tumors

Glomus cell tumor or glomangioma

This uncommon, benign vascular tumor arises from the glomus cells controlling tiny vascular shunts between arterial and venous capillaries at the periphery, having a close relation to the Sucquet-Hoyer canal. The constituent cells have a characteristic cuboidal appearance.

TABLE 12.1

Treatments for benign tumors

Tumor	Treatment
Dermatofibroma	• Poses only cosmetic problem: treatment unnecessary • Surgical excision can be done
Glomus cell tumor	• Surgical excision • local recurrence rare
Pyogenic granuloma	• Curettage and cautery under local anaesthesia • Recurrences common
Senile angioma	• Requires no treatment • For cosmesis, larger lesions can be excised • Vascular laser under local anaesthesia
Spider naevus	• Lesions developing in pregnancy disappear spontaneously • In healthy children, they persist • Respond quickly to the tuned dye 595 nm laser
Neurofibroma	• Genetic counselling • Treatment is symptomatic • Lesions causing disfigurement can be excised • Carbon dioxide laser is used
Neurilemmomma	• Surgical excision
Leiomyoma	• Surgical excision
Lipoma	• Surgical excision
Seborrhoeic keratoses	• Removal by curettage, cautery, or diathermy • Recurrence is the rule
Syringoma	• Cauterisation or diathermy for cosmesis
Cylindroma	• Surgical excision
Apocrine hidrocystoma	• Surgical excision
Eccrine hidrocystoma	• Surgical excision • Cauterisation or diathermy • Carbon dioxide laser and pulse dye laser
Eccrine poroma	• Surgical excision
Pilomatrixoma	• Surgical excision
Trichoepithelioma	• For cosmetic reasons: Surgical excision, curettage, pulsed carbon dioxide laser, cryotherapy, and dermabrasion • If malignancy is suspected adequate excision and histological examination
Sebaceous gland hyperplasia	• For cosmetic purpose, gentle cautery, cryotherapy, carbon dioxide, and pulsed dye laser and trichloroacetic acid
Clear cell acanthoma	• Surgical excision

Clinical features

The lesion is an exquisitely tender pink or purple nodule, which often presents in adults. It occurs usually on the hands, commonly around the fingertips, on the head, neck, and penis.

Vascular tumors

Senile angioma (Campbell De Morgan spot, cherry angioma)

As with seborrhoeic warts and skin tags, senile angioma is a frequent accompaniment of skin ageing. Abrupt onset of numerous lesions has been reported with chemotherapy, mostly nitrogen mustards. Histologically, it resembles the capillary angioma.

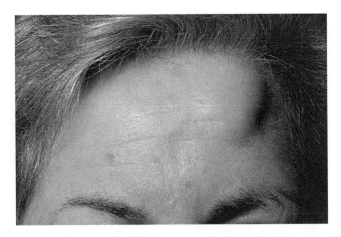

FIGURE 12.3 A lipoma situated deep to the frontalis muscle (from Marks and Motley, 18th edition).

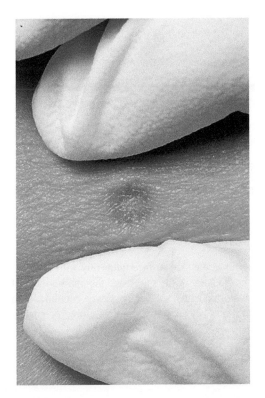

FIGURE 12.4 Dermatofibroma: demonstrating characteristic 'dipping' on lateral pressure (from Marks and Motley, 18th edition).

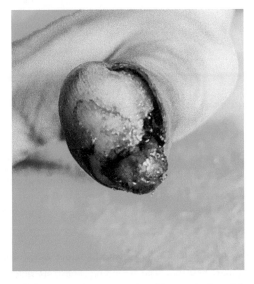

FIGURE 12.5 Dome-shaped, red-haemorrhagic nodule of pyogenic granuloma.

Clinical features

These are smooth-surfaced, dome-shaped, purplish, or cherry-red papules on the trunk of the middle-aged or the elderly (Figure 12.6). Many lesions may appear over a period of some months, but apart from the distress that their appearance seems to cause, they have no special significance for general health.

Capillary aneurysm

Since the most common presentation of this tiny vascular lesion is of a suddenly appearing black pinhead spot, it is sometimes mistaken for an early malignant melanoma. If left, it gradually fades.

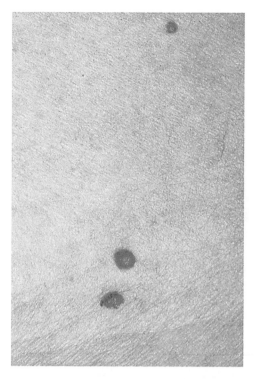

FIGURE 12.6 Senile angioma on the trunk in a man aged 63 years (from Marks and Motley, 18th edition).

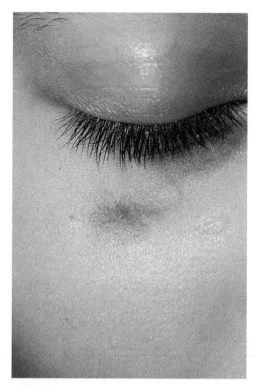

FIGURE 12.7 Spider naevus (from Marks and Motley, 18th edition).

Spider naevus (spider telangiectases, naevus araneus, spider angioma)

It is found in association with liver disease and pregnancy. It is thought to be related to increased oestrogen.

Clinical features

This is a small prominent pulsatile blood vessel, which appears at the skin surface frequently with radiating capillary branches. The ascending central arteriole represents the body of the spider and the fine vessels that radiate from the centre represent the legs of the spider. It is frequently solitary or maybe multiple, seen usually on the upper half of the body in children, and may develop in women during pregnancy (Figure 12.7).

Neural tumors

Neurofibroma and von Recklinghausen's disease

The neurofibromas can be solitary or multiple. Multiple neurofibromas are present in several distinct genetic disorders. The two main forms are NF1 (Neurofibromatosis 1 or von Recklinghausen's disease) and NF2 (Neurofibromatosis 2). It is inherited as an autosomal dominant condition, but 30–50% of patients do not give a family history, suggesting that there is a high rate of new gene mutation.

Histologically, the typical picture is of a non-encapsulated dermal mass composed of interlacing bundles of spindle-shaped cells, often in a 'nerve-like' arrangement, set in a homogeneous matrix amid which mast cells may be seen.

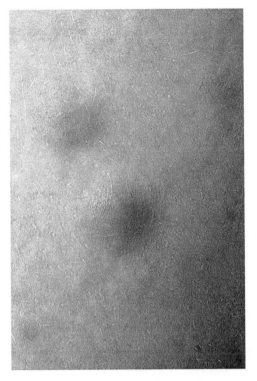

FIGURE 12.8 Soft mauve or pink, compressible lesions of neurofibroma (from Marks and Motley, 8th edition).

Clinical features

Individual lesions are often quite large, soft, compressible, and skin-colored (Figure 12.8). Neurofibromata start to appear in childhood and increase in number during adolescence. They are cosmetically very disabling and, in the worst cases, result in gross deformity. Ultimately, large numbers may be present. Some of these lesions become very large, soft, diffuse swellings; others become pedunculated and pendulous. Alongside the neurofibromata, light-brown, uniformly pigmented, irregular macular patches appear (café-au-lait patches) over the trunk and limbs (Figure 12.9). A useful diagnostic point is the presence of small pigmented macules at the apices of the axillae (so-called axillary freckling). There is a greatly increased risk of tumors affecting the central and peripheral nervous systems as well as of tumors of sympathetic tissue, such as phaeochromocytoma.

The National Institute of Health Consensus Development Conference Statement requires two or more of the following criteria to be fulfilled to be called NF-1:

1. Six or more café-au-lait macules of over 5 mm in greatest diameter in prepubertal individuals and over 15 mm in greatest diameter in postpubertal individuals
2. Two or more neurofibromas of any type or one plexiform neurofibroma
3. Freckling in the axillary or inguinal regions (Crowe's sign)
4. Optic glioma
5. Two or more Lisch nodules

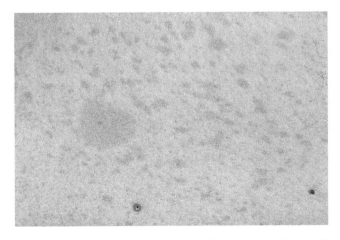

FIGURE 12.9 Café-au-lait patch in von Recklinghausen's disease (from Marks and Motley, 18th edition).

6. A distinctive osseous lesion such as sphenoid dysplasia or thinning of the long bone cortex with or without pseudoarthrosis

7. A first-degree relative (parent, sibling, offspring) with NF1 by the preceding criteria

Neurilemmoma (Schwannoma)

The neurilemmoma is an uncommon benign tumor of neural connective tissue and is composed of Schwann cells.

Microscopically, they consist of thin, spindle-shaped cells arranged in a stacked or 'storiform' manner.

Clinical features

The lesions vary in size, are usually slow-growing, and occur anywhere on the skin surface. They are usually pink-grey or yellowish, firm, well-circumscribed, rounded nodules, and sometimes painful.

Neuroma

This rare benign neural tumor is the most differentiated of all the neural connective tissue tumors and consists of well-formed nerve elements. It occurs at the site of nerve injury and occasionally seems to arise spontaneously and is frequently tender.

Muscle tumors

Leiomyoma

This is an uncommon benign tumor of smooth muscle that arises either from arrector pili muscle of hair follicles or from the smooth muscle of blood vessel walls. It can be confused histologically because of its spindle-shaped and strap-shaped plain muscle cells, which may look like fibrous or neural tissue. They are classified into piloleiomyomas, genital leiomyomas, and angioleiomyomas. Eruptive leiomyomas are reported in patients with haematological malignancies, especially chronic lymphocytic leukaemia.

Clinical features

It is mostly smooth, tender, oval, and bluish red in color nodules or plaques, varying in size from 1 cm to 3 cm in length and 0.5 cm to 1.5 cm in breadth, present usually on extremities and trunk. It may be spontaneously painful, especially in the cold, and indeed can sometimes be seen to contract when cooled. Leiomyomas have been associated with type II papillary renal carcinomas and Alport syndrome.

Tumors of epidermal origin

Seborrhoeic keratoses (basal cell papillomas, seborrhoeic warts)

They are extremely common benign tumors of ageing skin. Most patients are over 40 years, have multiple lesions, and may have a familial tendency. They seem to be most common in Caucasians, but similar lesions are seen in black-skinned and Asian peoples.

Histologically, there is epidermal thickening, with the predominant cell being rather like the normal basal epidermal cell. Surmounting the thickened epidermis, there is a warty hyperkeratosis whose

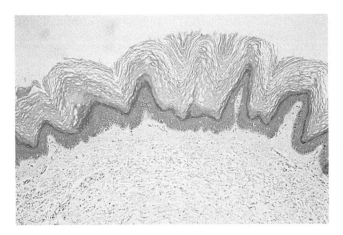

FIGURE 12.10 Pathology of a flat seborrhoeic wart showing 'church spire' arrangement (from Marks and Motley, 18th edition).

arrangement has been likened to a series of church spires (Figure 12.10). Within the lesion are foci of keratinization and horn cysts.

Clinical features

They are solitary or multiple brownish, warty nodule, or plaque on the upper trunk or head and neck regions; their pigmentation varies from light fawn to black (Figure 12.11). They often have a greasy and 'stuck on' look. In black-skinned people, they may appear as multiple, blackish, dome-shaped warty papules over the face, a condition known as *dermatosis papulosa nigra*. The differential diagnosis of warty lesions is given in Table 12.2. When deeply pigmented, they are sometimes mistaken for malignant melanoma.

They usually cause no symptoms, but patients complain that they catch in clothing and are un-sightly. They may also irritate and, less frequently, become inflamed and cause soreness and pain and may be mistaken for a squamous cell carcinoma. Eruptive seborrhoeic keratoses have been referred to as Leser Trelat sign, and this is a marker of an underlying malignancy. The changes are referred to as an irritated seborrhoeic keratosis and are a common reason for patient anxiety and referral for specialist advice.

Benign tumors of sweat gland origin

The more common benign tumors of sweat gland origin are listed in Table 12.3. The most common are described next.

Syringoma (Syringocystoma)

They are benign skin tumors, usually multiple. Histologically, there are tiny, comma-shaped (tadpole-like) epithelial structures, some of which appear cuticle-lined, forming microcysts (Figure 12.12).

Clinical features

They are multiple small white or skin-colored papules that are typically seen on the skin below the eyes (Figure 12.13) in young adults. Occasionally, they are also evident on the arms and lower trunk. They may be associated with Down's syndrome.

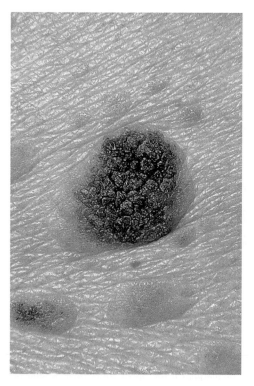

FIGURE 12.11 Typical brown/black, 'stuck-on' warty lesions known as seborrhoeic warts (from Marks and Motley, 18th edition).

Cylindroma (Turban tumor, Spiegler's tumor)

This is a slow-growing benign tumor arising from apocrine sweat glands that, like syringoma, is often multiple. It has an autosomal dominant inheritance in familial cases. Oval and rounded masses of basaloid epidermal cells surrounded by an eosinophilic band of homogeneous connective tissue characterize the histological appearance ('jigsaw-puzzle' appearance).

Clinical features

Smooth pink and skin-colored nodules and papules occur over the scalp and face in young adults, which are sometimes painful. Multiple tumors may arise and cause considerable cosmetic distress.

Apocrine hidrocystoma

A benign tumor arising from cystic dilatation of the apocrine gland.

Clinical features

It is an uncommon cyst, usually solitary, and may have skin to greyish-blue color, usually seen around the eyelids. It is often confused with basal cell carcinoma (Figure 12.14).

TABLE 12.2

Differential diagnosis of warty tumors

Lesion	Comment
Seborrhoeic keratosis	Mostly in elderly individuals and multiple; may have a greasy, 'stuck-on' appearance
Viral wart	Not usually pigmented; mostly in younger individuals on hands, feet, face, and genitalia
Solar keratosis	Flat, pink, and scaly usually, but can have a horny or warty surface; mostly on the backs of hands and face
Epidermal naevus	Usually since birth; anywhere on the body; often a linear arrangement

TABLE 12.3

Benign tumors of sweat gland origin

Lesion	Comment
Syringoma	Multiple white papules beneath eyes; composed of tiny cysts and comma-shaped epithelial clumps
Cylindroma	Solitary or multiple nodules on face or scalp; clumps of basaloid cells with eosinophilic colloid material
Syringocystadenoma papilliferum	Mostly develop in naevus sebaceous on the scalp or on mons pubis
Apocrine hidrocystoma	Small thin-walled, bluish cyst found around eyelids
Eccrine poroma	Solitary nodule on palms or soles or, rarely, elsewhere; basaloid clumps in the upper dermis
Eccrine spiradenoma	Tender and painful solitary nodule

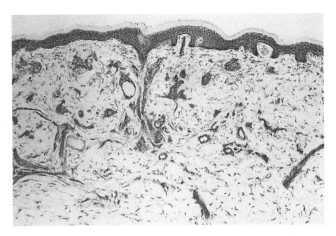

FIGURE 12.12 Pathology of syringoma showing many comma-shaped epithelial structures and tiny cysts (from Marks and Motley, 18th edition).

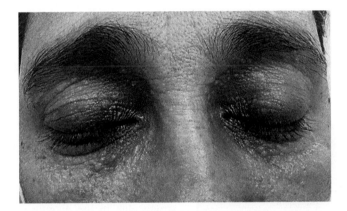

FIGURE 12.13 Syringoma lesions around the eyes.

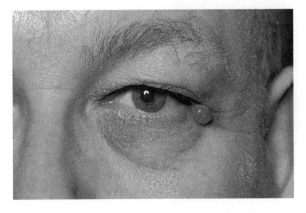

FIGURE 12.14 An apocrine hidrocystoma: this example is larger than usually seen in the periorbital skin (from Marks and Motley, 18th edition).

Eccrine hidrocystoma

A benign tumor arising from dilatation of eccrine gland units.

Clinical features

This is also a solitary, uncommon cyst and a close differential of apocrine hidrocystoma. It has the skin of greyish-blue color, usually seen around the eyelids and cheeks. A history of an increase in size on exposure to heat and improvement when the skin is exposed to cold is present.

Eccrine poroma

It is an eccrine sweat duct-derived tumor. Histologically, the lesion appears contiguous with the surface epidermis and consists of basaloid cells in which there are cuticularly lined duct-like structures.

Clinical features

They are pink-red, moist exophytic lesions arising predominantly on the palms and soles in adults.

Benign tumors of hair follicle origin

Pilomatricoma (calcifying epithelioma of Malherbe, trichomatricoma)

It is a benign tumor of hair matrix cells. Clumps of basal cells progressively become calcified and eventually ossified, leaving behind their cell walls only (ghost cells).

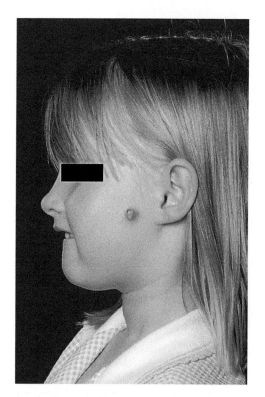

Clinical features

It is a solitary, smooth, skin-colored or bluish nodule present around the head, neck, and upper trunk in children and young adults (Figure 12.15). The hard nature of the lesion is a strong clue to the diagnosis. Stretching of the skin over the tumor with multiple angles results in a 'tent sign'.

Trichoepithelioma (Brooke's tumor)

It is a benign tumor of hair germ cells. There may be a familial tendency to develop these lesions.

Histologically, it consists of the most part of clumps of epithelial cells and horn-filled cysts; it may transform into basal cell carcinoma.

Clinical features

Trichoepithelioma are small, pearly papules more often multiple than solitary and usually occur over the scalp and central face with a predisposition to the skin around the nose (Figure 12.16).

FIGURE 12.15 Pilomatrixoma (from Marks and Motley, 18th edition).

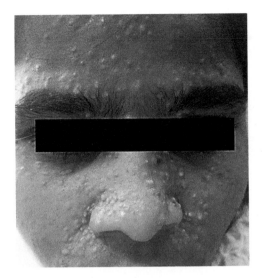

FIGURE 12.16 Trichoepithelioma.

Sebaceous gland hyperplasia

It is a common feature of elderly skin representing benign proliferation of sebaceous gland and has been suspected to be due to chronic solar damage rather than ageing.

Histologically, it consists of hypertrophied lobules of normal sebaceous gland tissue.

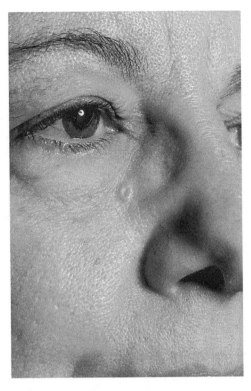

FIGURE 12.17 Sebaceous gland hyperplasia. Note the central 'punctum' within a yellowish papule on the face (from Marks and Motley, 18th edition).

Clinical features

One or, more often, several yellowish, skin-colored papules develop over the skin of the face, some of which have central puncta (Figure 12.17). They are often mistaken for basal cell carcinomata or dermal cellular naevi.

Clear cell acanthoma (Degos acanthoma)

The name derives from the epidermal thickening composed of large cells that, when stained with periodic acid–Schiff reagent, are found to be stuffed with glycogen (Figure 12.18) and infiltrated with polymorphonuclear leucocytes.

Clinical features

This is usually a solitary moist, pink papule or nodule on the upper arms, thighs, or trunk that has been present, unchanging, for several years in adults.

Naevi

The term 'naevus' is used for a fixed lesion present at or soon after birth. These are developmental anomalies consisting of immature melanocytes in abnormal numbers and sites within the skin. They are very common and, on average, white-skinned Caucasians have 16 over the skin surface. Melanocytic

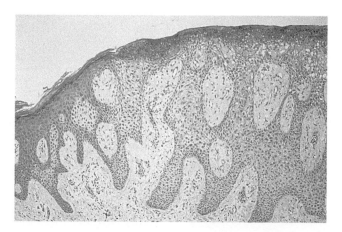

FIGURE 12.18   Pathology of clear cell acanthoma showing hypertrophied epidermis with areas of large, pale epithelial cells (from Marks and Motley, 18th edition).

naevi come in a wide variety of shapes and sizes and the main types are summarized in Table 12.4. The treatment of various naevi is provided in Table 12.5.

Congenital naevi

They are deeply pigmented lesions present at birth or appear a few months after birth and grows in proportion to the growth of the child. The size of the naevi determines the risk of development of melanoma. American National Institutes of Health (NIH) consensus definition categorizes these naevi into small (<1.5 cm in diameter), large (1.5–20 cm in diameter), and giant naevi (>20 cm in diameter)

Histologically, these lesions consist of numerous 'packets' (theques) of naevus cells (Figure 12.19), which may be small and basophilic (lymphocytoid), large and less intensely staining (epithelioid), or spindle-shaped. They may also coalesce to form naevus giant cells or after they have been present for many years, may show degenerative changes, including fatty degeneration and calcification. Naevus cells tend to be faceted together in a rather characteristic way.

Clinical features

These lesions, which are present at birth, are usually solitary and dark brown and are more than 1 cm^2 in size. They are plaque-like or nodular and may contain hair (Figure 12.20). The surface of large naevus may become warty and develop nodules with the growth of the infant. They share with the limb-girdle naevus the increased tendency to malignant transformation. It has been suggested that 10% of the larger congenital naevi develop malignant melanoma. The most deforming congenital melanocytic naevi are those that cover large areas of skin in the pelvic region and adjoining back (bathing trunk naevi) or over the shoulder region and upper limb.

Acquired naevi (mole, naevocytic naevus, cellular naevus)

Acquired naevi appear after birth, usually during adolescence or young adult life. Potential difficulty arises when an adult notices a brown lesion for the first time. Has it been there for many years before being noticed? Or is it a new benign mole, some other pigmented lesion, or a malignant melanoma?

TABLE 12.4

Main varieties of melanocytic naevi

Type	Clinical features	Comment
Congenital/simple	Present since birth, tend to be larger than acquired naevi, often hairy	Compare with acquired naevi
Girdle	Cover large areas around pelvic or pectoral zone (bathing trunk or cape naevus)	Increased tendency for malignant transformation – especially if very large
Acquired	Develop mainly in late childhood and early adolescence	
Junctional	Macular, brown/black	Anywhere on skin or mucosae
Dermal cellular	Papular or nodular, may be hairy; usually light brown or skin-colored	Very common on face and scalp
Compound		Combination of dermal, cellular, and junctional
Naevus spilus	Large, speckled, light-brown naevus	Uncommon, increased risk of malignant change
Dysplastic naevus syndrome	Many moles with irregular margins and pigmentation; may be sporadic but also familial	Increased tendency to malignant melanoma
Juvenile melanoma	Orange–pink nodule or plaque in childhood; also known as 'Spitz' naevus	Histological picture may simulate melanoma
Blue naevus	Blue due to depth of pigment in dermis	
Cellular blue naevus	Bluish nodule on scalp, hands, or feet	
Mongolian spot	Large, flat, greyish blue macule	Present at birth over sacrum; may fade
Naevus of Ota or Ito	Flat, blue–grey areas on face and neck	Predominantly in Asians

They are benign proliferation of melanocytes at the dermal–epidermal junction. If the cluster remains in dermo-epidermal junction it is known as junctional naevus and migration of some of the cells to dermis gives rise to compound naevus. It is called dermal cellular naevi when the whole cluster lies in the dermis.

The differential diagnosis for this situation is given in Table 12.6.

Junctional naevi

These are flat, brown, or black moles. It is presumed that this is the first stage in the 'lifecycle' of the ordinary mole. This type of mole is seen most frequently on the palms and soles, especially in children.

Compound naevi

These have the characteristics of a dermal cellular naevus, but there are areas of 'junctional activity'. It is presumed that these lesions are intermediary in development between the junctional naevus and the dermal cellular naevus.

Dermal cellular naevi

They are fawn or light-brown or just skin-colored papular or nodular lesions. They are common on the face and are often 'hairy', accounting for occasional episodes of pain, redness, and swelling due to

TABLE 12.5

Treatment of naevi

Naevus	Treatment
Congenital naevi	• Aimed at improving cosmetic effect and to reduce the risk of malignant transformation • Various plastic surgery techniques are utilized. • Both these aims are difficult to attain in large melanoma • Choice of intervention has to be balanced, keeping in mind the need for cosmesis
Acquired naevi	• Aim is to differentiate benign from atypical naevi • History, examination, and dermoscopy should be utilized to differentiate • Excision should be followed by histopathology • Lasers and various surgical methods can be utilized if excision is done for cosmetic purpose
Spitz naevus	• Local excision with a narrow margin
Naevus of Ota	• Q-switch ruby laser is effective
Verrucous epidermal naevus	• Surgical excision, shave excision, dermabrasion can be done • Cryotherapy and lasers (Er:Yag and CO_2) can be utilized • Recurrence is common
Becker's naevus	• Q-switched Nd:YAG laser can be done
Naevus sebaceous	• Excision of scalp lesions with primary closure
Shagreen patch	• Surgical excision • Laser ablation
Naevus lipomatodes cutaneus superficialis	• Surgical excision • Laser ablation
Adenoma sebaceum	• Surgical excision • Laser ablation
Port wine stain	• Laser treatment (pulse dye laser) can be dramatically effective • Not all lesions respond equally to treatment
Lymphangioma circumscriptum	• Sclerotherapy • Laser ablation
Infantile haemangioma	• Depends on the location, stage of evolution, morphology, risk of functional or cosmetic disfigurement, and comorbidities • If situated on the face they have the potential to grow and interfere with vision (Figure 15.42) or upper airway haemangioma can cause breathing difficulties • Under these circumstances early intervention is necessary • Systemic and topical steroids have been replaced by oral propranolol with better efficacy and side effect profile • Topical timolol has been tried with some success • Surgery is rarely required. They are undertaken if results are likely to be superior and to restore the contour and anatomy of a structure • Tuned dye 595 nm lasers may have a minor role in 'toughening' the surface of these lesions, particularly those prone to bleeding • There has been some success using Nd:YAG lasers
Angiokeratoma	• Smaller lesions to be treated with curettage and cautery • Larger lesions are excised surgically or by laser

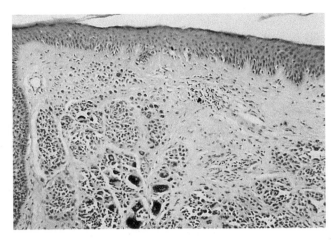

FIGURE 12.19   Pathology of congenital melanocytic naevus showing packets or theques of naevus cells, some of which are 'naevus giant cells' (from Marks and Motley, 18th edition).

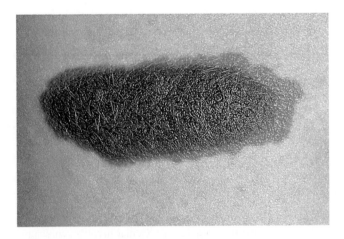

FIGURE 12.20   Large congenital melanocytic naevus (from Marks and Motley, 18th edition).

TABLE 12.6

Differential diagnosis of an acquired naevus

Diagnosis	Comments
Acquired naevus (mole)	Usually light brown, static
Seborrhoeic keratosis (basal cell papilloma)	Brown, warty
Dermatofi broma (histiocytoma)	Firm, light brown
Malignant melanoma	Enlarging, irregular, variegate
Pigmented basal cell carcinoma	Smooth, pigmented nodule

folliculitis. In some, there is a deep component with many spindle-shaped naevus cells that may superficially resemble the cellular component of a neurofibroma. In the elderly, when there is a little pigment, they may be misdiagnosed as basal cell carcinoma.

Degenerative changes in naevi

Naevus cell naevi gradually become fewer during the ageing process and it is believed that moles develop involutional changes before disappearing. Some develop lipid vacuoles in their substance, others develop a type of foamy change, and others appear to calcify before finally disappearing.

Dermal (blue) naevi

Cellular blue naevus

The melanin pigment and the bulk of the naevus cells are in the mid and deep dermis. The striking blue color given by the pigment is due to the red wavelengths being filtered out by the superficial dermis and epidermis known as the Tyndall effect.

Clinical features

A raised, smooth area of diffuse pigmentation is found to be present over the back of the hands or feet and scalp, usually appearing at puberty (Figure 12.21).

Mongolian spot

A type of blue naevus commonly found in Asians. It occurs as a greyish discoloration over the sacral area in the newborn, becoming less prominent in later life. The dermal melanocytes in persistent Mongolian spots have an extracellular sheath and are frequently associated with disorders of inborn errors of metabolism and vascular birthmarks.

Naevus of Ota

Blue-grey to brown pigmentation affecting face usually unilaterally in the area supplied by the ophthalmic and maxillary divisions of the trigeminal nerve. Ocular involvement is present, most commonly of the sclera (Figure 12.22).

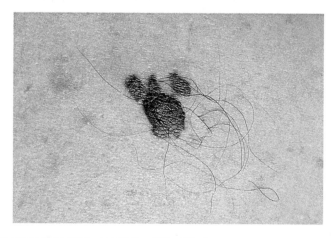

FIGURE 12.21   Blue naevus (from Marks and Motley, 18th edition).

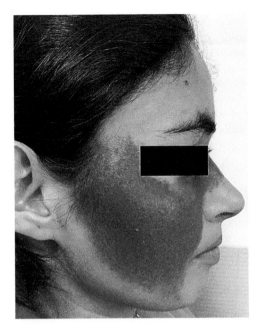

FIGURE 12.22   Naevus of Ota.

Naevus of Ito

Similar to naevus of Ota but situated in the distribution of posterior supraclavicular and lateral brachial cutaneous nerves.

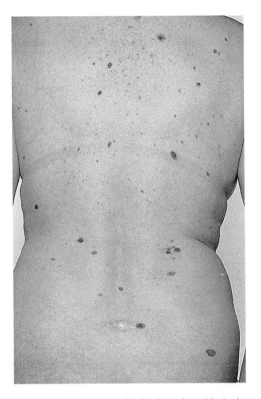

FIGURE 12.23   Multiple dysplastic moles with the irregularity of shape and pigmentation (from Marks and Motley, 18th edition).

Dysplastic naevus syndrome (atypical mole syndrome)

Recognition of this syndrome is important because of the increased frequency of malignant melanoma associated with it. The condition may occur sporadically but is also familial in many patients. It is said that the risk of a melanoma developing is approximately 1%, but it is certainly much more than that in the familial form if one of the affected members of the family has had a melanoma – perhaps 10%. It is even greater – possibly 100% – if the individual has already had one melanoma.

These lesions often have what the dermatopathologists call a 'worrying appearance', meaning that many have one or more features suggesting melanoma. There may be a degree of cytological atypia and excessive mitoses. These patients should be reviewed regularly and any suspicious moles removed for histological examination. It is helpful to take detailed clinical photographs and dermatoscopy photographs of their moles for future comparison.

Clinical features

The lesions are variable in number and may be quite large compared with ordinary moles. They have irregular margins and irregular brown pigmentation, some having an orange-red hue (Figure 12.23). The ABCDE algorithm is a quick way of obtaining a diagnostic clue to pick suspected melanoma lesions.

- Asymmetry
- Border irregularity
- Color variegation
- Diameter >6 mm
- Evolution

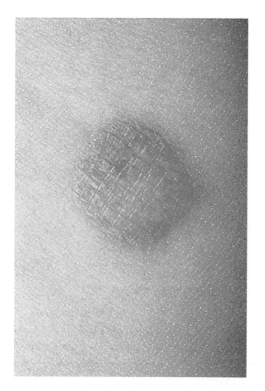

FIGURE 12.24 Juvenile melanoma: a red nodule on the arm of a 9-year-old boy (from Marks and Motley, 18th edition).

However, despite these clinical clues, the diagnostic accuracy remains low. In such a scenario, dermoscopy is a useful tool for the evaluation of skin lesions. It has increased sensitivity and specificity for melanoma, allowing detection at an early stage. It acts as a bridge between clinical suspicion and biopsy, thereby reducing the number of unnecessary biopsies of naevi.

Spitz naevus (juvenile melanoma)

This is an uncommon, benign lesion of childhood and adolescence; its alternative name derives from its histological appearance, which may look frighteningly like a melanoma to the uninitiated.

Clinical features

Usually, solitary, occasionally multiple red, pink, or orange papules, nodules, or small plaques (Figure 12.24), which may have a corrugated or peau d'orange surface present on the face, generally the cheeks, and the legs (in young adults).

Epidermal naevus

Epidermal naevi are an uncommon, localized malformations of the epidermis, composed of keratinocytes and classified as hamartomata. They are congenital in origin, represent genetic mosaicism, and are usually present at birth. Histologically, there is regular epidermal thickening and hyperkeratosis, often in a church-spire pattern.

Clinical features

Many epidermal naevi are arranged linearly and are warty, known as verrucous epidermal naevus (Figure 12.25). Sometimes they track along with a limb and adjoining trunk and are extensive and disfiguring. This type is known as naevus unius lateris (Figure 12.26).

Variants

Becker's naevus

Becker's naevus is an odd type of hamartomatous lesion that develops in adolescence or early adult life and sometimes shows increased androgen sensitivity. It consists of hypertrophy of all the epidermal structures, including the hair follicles and melanocytes.

Clinical features

A comparatively large area of skin is affected by a brownish and sometimes hairy plaque usually occurring around the shoulders or upper arms (Figure 12.27).

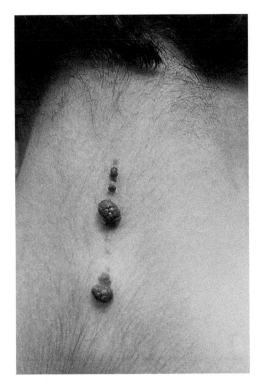

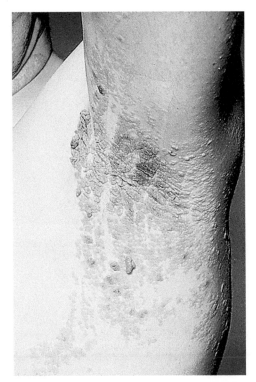

FIGURE 12.25   Verrucous epidermal naevus on the back of the neck.

FIGURE 12.26   Naevus unius lateris – linear warty lesion (from Marks and Motley, 18th edition).

Naevus sebaceous

These are epidermal hamartomas consisting of sebaceous glands (Figure 12.28).

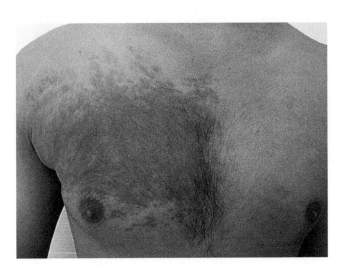

FIGURE 12.27   Becker's naevus on the upper back. The affected area is pigmented, thickened, and hairy.

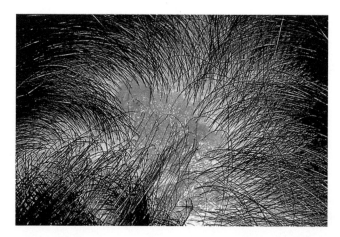

FIGURE 12.28   Typical orange plaque of naevus sebaceous on the scalp (from Marks and Motley, 18th edition).

Clinical features

Lesions are yellowish orange-brown plaques on the scalp, either present at birth or shortly afterwards, and may enlarge, thicken, and develop other lesions in them, such as basal cell carcinoma in adult life.

Connective tissue naevi

These are rare intracutaneous plaques and nodules, often with a knobbly or corrugated skin surface. They are very difficult to identify histologically because they are composed of normal connective tissue.

Shagreen patch

Plaque-type collagenoma most often occurring in the lumbosacral area (Figure 12.29).

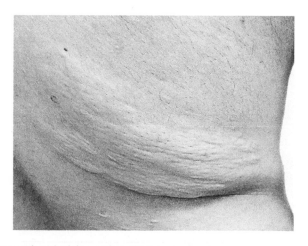

FIGURE 12.29   Shagreen patch on back in a patient of tuberous sclerosis.

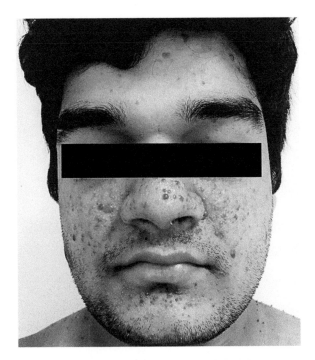

FIGURE 12.30   Skin colored to pink-red dome-shaped papules in a patient of adenoma sebaceum.

Adenoma sebaceum

'Adenoma sebaceum' is a misnomer as it is not an adenoma and is not derived from sebaceous glands. It occurs on the cheeks and the central part of the face of patients with tuberous sclerosis and consists of pink or red, firm papular lesions (Figure 12.30) in which vascular fibrous tissue is found rather than (as the name would suggest) an excess of sebaceous glands.

Tuberous sclerosis (epiloia)

This dominantly inherited syndrome is a neurocutaneous disorder.

Clinical features

The cutaneous components include shagreen patches, ash leaf-shaped hypopigmented patches on the trunk, subungual fibromata, which are fibrous nodules that develop beneath the toenails and fingernails, and adenoma sebaceum (see the earlier discussion).

Fat naevi

Naevus lipomatodes cutaneus superficialis

This is a rare disorder with ectopic collections of mature lipocytes in the dermis.

Clinical features

They can be either in form of clusters of soft, fleshy, yellow to skin-colored papules or nodules found commonly on the lower trunk and on the upper posterior thighs or as solitary, domed, or sessile papule at sites other than the lower trunk (Figure 12.31).

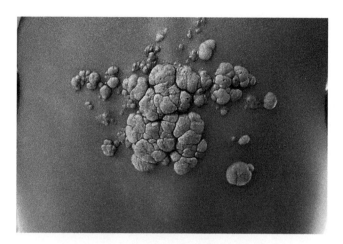

FIGURE 12.31   Naevus lipomatoses on the lower back.

Vascular naevi

According to the International Society for the Study of Vascular Anomalies (ISSVA), vascular birthmarks can be broadly divided into vascular tumors and vascular malformations (Table 12.7).

Vascular malformations

Soft, compressible, mauvish-blue swellings composed of large vascular spaces may occur. These lesions show little tendency to reduce in size in later life and may extend widely through the local tissues.

Capillary malformations

Stork mark (Salmon patch, Nuchal stain)

It is a popular name for the red discoloration at the back of the neck in a high proportion of newborns. It fades in later childhood and seems to be due to vasodilatation rather than due to an excess of blood vessels.

Port wine stain

This is a common low-flow vascular malformation. The lesions contain many dilated blood vessels but no other obvious histological abnormality.

Clinical features

The deep crimson color (of 'port wine') is distinctive and cosmetically very disfiguring, occurring most commonly on the face (trigeminal nerve distribution) (Figure 12.32a) and scalp. Facial lesions may be associated with mucosal and gingival involvement (Figure 12.32b).

The surface of the lesion becomes more thickened and rugose with age and even develops polypoid outgrowths, adding to the grotesque appearance. When on a limb, deep vascular malformations may also be present, which can cause limb hypertrophy. Over the ophthalmic region, the obvious skin malformation of blood vessels may be associated with an underlying meningeal angiomatous

TABLE 12.7

International Society for the Study of Vascular Anomalies (ISSVA) Classification of Vascular Anomalies (©2018) (available at issva.org/classification)

Vascular anomalies

Vascular tumors	Vascular malformations			
	SIMPLE	COMBINED	OF MAJOR NAMED VESSELS	ASSOCIATED WITH OTHER ANOMALIES
Benign	Capillary malformations	CVM, CLM	**Affect** lymphatics veins arteries	Klippel–Trenaunay syndrome
Locally aggressive or borderline	Lymphatic malformations	LVM, CLVM	**Anomalies of** origin course number length diameter (aplasia, hypoplasia, stenosis, ectasia/ aneurysm) valves communication (AVF) persistence (of embryonal vessel)	Parkes–Weber syndrome
Malignant	Venous malformations	CAVM		Sturge– Weber syndrome
	Arteriovenous malformations	CLAVM		Maffucci syndrome
				Microcephaly
				Macrocephaly
	Arteriovenous fistula			CLOVES syndrome
				Bannayan Riley Ruvalcaba
				Proteus syndrome

malformation. When this combination of lesions is associated with epilepsy, the disorder is known as the Sturge–Weber syndrome.

Lymphangioma circumscriptum

This lesion is a malformation of lymphatic channels, although there may also be an associated blood vessel anomaly. The lesions usually have a deep component, which is almost impossible to eradicate surgically.

Clinical features

The malformation is recognized as a diffuse skin swelling with what appears to be a cluster of tense vesicles with clear or blood-stained fluid, with a *frogspawn-like appearance*. It can be found anywhere but is common in lymphatic-rich areas (Figure 12.33).

(a)

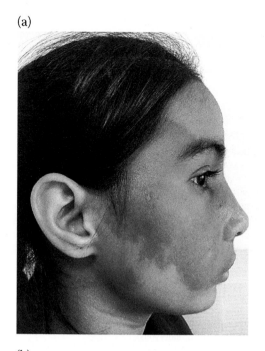

(b)

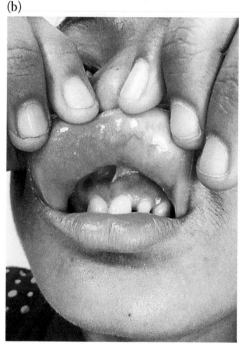

FIGURE 12.32 (a) Typical port wine stain in the distribution of trigeminal nerve and (b) mucosal involvement in the same patient.

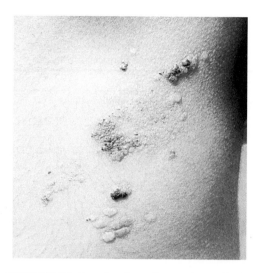

FIGURE 12.33 Lymphangioma circumscriptum affecting the abdomen.

Vascular tumors

Infantile haemangioma ('strawberry naevus')

The lesions are not usually visible at birth but develop in the first few weeks of life and undergo spontaneous involution. It has been suggested that they may represent an embolus of maternal placental vascular endothelial cells, which begin to proliferate in the child's skin. They may be segmental or multifocal involving the viscera.

Clinical features

They are raised, purplish nodules and plaques whose surface is often lobulated (supposedly like a strawberry), and they show an enormous range of sizes. The smaller lesions have little functional significance and usually flatten or disappear within a few years. The larger lesions may be very deforming and destructive and may cover quite a large area of skin (Figure 12.34). Periocular hemangiomas may lead to visual problems (Figure 12.35).

The larger lesions, particularly, may ulcerate after minor trauma, presumably due to ischaemia of the overlying superficial dermis and overlying epidermis because of the shunting of blood between the larger, deeper vessels of the angioma. Any bleeding can be stopped with gentle pressure and the eroded area gradually heals with routine care. One other rare complication only occurs with the largest of capillary angiomas. Blood platelets

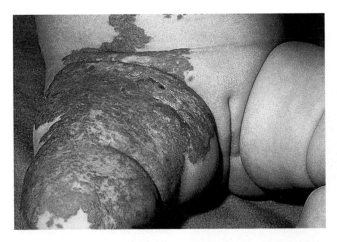

FIGURE 12.34   Large capillary naevus affecting the thigh and lower abdomen (from Marks and Motley, 18th edition).

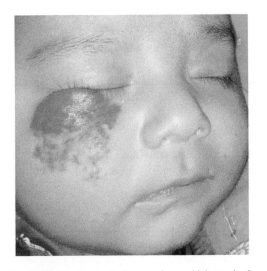

FIGURE 12.35   Periocular haemangioma which may lead to visual disturbance.

become sequestered in the abnormal vascular channels of the angioma, creating a consumption coagulopathy and uncontrolled bleeding (*Kasabach–Merritt syndrome*).

Angiokeratoma

There are several types of angiokeratoma, which all consist of a small, subepidermal vascular malformation surmounted by a hyperkeratotic epidermis.

Clinical features

They may occur as solitary red papules or, occasionally, as a crop of red spots over the scrotum (Figure 12.36). When literally hundreds of tiny red papules develop over the trunk in young men (bathing trunk distribution), the possibility of the very rare inherited metabolic abnormality known as angiokeratoma corporis diffusum or Fabry's disease must be considered.

Cysts

A cyst is an epithelium-lined cavity filled with fluid or semi-solid material. The distinguishing features of the commonly encountered cysts of the skin are summarized in Table 12.8. Their treatment is briefed in Table 12.9.

Epidermoid cysts

These lesions are lined by the epidermis and produce stratum corneum (keratin).

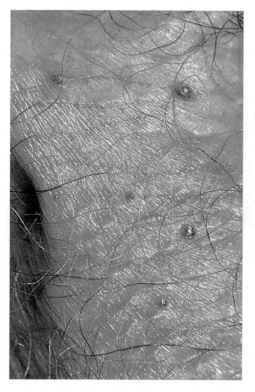

FIGURE 12.36 Angiokeratoma of the scrotum (from Marks and Motley, 18th edition).

Clinical features

Firm, skin-colored papules or nodules containing keratin that are surrounded by a tough, fibrous capsule, presumably stimulated by leakage of the cyst contents. A keratin filled punctum may be present (Figure 12.37). If the cyst contents find their way into the dermis, considerable inflammation results. The horny content may eventually degenerate, forming a foul-smelling, semi-solid material. The fancied resemblance of this to sebum has mistakenly led to the term 'sebaceous cysts' for these lesions. Epidermoid cysts may occur anywhere but are most common over the head, neck, and upper trunk. Gardner syndrome, an autosomal dominant disorder representing familial adenomatous polyposis (FAP), is associated with multiple epidermoid cysts.

Milia

They are tiny epidermoid cysts that occur spontaneously over the upper cheeks and beneath the eyes (Figure 12.38) and at the sites of subepidermal blistering, as seen in porphyria cutanea tarda.

Clinical features

They are small white papules usually no larger than a pinhead. They contain tiny accretions of the horn.

Pilar cysts (tricholemmal cysts)

They are often genetically determined as an autosomal dominant trait. The lining epithelium of these cysts, which are commonly seen on the scalp, is derived from a portion of the hair follicle neck and shows a

TABLE 12.8

Differential diagnosis of common skin cysts

Cyst type	Body site	Clinical features
Epidermoid	Virtually anywhere	Smooth-walled, firm lesions; may become inflamed if they leak; common
Milium	At sites of blistering, spontaneously on upper cheeks	Pinhead-sized, white, hard lesions
Pilar	Scalp and scrotum	May be inherited; often multiple; less common than epidermoid cysts; smooth-walled but not as firm as epidermoid cysts
Sebocystoma multiplex	Anywhere, but especially the upper trunk	May be inherited; always multiple; usually small, smooth-walled; contents less firm than other types; may become inflamed and develop acne-like lesions; uncommon
Dermoid	Face, particularly around the eyes	Deep-set in skin; may be oval and less mobile than other cyst types

TABLE 12.9

Treatment of cysts

Cyst	Treatment
Epidermoid cysts	• Uninflamed cyst: dissected out
	• Inflamed cyst: incised and drained followed by phenolization
Milia	• Expressed by slitting the thin epidermis over them with a needle tip
Pilar cysts	• Uncomplicated cysts: dissected out
	• Proliferating cysts: excised with a margin
Sebocystoma multiplex	• Due to their large number, surgical excision is impractical
Dermoid cysts	• Surgical excision

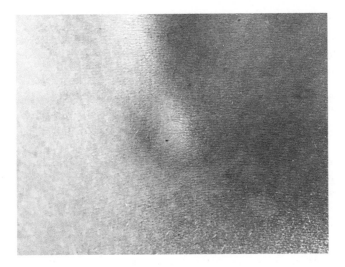

FIGURE 12.37   Epidermal inclusion cyst.

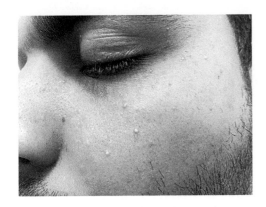

FIGURE 12.38   Milia.

quite characteristic type of keratinization in which there is an abrupt formation of a glassy-appearing type of horn without a granular cell layer.

Clinical features

Pilar cysts are solitary or multiple smooth, firm, and rounded nodules. They occur on the scalp and on the scrotum in particular. Inflammation can cause tenderness.

Sebocystoma multiplex (steatocystoma multiplex)

These cystic malformations are formed from sebaceous gland tissue and other hair follicle-derived epithelium. They are inherited as an autosomal dominant trait. Their content is sometimes pure sebum. The familial forms are associated with pachyonychia congenita type 2 (hypertrophic nail dystrophy, focal keratoderma, multiple pilosebaceous cysts).

Clinical features

They are small cysts, always multiple, often in very large numbers, and distributed over the body, particularly over the upper trunk and sternum. They usually have no punctum and comedones can be present.

Dermoid cysts

Dermoid cysts are uncommon lesions that are present from birth but may only become apparent several years later. They seem to contain embryonic epithelium capable of forming a wide spectrum of tissue types.

Clinical features

These cysts may occur anywhere but are especially often found around the eyes as oval, firm, smooth-walled swellings. They may extend deeply into the tissue and occasionally are associated with defects in the underlying bone.

Follicular retention cysts

When large hair follicles develop a hard, immovable comedonal plug in the follicular neck or at the skin surface, the follicle distends because of the continuing secretion of sebum and production of horny material. Often, these cysts rupture, causing inflammation, but sometimes this does not happen and quite large swellings are produced. This seems to occur particularly frequently over the back in the elderly when they appear as giant comedones.

13

Malignant diseases of the skin

Yasmeen Jabeen Bhat
Anupam Das

Malignant diseases of the skin are becoming more common, the reason being increased cumulative exposure to ultraviolet radiation (UVR), which is due to an increasingly elderly population, increased outdoor activities, clothing styles, depletion of atmospheric ozone, and environmental pollutants.

Non-melanoma skin cancer

Non-melanoma skin cancers (NMSCs) are epithelial cancers that originate from the epidermal keratinocytes or adnexal structures.

Premalignant lesions

Various precancerous lesions include actinic keratosis, Bowen's disease, HPV-induced intraepithelial neoplasia, and bowenoid papulosis, arsenical keratosis, thermal keratosis, radiation keratosis, etc.

Actinic keratosis

Actinic or solar keratosis is common. It includes localized areas of rough scaling of the skin surface caused by chronic solar exposure leading to dysplasia.

- **Incidence:** More common in white males beyond middle age. In the subtropical parts of Western countries, solar keratosis has been found in more than 50% of the population over the age of 40 years. However, dark-skinned subjects from Asia develop these, if they are excessively exposed to the sun.
- **Pathogenesis:** Chronic exposure to solar UVR is the most important cause, followed by chronic heat damage, X-ray irradiation, and chemical carcinogens.
- **Clinical features:** Single or multiple discrete raised, rough, pink or grey, scaly, or warty hyperkeratotic plaque are found for months to years on the exposed areas of the skin of elderly, fairskinned subjects who show other signs of solar damage (Figure 13.1). The lesions are better felt than seen, and the scales are adherent.
- **Investigations:** Dermoscopy of the lesion helps in diagnosis.
- **Pathology:** Paraketatosis and hyperkeratosis surmount the variably thickened epidermis, mild to moderate pleomorphism in the basal layer, heterogeneity of cell and nuclear size, shape, and staining (epidermal dysplasia).
- **Differential diagnosis:** Seborrheic keratosis, flat warts, discoid lupus erythematosus, and superficial basal cell carcinoma.
- **Course and complications:** A small proportion of solar keratoses disappear spontaneously over years, but a few can transform to squamous cell carcinoma (0.2%).
- **Treatment:** Sunscreen application on the exposed sites may prevent the occurrence.

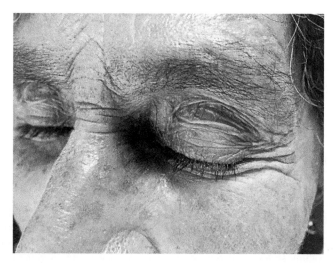

FIGURE 13.1   Multiple actinic keratosis presenting as rough scaly lesions in an elderly woman.

- **Topical therapy:** Curretage or cryotherapy for single lesions; topical chemotherapy for multiple lesions. Topical 5-fluorouracil 5% is applied as a single application daily for 2 weeks or on alternate days for 2 months. Daily doses may cause erythema and erosions of the skin. Imiquimod 5% cream, an immune response-modifying agent, is applied three times per week for 16 weeks. Topical diclofenac 3% gel appears to be quite effective and is applied twice daily for 3–4 months to the affected skin with mild skin reactions. Topical retinoids have a prophylactic as well as a therapeutic effect when used over long periods.
- **Photodynamic therapy:** Is effective and useful for large areas – such as the bald scalp. A topical photosensitizer – methyl amino laevulinic acid – is applied to the skin for several hours and the skin is exposed to an intense light – which activates the photosensitizer and destroys superficial areas of keratosis. Laser therapy with erbium or carbon dioxide lasers may be helpful.
- **Systemic therapy:** Retinoids like acitretin or isotretinoin can be used for extensive lesions.

Bowen's disease

Bowen's disease or intraepidermal epithelioma or squamous cell carcinoma in situ (SCCIS) is a localized area of epidermal neoplasia remaining within the confines of the epidermis.

- **Incidence:** Increasing.
- **Pathogenesis:** UVR, HPV, tar, chronic heat, chronic radiation.
- **Clinical features:** The most typical type of lesion of Bowen's disease is a well-defined, raised, red, scaling plaque, and lesions are often very psoriasiform in appearance. They are mostly present on light-exposed areas of skin and are often seen on the legs of women who are more commonly exposed to UV light or chronic heat (Figures 13.2 and 13.3). Single lesions are most common, but multiple lesions also occur.
- **Investigations:** Dermoscopy shows glomerular capillaries with diffuse erythema (strawberry appearance).
- **Pathology:** The histological appearance is as an exaggerated version of an actinic keratosis in which there is marked thickening and marked heterogeneity of the epidermal cells in the form of atypical keratinocytes, single-cell dyskeratosis, and increased mitotic rate (Figure 13.4).
- **Differential diagnosis:** Psoriasis, discoid eczema, superficial BCC, seborrheic keratosis.
- **Course and complications:** Untreated, it will progress to invasive SCC.

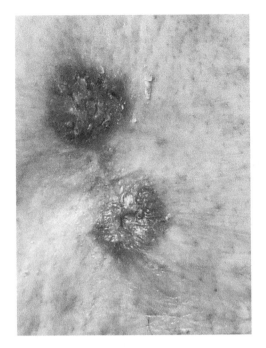

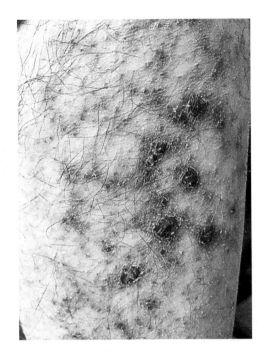

FIGURE 13.2   Psoriasiform patch of Bowen's disease on the abdomen of an elderly man.

FIGURE 13.3   Pigmented Bowen's disease on the leg of a patient with erythema ab igne.

- **Treatment:** Bowen's disease may be treated with local destruction by curettage, cautery, and cryotherapy, with topical agents such as 5-fluorouracil or imiquimod, or with photodynamic therapy. Surgical excision should be done in lesions where invasion cannot be excluded by biopsy.

Erythroplasia of Queyrat

This is the term used for squamous cell carcinoma in situ affecting the glans penis and vulva. It presents as a red, velvety patch that slowly progresses, eventually transforming into a squamous cell carcinoma if left untreated. Surgical excision of the affected area is the best form of treatment. Anogenital HPV-induced scc *in situ* is referred to as bowenoid papulosis.

Squamous cell carcinoma/Squamous cell epithelioma

Squamous cell carcinoma of the skin is a malignant tumor of keratinocytes.

- **Incidence:** In the United States, 12 males and 7 females per 100,000 white population. Organ transplant recipients have a markedly high incidence of SCC, about 40–50 times that in the general population.
- **Pathogenesis:** Chronic UVR damage from solar exposure, phototherapy, and tanning beds in fair-skinned persons is the most important aetiological factor in SCC development with chronic immunosuppression as a very significant disease-modifying factor. Other factors include irradiation damage to the skin; persistent heat injury (as in erythema ab igne); chronic inflammatory and scarring disorders of the skin, such as discoid lupus erythematosus, hypertrophic lichen planus, and dystrophic epidermolysis bullosa; chronic wounds, ulcers, and burns; certain genodermatoses and localized congenital malformations such as xeroderma pigmentosum, epidermodysplasia verruciformis, and epidermal naevus; human papillomavirus infection – certain oncogenic types (e.g. HPV types-5, -16, -18, -31, -33) seem particularly likely to cause malignant

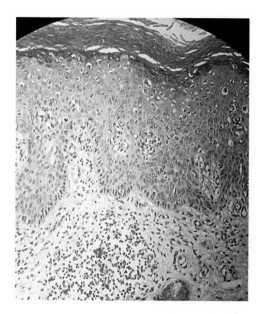

FIGURE 13.4   Histopathology of Bowen's disease showing occasional dyskeratotic cells.

transformation in immunosuppressed renal transplantation patients and those with HIV; exposure to chemical carcinogens, such as industrial contact with tars and pitch or systemic administration of arsenic.

- **Clinical features:** The majority of lesions of squamous cell carcinoma are asymptomatic warty nodules or plaques that evolve gradually or, in some cases, rapidly enlarge to form exophytic eroded nodules or ulcerated plaques. The lesion is in most cases solitary and occurs against a background of solar damage with multiple solar keratosis in sun-exposed sites such as the scalp, ears, lips, and dorsa of the hands. In differentiated SCC, indurated papule, plaque, or nodule with adherent keratotic scale, central ulceration, and elevated margins can be seen (Figures 13.5a and 13.5b). In undifferentiated SCC, pap-illomatous, cauliflower-like growths occur with central necrotic ulcerations and fleshy margins, bleeding easily on touch (Figure 13.6). Regional lymphadenopathy due to metastasis is common.

Investigations

- **Dermoscopy:** A red starburst pattern may point to the aggressive growth of the tumor.
- **Histopathology:** There is marked epidermal thickening with cellular and nuclear heterogeneity and atypia and evidence of abnormal mitotic activity. There is also evidence of focal and inappropriate keratinisation so that so-called horn pearls are formed (Figure 13.7). There is usually evidence of invasion of surrounding tissue by epithelial clumps and columns.

Several innovative optical imaging techniques, such as Raman spectroscopy, confocal microscopy, and fluorescence imaging may help intraoperatively for margin assessment and tumor detection.

- **Differential diagnosis:** Squamous cell carcinoma has to be distinguished from the massive but benign epidermal thickening known as pseudoepitheliomatous hyperplasia, which is seen in hypertrophic lichen planus, prurigo nodularis, and lichen simplex chronicus. Keratoacanthoma may be indistinguishable from well-differentiated SCC.
- **Course and complications:** Local tissue destruction and metastases occur if the primary lesions are left untreated, spreading to local lymph nodes, and ultimately lungs, bone, and brain. Most squamous cell carcinomas are removed before they metastasize, but patients who are

(a)

(b)

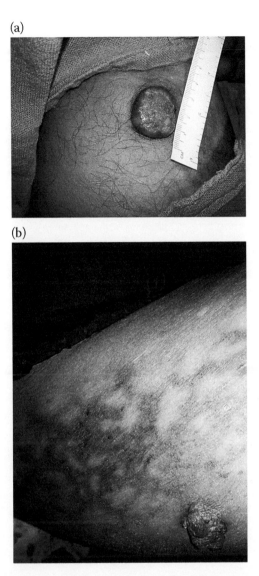

FIGURE 13.5   (a) Well-differentiated squamous cell carcinoma with raised margins and central ulceration; (b) Well-differentiated SCC on the background of erythema ab igne due to Kangri (Kangri cancer).

immunosuppressed are at a much higher risk of developing a metastatic disease. SCCs that are large, recurrent, and involve cutaneous nerves metastasize more.

Treatment

- **Surgical:** Excision – with an adequate margin to ensure inclusion of all neoplastic tissue and some healthy tissue all around the lesion, with primary closure, skin flaps or grafting – is sufficient for cure in more than 95% of patients. Moh's micrographic surgery can be done in difficult sites. This involves taking a thin saucer-like layer of tissue from beneath the tumor and then examining the undersurface of the tissue using frozen histological sections. Residual tumor is identified and localized in the wound and the process is repeated until the wound is tumor-free.

For the very elderly with solitary, large, difficult to remove lesions, treatment by radiotherapy may be more appropriate.

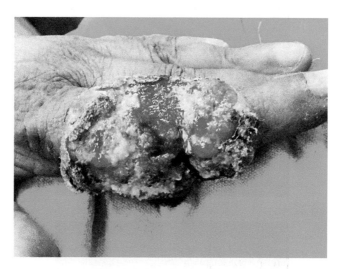

FIGURE 13.6   Undifferentiated SCC with fragile and necrotic tissue.

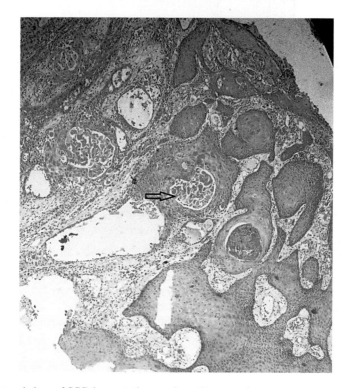

FIGURE 13.7   Histopathology of SCC demonstrating, atypia, and horn pearls.

For high-risk lesions involving deeper tissues, patient immunosuppression, location on ear and lip, oral 5-fluorouracil, retinoids, and interferons are given.

Cetuximab, a monoclonal chimeric IgG1 antibody that binds and blocks the epidermal growth factor receptor, acts in metastatic or unresectable squamous cell carcinoma when combined with radiotherapy.

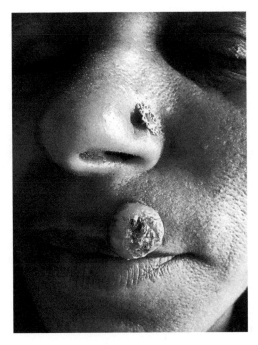

FIGURE 13.8   Keratoacanthoma on the upper lip presenting as a nodule with central crater.

Keratoacanthoma (molluscum sebaceum)

This term describes a rapidly growing epidermal tumor with many of the characteristics of a squamous cell carcinoma, but which may resolve spontaneously after many months.

- **Incidence:** Seen in people above 50 years of age, twice as common in males as females.
- **Pathogenesis:** It seems to be provoked by the same stimuli that cause solar keratoses, but is much less common. It has been suggested that keratoacanthomas develop from hair follicle epithelium.
- **Clinical features:** It usually appears within a week or two on light-exposed skin as a solitary crateriform nodule (Figure 13.8). It then gradually enlarges for a few weeks and stays at that size for a variable period before finally remitting after several months, leaving a crater-like scar. Rarely, it may be multiple and eruptive. Multiple self-healing squamous epithelioma of Ferguson-Smith (MSSE) is a rare autosomal dominantly inherited disease with recurrent, histologically malignant tumors that undergo spontaneous regression.
- **Investigations:** The keratoacanthoma is diagnosed on clinical grounds. On histopathology, keratoacanthoma has a characteristic, symmetrical, cup-shaped, or flask-shaped structure with epidermis extending over the sides of the crater. There is a minor degree of epidermal dysplasia and little evidence of tissue invasion.
- **Differential diagnosis:** SCC, hypertrophic actinic keratosis, verruca vulgaris.
- **Course and complications:** Spontaneous regression occurs in months. Untreated, these lesions may often reach 2–3 cm in diameter and become offensive due to necrotic infected tissue. Occasionally true squamous cell carcinomas may also arise rapidly and be indistinguishable.
- **Treatment:** Although spontaneous resolution may occur, this does not happen for many months – and frequently leaves an unsightly scar. For these reasons, therapeutic intervention is usually indicated. Surgical excision or curettage and cautery may be employed. Intralesional methotrexate and prednisolone have also been reported to be effective. Systemic retinoids can be given for multiple lesions.

Basal cell carcinoma (basal cell epithelioma)

Basal cell carcinoma is a locally invasive but rarely metastasizing malignant epithelial tumor of basaloid cells without the tendency to differentiate into horny structures.

Incidence: Worldwide, BCC is the most common skin cancer with a higher incidence in countries closer to the equator. As with squamous cell carcinoma and other forms of photodamage, basal cell carcinoma appears to be increasing in incidence. In the United States, the rate of incidence is 500–1000 people per 100,000 white population.

Pathogenesis: Most lesions of basal cell carcinoma are due to chronic solar exposure and UVR damage, as they occur on light-exposed sites in photodamaged subjects. However, a larger proportion occurs in younger, non-light-exposed, non-photodamaged subjects than solar keratoses or other forms of NMSC. The explanation for this is uncertain.

Clinical features: There are several clinical types.

Nodular. These are by far the most common variety. Translucent or skin-colored, dome-shaped nodules (0.5–1.5 cm in diameter) slowly appear on the skin and remain static for long periods, often for several years, before ulcerating (Figure 13.9). They often have a telangiectatic overlying skin and maybe flecked with pigment. They usually occur as solitary lesions on the exposed areas of the skin of the head and neck and are uncommon on the limbs. Some 20% occur on the trunk.

Ulcerative. The nodulocystic type eventually breaks down to form an ulcer with a raised, smooth, pearly border (Figure 13.10). This type is known colloquially as 'rodent ulcer'.

Pigmented. Brown to black, firm nodules with smooth, glistening surface, and surface telangiectasia (Figure 13.11).

Morpheaform. These are often whitish, scar-like, depressed, firm plaques, and are so named because of their supposed resemblance to localized scleroderma.

Superficial. These take the form of variably sized, thin, pink, scaling plaques with a well-defined, fine, thread-like border and telangiectasia. They often occur on the trunk and limbs.

Fibroepithelioma of Pinkus. Resembling a skin tag, long strands of interwoven basiloma cells are embedded in fibrous stroma.

Investigations Dermoscopy: Shows arborizing vessels, starburst pattern at periphery, and leaf-like structures.

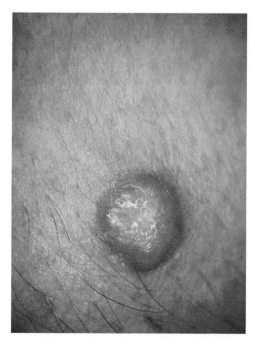

FIGURE 13.9   Nodular BCC presenting as an erythematous scaly nodule with telangiectasias.

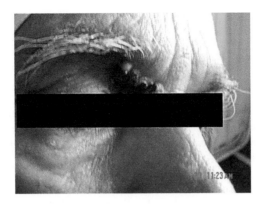

FIGURE 13.10   Ulcerative BCC (rodent ulcer) near the medial canthus of the eye.

Histopathology: Clumps of small basophilic epidermal cells occupy the upper dermis with the outermost cells often being more columnar and arranged in a palisaded pattern. Variable amounts of mucinous stroma can be seen. Many mitotic figures may be seen among the mass of basal cells, as may many degenerate cells. Laser-induced fluorescence spectroscopy is an emerging diagnostic technique for the diagnosis and demarcation of BCC.

Differential diagnosis: Dermal melanocytic nevi, trichoepithelioma, dermatofibroma for nodular type; SCC and painless firm ulcers for ulcerative type; superficial spreading and nodular melanoma for pigmented type; morphea or superficial scar for morphoeic; Bowen's disease for superficial type.

Course and complications: Basal cell carcinomas rarely metastasize, but untreated, they are progressively and inexorably destructive to local tissues. As a majority of lesions occur on the head and neck, especially the face, effective treatment of these lesions is essential to prevent unsightly and unnecessary destruction of facial features. Untreated periocular basal cell carcinomas may spread to involve the orbit and even extend into the brain.

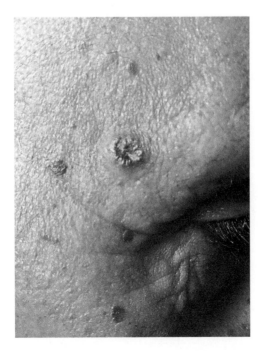

FIGURE 13.11   Pigmented BCC presenting as a pigmented plaque with raised beaded margin.

Treatment Depends upon the anatomic location and histologic features.

- Surgical: For the majority of facial lesions with clinically well-defined margins, the treatment of choice is surgical excision with a 3-mm margin around the tumor, which should be further defined by curettage prior to excision.

Where the margins of the tumor are ill-defined, when the tumor has recurred after previous treatment or where smaller surgical margins are desired for technical or aesthetic reasons, the tumor should be removed and the margins should be examined using Mohs' micrographic surgery, which has the highest cure rates for all forms of basal cell carcinoma.

Curettage and cautery or electrodessication is a common and successful technique for treating basal cell carcinomas on extremities and trunk and when tumor growth is non-aggressive. Cautery or electrodessication is used to obtain haemostasis and to destroy an additional layer of tissue.

Radiotherapy is an effective treatment but also depends on accurate identification of the clinical margins of the tumor. It is rather time-consuming, expensive and leaves a wound, which is slow to heal and with time becomes atrophic and unsightly. For these reasons, as the skills of dermatological surgeons have increased, radiotherapy has become a less popular choice.

At non-critical (non-facial) sites, a variety of additional therapeutic options exist, including topical chemo- or immunotherapy with 5-fluorouracil or imiquimod, cryotherapy with liquid nitrogen, or photodynamic therapy.

For metastatic BCC, good results have been seen with chemotherapy with cisplatin and paclitaxel.

Vismodegib, a specific oncogene inhibitor, is a new drug approved for the treatment of advanced BCC where radiation is contraindicated or lesions are inoperable.

Basal cell naevus syndrome (Gorlin's syndrome)

This is a rare, autosomal, dominantly inherited condition in which multiple pigmented basal cell carcinoma lesions develop as part of a multi-system disorder.

Incidence: Occurs mostly in whites but also occurs in people of color.

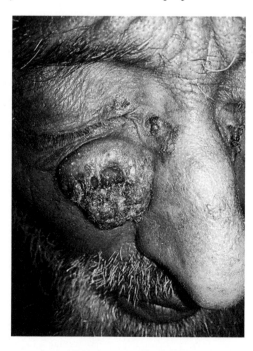

FIGURE 13.12   Basal cell naevus syndrome presenting as multiple BCCs on the face of an elderly man.

Pathogenesis: Mutations in the *PTCH1* gene are responsible for Gorlin's syndrome. The *PTCH1* gene is a tumor-suppressor gene, which prevents cells from proliferating too rapidly or in an uncontrolled way.

Clinical features: The three characteristic abnormalities are tumors like BCC, palmoplantar pits, and odontogenic cysts of the jaw. Multiple basal cell carcinomas may start to develop in the second decade of life and erupt in large numbers in succeeding years. Less severely affected individuals start to develop them later in life and develop fewer lesions (Figure 13.12). The lesions are mostly pigmented and may occur anywhere on the skin surface, to the inexperienced observer many of these basal cell carcinomas have the appearance of small naevi. Small pits may be found on the palms (more easily seen if the hands have been soaked in water for a few minutes beforehand), but otherwise, there are no skin abnormalities.

A series of skeletal anomalies are also present in the majority of patients, including mandibular cysts and bifid ribs. In addition, patients have a high incidence of benign ovarian, central nervous system, and spinal tumors.

Treatment: Individual lesions should be removed as necessary. In general, lesions on the face should be excised – if necessary with Mohs micrographic surgery. At non-facial sites, a variety of other treatments may be more practical, particularly when there are very large numbers present and new lesions are continuing to appear. Curettage and cautery, cryotherapy, photodynamic therapy, and topical chemotherapy – with products such as imiquimod – can be considered. Radiotherapy should be avoided – it may lead to more tumors in the periphery of the irradiated field. The administration of systemic retinoids will reduce the number of lesions and the rate of appearance of new basal cell carcinomas. Vismodegib is effective for the treatment of keratocystic odontogenic tumors and basal cell carcinomas.

Xeroderma pigmentosum

Xeroderma pigmentosum is the name given to a group of rare, inherited disorders in which there is a faulty repair of damaged DNA and the development of numerous skin cancers.

Incidence: It has been estimated that the incidence of xeroderma pigmentosum is 1 in 250,000 but in some areas, such as parts of the Middle East, the condition is unusually common.

Pathogenesis

Clinical features: The phenotypic expression depends on the particular genetic abnormality responsible, but in all types, pre-neoplastic and neoplastic lesions including actinic keratoses, squamous cell carcinomas, basal cell carcinomas, and melanomas develop from childhood, and in the worst cases cause death in late adolescence or early adult life. The development of skin cancers is accompanied by severe photodamage (Figure 13.13). In one severe recessive variety known as the de Sanctis–Caccione syndrome, there are also crippling neurological defects, including cerebellar ataxia and intellectual impairment.

Treatment

Management is directed to genetic counselling, removal of neoplastic lesions as they occur, and prevention of further photodamage by advice and sunscreens. Addition of DNA repair enzymes (photolyase and endonuclease) to traditional sunscreens may lessen UVR-induced molecular damage. The use of systemic retinoids may reduce the rate of development of new cancers.

Melanoma skin cancer

Melanoma is a malignant tumor of melanocytes, affecting most commonly the photoexposed parts. It accounts for less than 5% of all skin cancers diagnosed but the disease burden is significant as more than 50,000 deaths occur annually from it worldwide.

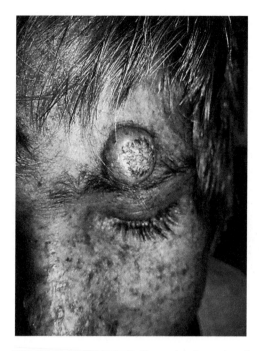

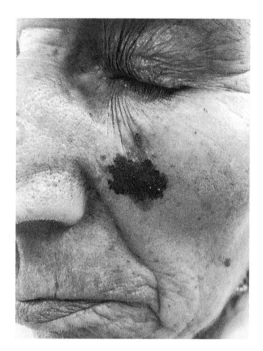

FIGURE 13.13 Multiple freckles, actinic keratosis and keratoacanthoma in a girl with xeroderma pigmentosum.

FIGURE 13.14 Lentigo maligna in a female presenting as a pigmented macule with variegated colors.

Lentigo maligna (Hutchinson's freckle)

Incidence: Equal in males and females; older populations and outdoor workers are affected.

Clinical features: Lentigo maligna is a slowly progressive, pre-neoplastic disorder of melanocytes, which develops insidiously on exposed areas of skin, particularly the skin of the face. The lesion itself is a pigmented macule with a well-defined, rounded or polycylic edge, which may be up to 5 cm in diameter or even larger (Figure 13.14). A characteristic feature is the varying shades of brown and black contained within the lesion – a feature known as variegation.

Investigations: Dermoscopy and skin biopsy help in diagnosis. There are many abnormal, often spindle-shaped, melanocytic clear cells at the base of the epidermis and clumps of melanin pigment in the upper part of the dermis. As the disease progresses, clumps of abnormal melanocytes appear, projecting into the dermis, and a dense infiltrate of mononuclear cells develops.

Differential diagnosis: Seborrhoeic wart, simple senile lentigo, and pigmented solar keratosis.

Course and complications: The disorder is usually slowly progressive over a period that may be in excess of 20 years. If left untreated, a true malignant melanoma develops within the lentigo maligna, which then has the characteristics of a typical malignant melanoma. Amelanotic melanoma may develop within lentigo maligna and so any nodular component, whatever the color, should be treated with suspicion.

Treatment: This is dictated by the size and exact site of the lesions. Wherever possible, surgical excision is the treatment of choice. However, they may be of a considerable size and alternative treatments may be required. These include locally destructive measures, such as curettage and cautery, and radiotherapy. Cryotherapy should be avoided because it may create non-functioning but viable melanocytes, which may recur without pigmentation to indicate their return. Imiquimod cream has been reported to be effective in some cases. Follow-up is advised after these non-excisional treatments in order to detect recurrence of the lesion; even after surgical excision, it is not uncommon for further lentigo maligna to develop in the vicinity of the original lesion or in other areas of skin. This can be considered part of a 'field effect' of susceptibility to the lentiginous atypia.

Malignant melanoma

Melanoma is an invasive, neoplastic disorder of melanocytes in which the tendency is for invasion either horizontally and upwards into the epidermis or vertically downwards. Different patterns are described: superficial spreading malignant melanoma (SSMM), nodular malignant melanoma (NMM), acral lentiginous malignant melanoma, and desmoplastic malignant melanoma.

Incidence: Malignant melanoma is rare before puberty but can occur at any age after that. It is seen in all racial types, but is more common in fair-skinned, Caucasian types. The rates of melanoma are 20 times more common in whites than in African-Americans with the overall lifetime risk of getting it being about 2.4% for whites, 0.1% for blacks, and 0.5% for Hispanics. Acral lentiginous melanoma seems most frequent in black-skinned individuals and subjects of Japanese or other Asian descents.

Pathogenesis: Solar UVR is believed to be the single-most important causative factor, but, as up to 50% of lesions of malignant melanoma occur on non-sun-exposed sites, other factors may play a role. The propensity for patients with the dysplastic mole syndrome and large congenital melanocytic naevi to develop this condition suggests that developmental factors may also be involved in some instances. Other risk factors for the development of melanoma include melanocortin-1 receptor genotype, childhood cancer history, immunosuppression, indoor tanning and Parkinson's disease. Mutations in the Kit gene stimulate various pathways like *MAPK, PI3K, PTEN,* and *MITF* in melanocyte proliferation.

Clinical features: Some 50% of lesions of malignant melanoma develop from a pre-existing melanocytic naevus, and the other 50% develop *de novo* on any part of the skin surface. Any pigmented lesion that suddenly develops or any change in the size, shape, or color of a pre-existing pigmented lesion should be suspected of being a malignant melanoma. Particular signs that are valuable in the recognition of these lesions are irregularity in the margin or in the degree of pigmentation, and erosion or crusting of the skin surface (Figures 13.15 and 13.16). Itchiness of the lesion is a not uncommon symptom in malignant melanoma.

Melanoma can be classified as in Table 13.1. Late local signs are the development of satellite pigmented (and non-pigmented) nodules and enlargement of the regional lymph nodes. Redness and other signs of inflammation may be present, but benign compound moles may also become inflamed, and inflammatory change *by itself* is not common in malignant melanoma.

The rate of progress of the disease seems largely determined by the inherent biology of the malignant melanoma. When the lesion spreads horizontally (SSM), they tend to be noted and treated earlier than when the predominant direction of growth is vertically downwards (nodular malignant melanoma – NMM). It is,

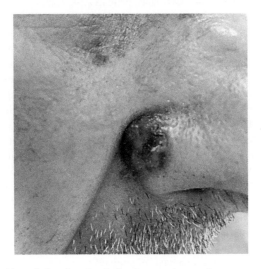

FIGURE 13.15   Melanoma with eroded surface developing in a previous mole.

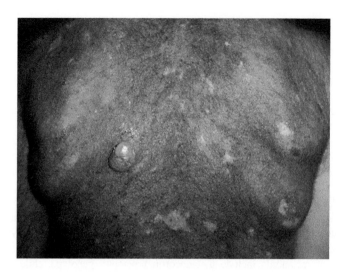

FIGURE 13.16   Nodular melanoma developing on the trunk in a boy with giant congenital melanocytic naevus.

TABLE 13.1

Classification of melanoma

De novo melanoma	Melanoma arising from precursors
Melanoma in situ (MIS)	Dysplastic naevomelanocytic naevi
Lentigo maligna melanoma (LMM)	Congenital nevomelanocytic naevi
Superficial spreading melanoma (SSM)	Common nevomelanocytic naevi
Nodular melanoma (NM)	
Acral-lentiginous melanoma (ALM)	
Melanoma of the mucous membrane	
Desmoplastic melanoma	

therefore, not surprising that the overall prognosis is much better for SSM than for NMM. The single most important determinant of prognosis appears to be the depth of invasion into the dermis, but this is really a proxy measurement for the overall tumor mass. Thus, patients with small lesions of less than 1 mm invading into the dermis have an expected 5-year survival rate of 95%. Because of the significance for the prognosis of the depth of invasion into the dermis, various classifications based on microscope measurements have been developed. The two most common are the Breslow thickness technique and the Clark staging method. In the Breslow technique, the maximum depth of malignant melanocytes is measured from the granular cell layer in the epidermis to the deepest cell in the dermis. Four categories are commonly described: <1 mm, 1–2 mm, 2.1–4 mm, and >4 mm. The Clark staging method recognizes five stages depending on where the tumor reaches: stage 1 being confined to the epidermis, and stage 5 including infiltration of the subcutaneous fat. Stages 2, 3, and 4 describe progressively deeper levels within the dermis.

Investigations: Melanomas can be detected early by the ABCDE rule (Table 13.2). Dermoscopy: plays a very important role in the early detection of melanoma. Skin biopsy: on histopathological examination, there are clumps of abnormal melanocytes at the dermoepidermal junction. In SSMM, abnormal melanocytes tend to invade upward into the epidermis and horizontally along the epidermis. In NMM, there are groups of abnormal cells invading vertically downwards (Figure 13.17). There is usually some accompanying inflammatory cell infiltrate. Immunohistochemistry and fluorescent in situ hybridization, utilizing various antibodies like S100, HMB-45, Melan-A, and MART-1 help in the diagnosis of cutaneous melanoma.

Differential diagnosis: Melanocytic naevus, pigmented basal cell carcinoma, dermatofibroma, and vascular malformation.

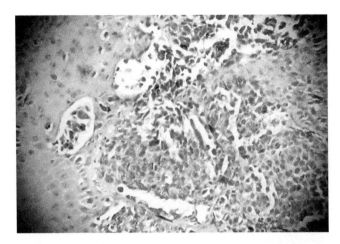

FIGURE 13.17   Clusters of melanin-producing tumor cells infiltrating the dermis in a melanoma. (H&E×100).

Course and complications: Spread of malignant melanoma is local, regional, and distant. Distant metastases occur by haematogenous spread. Haematogenous metastases may occur anywhere, but quite commonly they develop in the lungs, liver, and brain. Regional spread is via the lymphatics to regional lymph nodes. When regional lymph node metastases have been found, the 5-year survival rate is less than 25%, and when distant metastases have occurred, the comparable figure is around 5%.

Secondary satellite lesions develop around the primary malignant melanoma in many instances. When metastases are widespread, the production of melanin pigment and its subsequent release into the circulation may be sufficiently great to result in a generalized darkening of the skin and even excretion of melanin in the urine (melaninuria), although this is quite rare. Occasionally, regression of part of the lesion occurs and, rarely, the entire lesion and metastases may undergo spontaneous resolution.

Overall, men have a worse prognosis than women. Back lesions in men and leg lesions in women have the least favorable prognoses.

Treatment: Melanoma development can be prevented by limiting exposure to UVR by using sunscreens and protective clothing. Regular screening of the moles by ABCDE rule and dermoscopy is advisable. Long-term use of aspirin may be associated with a reduced risk of melanoma.

Surgery: The definitive treatment is wide surgical excision with a generous margin of normal skin (Table 13.3). Sentinel lymph node biopsy is an experimental technique in which a radioactive tracer is injected at the site of the previous melanoma and then followed to the first 'sentinel' lymph node. This node is excised and examined for evidence of melanoma. If present the other lymph nodes within the lymph node basin are removed. It is proposed that early removal of the lymph nodes in patients in whom the sentinel node is involved may be advantageous compared with later removal of clinically involved lymph nodes.

Immunotherapy: Various immunomodulators include phosphodiesterase-1 inhibitors (pembrolizumab, nivolumab), cytokines (interferon-α, interleukin 2), BCG vaccine, and imiquimod cream.

Targeted therapy for melanoma by BRAF inhibitors (sorafenib), MEK inhibitors (trametinib), c-kit inhibitors (imatinib), CTLA-4 inhibitors (ipilimumab) Chemotherapy by isolated limb perfusion and radiotherapy have also been used.

TABLE 13.2

ABCDE rule for melanoma detection

A (asymmetry)	One-half of the mole does not match the other
B (border)	Borders are irregular, ragged, notched, or blurred
C (color)	The color is not uniform, includes shades of brown and black
D (diameter)	The spot is larger than 6 mm across
E (evolving)	The mole is changing in size, shape, or color.

TABLE 13.3

Recommended margins for surgical excision

Tumor thickness	Recommended margins
In situ	0.5 cm
1 mm	1 cm
1–2 mm	1–2 cm
2–4 mm	2 cm
Over 4 mm	2 cm

Neoplastic disorders of mesenchymal elements

Kaposi's sarcoma

Kaposi's sarcoma is a rare, multifocal, malignant vascular tumor of skin and other organs, which occurs either as an endemic, slowly progressive disease or as a rapidly progressive disorder in the immunosuppressed.

Incidence: The endemic type occurs predominantly in elderly males of either Jewish origin from central Europe or of Italian origin. The rapidly progressive type occurs in patients with AIDS, particularly male homosexuals, renal transplant patients, and in areas of Africa – notably Uganda.

Pathogenesis: Human herpesvirus 8, also known as Kaposi's sarcoma-associated herpesvirus (KSHV) is involved and causes proliferation of B cells and endothelial cells.

Clinical features: Mauve or purplish-red nodules and plaques and brownish macules develop over the dorsa of the feet and the lower legs. These lesions are usually accompanied by swelling of the lower legs. In AIDS patients, the clinical manifestations are similar to those of endemic Kaposi's sarcoma, but are much more extensive and much more rapidly progressive. Four clinical types are classic, endemic, iatrogenic, and HIV-related.

Investigations: Histopathology: the lesions consist of abnormal, slit-like vascular channels lined with spindle-shaped cells, a mixed inflammatory cell infiltrate, haemorrhage, and fibrosis.

Differential diagnosis: Vascular naevi, pyogenic granuloma.

Course and complications: They are slowly progressive and may not appear in other sites for many years. It has been estimated that the mean survival time after the appearance of the first lesions is approximately 12 years. Eventually, lesions disseminate to other parts of the skin and to the viscera.

Treatment: Wide excision, cryotherapy, radiotherapy and mTOR inhibitors like sirolimus or rapamycin have been used. In patients with HIV-associated Kaposi's sarcoma, highly active antiretroviral drugs appear to be effective at controlling the condition. Patients who are taking immunosuppressive drugs may respond to chemotherapy with interferons, paclitaxel, doxorubicin, and etoposide.

Dermatofibrosarcoma

This is a slowly progressive neoplastic disorder of fibroblasts. It looks quite similar to a dermatofibroma histologically and is an intracutaneous form of plaque clinically. These lesions often extend widely into the skin and subcutaneous tissues and the clinical margins may be difficult to detect. Wide surgical excision is necessary or Mohs' microscopically controlled excision.

Lymphomas of skin (cutaneous T-cell lymphoma)

Mycosis fungoides

It is a multifocal, neoplastic disorder of T-lymphocytes that primarily affects the skin.

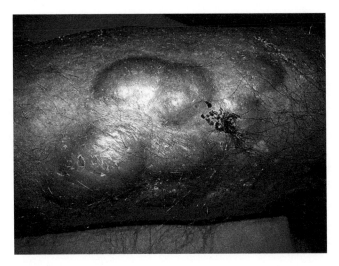

FIGURE 13.18   Infiltrated erythematous plaques on the leg in a patient with mycosis fungoides.

Incidence: Mycosis fungoides and Sezary syndrome together comprise 53% of primary cutaneous lymphomas that occur in 1/100,000 people.

Pathogenesis: Various chemokines, cytokines, and adhesion molecules lead to lymphocyte extra-vasation and skin homing of malignant T cells.

Clinical features: This uncommon disorder starts off as a series of red macules and scaly patches over the trunk and limbs, which gradually extend and become more prolific, but at first only cause inconvenience because of their appearance and mild pruritus. The red patches persist, although they may fluctuate in intensity, and eventually start to thicken and become plaques and, later still, eroded tumors (Figure 13.18). The ringworm-like appearance of some of the early patches and the fungating plaques in the late stages was presumably responsible for the term mycosis fungoides. In the later stages of the disorder, lymph node enlargement, hepatosplenomegaly, and infiltration of other viscera occur.

Histopathology: Epidermotropism of the malignant lymphocytes containing cerebriform nuclei (Pautrier's microabscess) in the absence of spongiosis is diagnostic. Immunohistochemistry and flow cytometry help in the identification of neoplastic T cells.

Differential diagnosis: Depends on the stage.

Course and complications: The disorder is inevitably fatal, although the rate of progress is quite variable, with survival ranging from 2 or 3 years in some patients to 20 years in others.

Treatment: Depends on the stage. Topical steroids, nitrogen mustard, bexarotene, phototherapy, interferons, and biologicals may be used.

Sézary syndrome

This is marked by an erythroderma that has a particularly intense erythematous color, a picture sometimes referred to as *l'homme rouge*. It is accompanied by thickening of the tissues of the face, neck, and palms. It is also characterized by the appearance of abnormal mononuclear cells circulating in the peripheral blood. These cells, which are identified in the 'buffy coat', are large and have a large, dense, reniform nucleus.

Other forms of T-cell lymphoma

    i. Parapsoriasis
    ii. Lymphomatoid papulosis

14

Skin problems in infancy and old age

Sumit Sethi
Rashmi Sarkar

Infancy

Functional differences

In the neonatal period and early infancy, the skin's defences are not yet fully developed, and it is much more vulnerable to chemical, physical, and microbial attack. The surface area–to–weight ratio is higher, thus a greater hazard from increased absorption of topically applied medicaments. There is also a greater rate of transepidermal water loss through intact, non-sweating skin in the newborn compared with the adult, indicating immaturity of the skin's barrier function.

During the early weeks of life, newborns possess the blood levels of hormones found in the mother at birth. This may be of special significance for the sebaceous glands, which react to circulating androgenic compounds by enlargement and increased sebum secretion.

Management problems in infancy

Medicaments are absorbed by infant skin far more easily and are more likely to cause systemic toxicity. Topical agents that are well tolerated by adults may cause quite severe reactions in infancy because of the lack of maturity of the skin barrier.

The ability to scratch does not seem to fully develop until around the age of 6 months, and when it does, a rash may alter substantially because of the secondary lesions and the physical effects of persistent scratching on the skin (lichenification) as well as the presence of infective lesions. The inability of the infant to complain of discomfort and irritation leads to general irritability and persistent crying. When this continues for long periods, the parents cannot sleep and the intra-familial emotional tension spirals upwards within the family home, necessitating attention to all those involved.

Widespread rashes may rapidly lead to dehydration in infancy because of the greatly increased rate of water loss through the abnormal skin. Hypothermia can develop very rapidly in young infants who have a widespread inflammatory skin disorder. These two complications, dehydration and hypothermia, may be prevented by anticipating and monitoring water loss with an evaporimeter and monitoring body temperature by taking the rectal temperature. Nursing infants with severe widespread skin disease are kept in an incubator for maintaining body temperature and hydration.

Napkin rash

This term is applied indiscriminately to any rash localizing in the napkin area. Several disorders focus on this area, which is perhaps not surprising when we consider the physical assault provided by wearing of napkins.

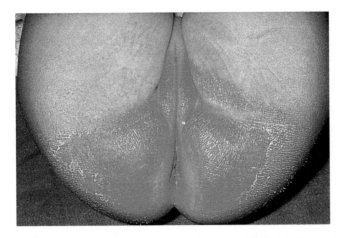

FIGURE 14.1   Erosive napkin dermatitis; note sparing in the flexures (from Marks and Motley, 18th edition).

Erosive napkin dermatitis

This is the most common type of napkin dermatitis. Red, glazed, fissured and even eroded areas develop on the skin at sites in contact with the napkin (Figure 14.1). The flexures are mostly spared, because the skin in these sites is less exposed to the foul soup of urine and feces, with the convexities commonly affected. There is often a strong ammoniacal smell when a soaked napkin is removed after a long time. This is due to the release of ammonia as a result of the action of the urease in fecal bacteria on the urea in the urine.

The condition responds to nursing without napkins for 2 or 3 days, but if this is not possible, more frequent napkin changes, the use of soft muslin napkins and avoidance of abrasive towelling napkins help, as do efficient disposables that maintain the skin surface dry. An emollient cleansing agent and a moisturizer used two or three times per day also help. Topical 1% hydrocortisone ointment twice daily could be used if the condition proves resistant.

Seborrhoeic dermatitis

This is less common than erosive napkin dermatitis. Scaling, red areas develop, mainly in the folds of the skin, although the eruption 'overflows' on to other areas in the napkin area. When the condition is severe', other sites such as the scalp, face, and neck may be affected. The involved sites may also crack and become exudative. The same kind of care of the napkin area as outlined earlier for erosive napkin dermatitis should be advised. In addition, a weak topical corticosteroid in combination with broad-spectrum antimicrobial compounds such as an imidazole (e.g. miconazole or clotrimazole) should be used twice daily.

Napkin psoriasis

This is an uncommon, odd, psoriasis-like eruption that develops in the napkin area and may spread to the skin outside – the flexural areas in particular. Treatment should once again be directed to better hygiene. Weak topical corticosteroids and emollients used as indicated earlier usually improve the condition quite quickly. The relationship with adult plaque-type psoriasis is uncertain.

Atopic dermatitis

The condition rarely starts before 4–6 weeks of age and usually begins between the ages of 2 and 3 months. It may first show itself on the face but spreads quite quickly to other areas, although the napkin area is conspicuously spared – presumably as a result of the area being kept moist. The ability to scratch develops after about 6 months of age and the appearance of the disorder alters accordingly, with excoriations and lichenification. At this time, the predominantly flexural distribution of the disorder begins, with thickened, red, scaly, and excoriated (and sometimes crusted and infected) areas in the popliteal and antecubital fossae. The eyes are often affected, eye rubbing being the probable cause of sparseness of eyebrows and eyelashes. It may also be the cause of corneal softening (keratomalacia) and its deformity (keratoconus). Emollients are important in management and mothers should be carefully instructed on their benefit and how to use them. Similarly, bathing should be in lukewarm water, with patting dry, rather than long-lasting hot scrubs with vigorous towelling afterwards. Weak topical corticosteroids only should be used – 1% hydrocortisone and 0.1% clobetasone butyrate are appropriate. For more severely affected infants, topical tacrolimus (Protopic) or pimecrolimus (Elidel) has proved a useful alternative to steroids.

Cradlecap

The newborn often develop a yellowish scale over the scalp with very little other abnormality apparent. This has no special significance and usually disappears after a few weeks.

Infantile acne

It is not uncommon for infants a few months old to develop seborrhoea, comedones, superficial papules, and pustules on the face (Figure 14.2). Deep inflammatory nodules or cysts are very uncommon but occur rarely. These maternal androgens cause the infant's sebaceous glands to enlarge and become more active. When the disorder develops after infancy and is severe, the possibility of virilization due to an endocrine tumor or adrenocortical hyperplasia has to be considered. Other signs of androgen overactivity, such as precocious muscle development and male distribution of facial and body hair, should be sought as indicators of this much more serious problem. Although the disorder usually subsides within a few weeks, it can be unpleasantly persistent.

Treatment with mild topical agents is usually sufficient to control the problem, e.g. 0.25% tretinoin gel or 2.5% benzoyl peroxide gel. Tetracyclines should not be given as they can cause bone and tooth dystrophy in childhood and adolescence.

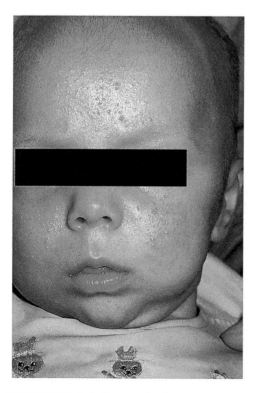

FIGURE 14.2 Infantile acne showing numerous acne spots on the cheeks and forehead (from Marks and Motley, 18th edition).

Staphylococcal scalded skin syndrome

This affects infants in the first few weeks of life but can occur in older children. There is a widespread erythematous eruption with striking desquamation of large areas of skin, as in a scald or burn. There may be a slight fever and some systemic disturbance, but usually, the children are not severely ill, although there is a 2–3% mortality rate. The disorder is due to a particular phage-type of *Staphylococcus aureus* (phage type II), which releases an erythematogenic exotoxin. This toxin can be shown experimentally to cause shedding of the most superficial part of the epidermis and stratum corneum in the skin of the newborn.

Treatment should be with an appropriate systemic antibiotic such as flucloxacillin. The skin should be managed as for a burn, and concern over heat loss, dehydration, and severe infection is necessary.

Lip-licking cheilitis

Children aged 4–8 years sometimes develop an area around the mouth contiguous with the lips, which becomes sore, red, scaly, and cracked (Figure 14.3). It is due to licking the lips and the skin around the lips, which become irritated and dry and are then licked to moisten them, making the situation worse. The treatment is to explain patiently the nature of the problem to mother and child and to use an emollient on the affected area. It is often mistaken for perioral dermatitis.

Juvenile plantar dermatosis

This disorder has apparently become more common in recent years, predominantly affecting children aged 6–16 years. It is a type of eczema that affects the soles of the forefeet and the toes. The affected skin becomes 'glazed', red scaly, and cracked, and the condition tends to be very persistent. Treatment with emollients, topical corticosteroids, and weak tar preparations is recommended, but the disorder tends to resist treatment and eventually remits spontaneously. The exact cause of this odd skin disorder is obscure but is been suspected to be due to the occlusive footwear (towards sports or training shoes).

Old age

There is a growing acreage of elderly skin because of the staggering increase in the proportion of the population over the age of 60 years. The increase in longevity since the beginning of the twentieth century is approximately equal to that seen in the human race in the previous 5000 years. We certainly need to know more about the ageing process and its effects on the skin.

The ageing process

Generally, we distinguish between intrinsic ageing and extrinsic ageing. The latter is not true ageing, i.e. the effects of the passage of time alone on the tissues, but the results of cumulated environmental

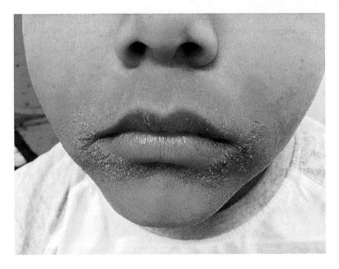

FIGURE 14.3 Lip-licking cheilitis.

trauma. As far as the skin is concerned, the most significant environmental trauma stems from solar radiation in the form of ultraviolet radiation.

There are many hypotheses to account for intrinsic ageing, which range from a kind of built-in obsolescence within the DNA molecule itself to the cumulated results of metabolic damage from the inevitable generation of active oxygen species and free radicals. Another inexplicable aspect of ageing is its variability. There are enormous variations in the rates at which different individuals age, as well as major differences in the rates at which individual organs and systems age within one individual.

Skin changes in the elderly

Structural changes

Both the epidermis and the dermis become thinner at non-light-exposed sites with the passing of the years. The degree of thinning is variable, but, between the ages of 20 and 80, dermal thickness on the flexor aspect of the forearm changes in men from a mean of 1.1 to 0.8 mm. The epidermis thins down from four to five cells thick at age 20 to approximately three cells thick at age 80. The individual keratinocytes also shrink with age, although the horn cells at the surface inexplicably increase in area. Interestingly, the stratum corneum does not appear to change substantially in thickness during ageing remaining approximately 15–20 µm. The papillary structure is gradually lost, and the dermoepidermal junction flattens.

Blood vessels decrease in number with age, but thicken. Adnexal structures also decrease in size and number with increasing age. This applies also to the hair but not always to the sebaceous glands, as on the face they may, paradoxically, enlarge, which is sometimes clinically evident in the condition of sebaceous gland hyperplasia.

The dermal connective tissue loses much of its proteoglycan ground substance and the collagen fibres become mainly tough, insoluble, and heavily cross-linked biochemically. Pigment cells become fewer in number and smaller, and Langerhans cells are also less in evidence in the skin of the elderly.

Functional changes

Wound healing is slower and may be less complete in the elderly. The aged also respond less vigorously to chemical and physical trauma – the erythema and swelling are less marked and slower to develop. However, it does not seem to apply to immediate hypersensitivity. Delayed hypersensitivity is depressed and this also applies to other components of the immune response. Skin surface markings become less prominent in the elderly and overall the surface flattens at non-exposed sites.

The activity of the pigment cells is depressed, and non-exposed areas of skin are in general paler in the elderly than in young and mature subjects. On exposed areas of skin, melanocytes show irregular increases in pigmentation. Sweat gland responses to heating decrease and the rate of sebum secretion also decreases, although this is less marked than many other functions in the elderly. Sensory discrimination decreases in the elderly, but, unfortunately, not the sensations of itch or pain!

Skin disease in the elderly

There are very few skin disorders that are specific to the elderly. However, there are many disorders that are more common in the aged, and others that have a different natural history and appearance.

Dry and itchy skin

As the skin ages, it becomes drier (i.e. tends to be scaly and rough) and tends to become itchier. This tendency is heightened by:

- Low relative humidity
- Frequent hot bathing and vigorous towelling
- Low ambient temperature

The itchiness can be disabling and it is important to try to reduce the desiccating stimuli to which the skin is exposed. The generous use of emollients as topical applications, as cleansing agents, and in bath additives is mandatory.

Although itchiness due to dry skin in the elderly is quite common, it has to be remembered that scabies and the other causes of generalized pruritus also occur in this age group and should be diligently sought.

Eczema

Eczema is a common problem in one form or another in the elderly. In most cases, no cause is found for the development of eczema, particularly in elderly people, in whom it can spread rapidly and become extremely disabling.

- *Atopic dermatitis* is uncommon in the elderly.
- *Discoid eczema* is a form of constitutional eczema that is more common in the elderly, which typically occurs as round coin-sized scaling patches.
- *Eczema craquelée/Asteotic dermatitis* is an eczematous disorder that is virtually specific to the skin of the elderly, occurring against a background of generalized xerosis, or drying of the skin surface.
- *Photosensitive eczema* is more common in elderly men and is often very persistent, causing great difficulties in its management.
- Mild cases *seborrhoeic dermatitis* are very common in the elderly, and occasionally the disorder can spread to become generalized.

Treatment

The treatment of eczema in the elderly is similar to that in other age groups but it can spread and become generalized more quickly than in other age groups. However, emollients are even more important and there should be greater readiness to use systemic remedies, including ciclosporin, azathioprine, and corticosteroids.

Skin tumors

Skin tumors are a frequent reason for the elderly consulting a physician. Seborrhoeic warts are found in virtually everyone over the age of 60 years and, although benign, often result in minor symptoms and some cosmetic embarrassment. They can easily be removed by curettage and cautery, but when present in large numbers, can present an insoluble problem. Although very few progress to squamous cell cancer, they indicate that serious solar damage has occurred and that more significant lesions may develop. They are uncommon below the age of 45 years and very common over the age of 60 years. As with seborrhoeic warts, solar keratoses may also cause minor symptoms and some cosmetic problems.

Basal cell carcinomas are almost as common as solar keratoses. Because of their capacity for local invasion and tissue destruction, they cause considerable morbidity. Squamous cell carcinomas are much less common, but can metastasize as well as cause local tissue destruction. Squamous cell carcinomas of the penis, lips, and ears have a bad reputation for metastasis. Malignant melanoma is slightly more common in the elderly compared with young age groups, but lentigo maligna is virtually restricted to the elderly.

Management of skin disorders in the elderly

Through no fault of their own, the elderly are often physically, socially, and economically deprived. Their housing, hygiene, nutrition, clothing, and means of heating may all be deficient, and this should be taken into account when designing treatments. If they live alone, as is often the case, they may well be unable to find anyone to help with the application of ointments to body parts they cannot reach themselves or to assist with bandages because of lack of mobility.

Older patients suffer from pruritus more severely and more frequently than patients of younger age groups. It must be remembered that the elderly may also have difficulty in hearing, understanding, and/ or remembering instructions, especially if these are complex and involve more than one medicament. If possible, instructions on the medications should also be given to an accompanying relative or legibly written out.

The previously mentioned potential difficulties need to be taken into account when trying to help an elderly patient with a skin problem.

15

Disorders of keratinization and other genodermatoses

Aparajita Ghosh
Anupam Das

Introduction

Epidermal differentiation

The epidermis is the outermost layer of the skin and is composed almost entirely of keratinocytes with a few other cells, like melanocytes, Merkel cells, and Langerhans cells interspersed among them.

The keratinocytes transform from metabolically active, cuboidal basal cells (stratum basale) to polyhedral cells of stratum spinosum to terminally differentiated, flattened, dehydrated, and dead corneocytes (stratum corneum) that are programmed to be shed off (desquamation). This complex and finely regulated process of differentiation is called keratinization. A human keratinocyte takes about 14 days to transit from the basal layer to stratum corneum. During this transit, the cell progressively loses its organelles and water content; there is polymerization and deposition of keratin filaments and filaggrin in the cytoplasm just beneath the plasma membrane and dissolution of the nucleus in the terminal stage. The end result, the stratum corneum, is a chemically and mechanically resistant barrier composed of stacks of protein-rich, anucleate, dead cells in a continuous matrix of extracellular lipid. Further, 14 days are required by these corneocytes to traverse the layers of stratum corneum and subsequently desquamate (Figure 15.1). Desquamation normally leads to inconspicuous shedding of individual corneocytes and is a controlled process involving degradation of corneodesmosomes by various lytic enzymes.

"Scaling" is the result of abnormal desquamation leading to conspicuous, visible shedding of corneocytes which have failed to separate from each other.

The function of the epidermis

The epidermis, particularly the stratum corneum, acts a barrier to physical, chemical, and microbiological insult. It prevents water loss from the underlying tissue, protects against solar injury, and effectively prevents penetration by microbes. It provides partial protection against mechanical shearing or stress.

Disability in disorders of keratinization

Epidermal differentiation and keratinization are complex processes, and various genetic mutations can disrupt the usual course of maturation. The resultant altered epidermis is unable to perform its normal functions or serve as an effective barrier. There is an increase in transepidermal water-loss, making the skin dry and prone to irritation. Impaired immunity to microbial infections can result in frequent infections. The defective epidermis is also considerably less compliant and pliable compared to normal

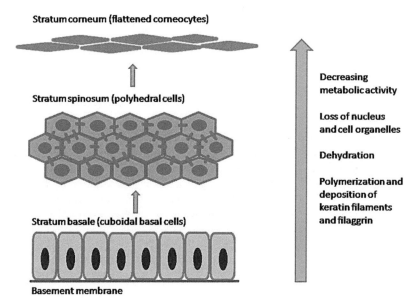

FIGURE 15.1   Schematic diagram of keratinization.

epidermis, and this can often cause blistering over pressure points or limitation to movements accompanied by pain and fissuring. However, the greatest impact of these disorders is possibly because of the significant cosmetic disability that they cause. The skin is of primary importance in determining the appearance of an individual, and abnormal skin can hamper the socio-economic and emotional aspects of the life of the affected individual.

Xerosis

The term 'xerosis' refers to dryness of the skin, and as such does not signify any particular disease. Xerosis often occurs or increases with age, and in the dry season. It may be worsened by repeated washing with soaps. Xerotic skin is often more prone to pruritus and is sometimes associated with atopy. Adequate use of emollients is helpful.

Ichthyosis

It is the name given to a heterogeneous group of non-inflammatory disorders of the skin presenting with generalized scaling. The word is derived from the Greek word *ichthys*, meaning 'fish', and refers to the similarity in appearance of the characteristic scales of the affected skin to the scales of a fish. The various ichthyoses are listed in Table 15.1.

TABLE 15.1

Common ichthyoses with their mode of inheritance

Autosomal dominant ichthyoses	Autosomal recessive ichthyoses	X-linked ichthyoses
• Ichthyosis vulgaris • Epidermolytic hyperkeratosis • Ichthyosis bullosa of Siemens	• Lamellar ichthyosis • Congenital ichthyosiform erythroderma • Harlequin ichthyosis	• X-linked recessive ichthyosis (steroid sulfatase deficiency) • Chondrodysplasia punctata

Ichthyosis vulgaris (autosomal dominant ichthyosis)

This is the commonest form of ichthyosis and is inherited in an autosomal dominant fashion. The cause is a mutation in the gene-encoding profilaggrin. The disease is more severe in individuals in whom both alleles are affected (homozygotes or compound heterozygotes) than in those who have a single defective allele.

Clinical features

The disease is characterized by scaling, which is prominent over extensors, particularly over the shins (Figure 15.2). The scales here are often dark-colored and polygonal in shape. A fine white scaling is usually present over other areas of the body, like the trunk. The flexures are mostly spared. The affected individuals often have hyperlinear palms, thickening of the skin (keratoderma) of palms and soles, and keratosis pilaris (Figure 15.3). Asthma, atopic dermatitis, and other manifestations of atopy are frequently associated. Symptoms are worse during the winter when the climate is dry.

Pathology and aetiopathogenesis

Profilaggrin is a precursor of the protein filaggrin, which is important for aggregation of keratin filaments and retention of water in the keratinocytes. Filaggrin is a component of the keratohyaline granules. Mutations in the profilaggrin gene lead to decreased synthesis of profilaggrin with a resultant decrease or absence of filaggrin in the keratinocytes. Histopathology shows mild hyperkeratosis with a diminished or absent granular layer. The keratohyalin granules are absent or are abnormal in shape and small, as shown by electron microscopy.

Treatment

Emollients and humectants are the mainstays of treatment. Topical keratolytic agents like urea and salicylic acid preparations increase desquamation and decrease the prominence of scales.

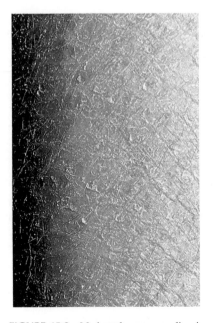

FIGURE 15.2   Moderately severe scaling in autosomal dominant ichthyosis (from Marks and Motley, 18th edition, with permission).

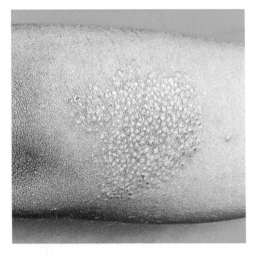

FIGURE 15.3   Keratosis pilaris with plugging of the hair follicle.

X-linked recessive ichthyosis

This is a relatively uncommon form of ichthyosis caused by the deficiency of the enzyme steroid sulfatase. Because of an X-linked recessive pattern of inheritance, a majority of the affected individuals are males. Females act as carriers of the mutation.

Clinical features

The disease is usually more severe than ichthyosis vulgaris. Scales are larger and dark brown in color and predominantly affect extensors. However, there might be significant involvement of the flexures in many cases. The face and neck are often involved, leading to significant cosmetic impairment. Corneal opacities, cryptorchidism, and increased incidence of testicular cancer are observed in affected males.

Pathology and aetiopathogenesis

The cause is a mutation in the steroid sulfatase gene located on Xp22 chromosome. This leads to a decreased or absent activity of the enzyme steroid sulfatase in most tissues. In the epidermis, this results in the accumulation of cholesterol sulfate, leading to abnormal desquamation. The fetal adrenal hormones are desulfated to estrogens by the steroid sulfatase present in the fetal placenta. Deficiency of the enzyme in the fetal placenta leads to decreased levels of estrogen and failure or difficulty in initiation or progress of labor in case of a male fetus.

Histopathology shows orthokeratotic hyperkeratosis. The granular layer is increased. The epidermis shows acanthosis and papillomatosis.

Treatment

Emollients and keratolytics may be used in the management of milder cases. More severe cases can benefit from the use of systemic retinoids.

Autosomal recessive congenital ichthyosis (ARCI)

It is a spectrum of disorders inherited in an autosomal recessive pattern. In the majority of the cases, the disorder manifests at birth. The baby may be born encased in a taut, parchment-like membrane (collodion baby). Subsequently, the individual may develop large, plate-like scales without any redness of skin (lamellar ichthyosis) or generalized fine white scaling with erythroderma (congenital ichthyosiform erythroderma). However, many individuals develop features overlapping with both these entities.

The underlying genetic defect is not well-characterized, and several different genes encoding for proteins involved in cornified envelope formation, membrane transport, etc., have been implicated. As such, ARCI appears to be a genetically heterogeneous group.

Lamellar ichthyosis (LI)

The disorder is characterized by large dark plate-like scales with minimal erythema of the skin (Figure 15.4). The scales are tightly adherent to the skin, and, in severe cases, cause scarring alopecia with loss of scalp hair, ear deformity, and ectropion and eclabium due to traction on eyelids and lips. Sweating may be impaired, leading to heat intolerance.

Histopathology shows mild to moderate acanthosis with orthokeratotic hyperkeratosis.

Treatment

Oral retinoids are the only effective modality of treatment and have to be given for long periods. Emollients provide symptomatic relief. Patients with ectropion also require eyecare with lubricants and artificial tears to prevent corneal ulcers.

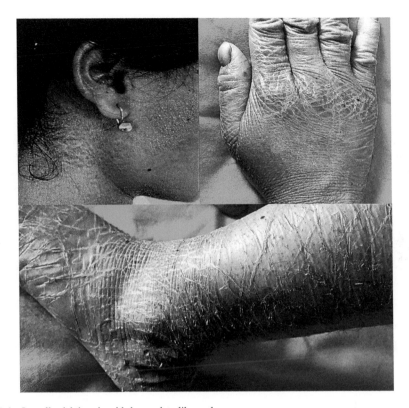

FIGURE 15.4   Lamellar ichthyosis with large plate-like scales.

Congenital ichthyosiform erythroderma (CIE)

This condition presents with generalized redness of the skin with fine, white scales (Figure 15.5). Large, plate-like scales, as seen in lamellar ichthyosis, are usually absent. Histopathology shows acanthosis and hyperkeratosis with parakeratosis.

Epidermolytic hyperkeratosis (EHK)

This condition, earlier known as bullous ichthyosiform erythroderma, is inherited in an autosomal dominant pattern. The cause is usually a mutation in genes encoding for keratin 1 or keratin 10.

The disease becomes apparent at birth with blistering, redness, and peeling of skin at sites of trauma. With age, the blistering improves but hyperkeratosis develops. The hyperkeratosis is usually severe and malodorous due to infection by mixed microbial flora and is more prominent over joints (Figure 15.6). There are several clinical phenotypes of the disease. The disease may present in generalized, localized, or nevoid forms. Palms and soles may be involved in certain clinical types.

Histopathology is classical. There is vacuolar degeneration (epidermolysis) of the suprabasal keratinocytes accompanied by severe hyperkeratosis.

Systemic retinoids are the only effective treatment, especially for the generalized or severe forms of the disease.

The comparative features of various ichthyoses have been summarized in Table 15.2.

Collodion baby

This is a condition where the baby is born encased in a taut, parchment-like membrane. The similarity of the membrane to 'collodion' lends the name to this condition. The membrane subsequently fissures and peels off but leads to impaired barrier function, water loss, and improper temperature regulation. The

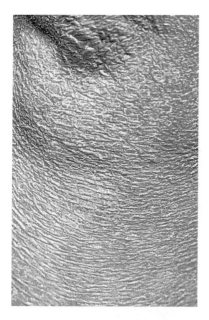

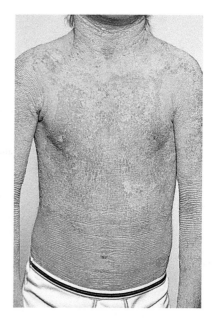

FIGURE 15.5 Non-bullous ichthyosiform erythroderma (from Marks and Motley, 18th edition, with permission).

FIGURE 15.6 Epidermolytic hyperkeratosis showing typical severe hyperkeratosis and scaling (from Marks and Motley, 18th edition, with permission).

tightness of the membrane sometimes leads to restrictions in movement, respiration, and sucking. The condition is classically associated with autosomal recessive ichthyosis but may be the presenting feature in certain other keratodermas and Gaucher's disease. Very rare cases of self-healing collodion baby have been described wherein after peeling off the collodion membrane the skin develops normally. The various conditions associated with collodion membrane at birth are listed in Table 15.3.

Treatment

Such babies need to be carefully monitored for any signs of dehydration, infection, and hypo- or hyperthermia. They are preferably nursed in a warm and humidified environment. Bland emollients may be used to keep the membrane soft and pliable and facilitate desquamation and healing.

Harlequin fetus

The child is born encased in thick plates of skin with deep fissures, which form a geometric pattern. There is striking ectropion and eclabium and the ears are poorly developed. The condition is fatal and most die within a few days after birth, though very rare cases of survival with oral retinoid therapy have been reported.

Acquired ichthyosis

Ichthyosis may sometimes develop later in life, secondary to various systemic causes. The causes of acquired ichthyosis are summarized in Table 15.4.

TABLE 15.2

Comparative features of certain common ichthyoses

	Ichthyosis vulgaris	X-linked recessive ichthyosis	ARCI (lammellar ichthyosis and congenital ichthyosiform erythroderma)	Epidermolytic hyperkeratosis
Mode of inheritance	Autosomal dominant	X-linked recessive	Autosomal recessive	Autosomal dominant
Mutation	Filaggrin gene – absence of filaggrin	Steroid sulfatase	TGM1, ABCA12, ALOXE3, ALOX12B	Keratin 1,10
Characteristics of scales	Fine, white, flaky, and larger on lower limbs	Fine to large scales	Large, thick, plate-like brown scale (LI) fine, white, generalized scales with erythroderma (CIE)	Brown verrucous scales, may be porcupine-like (hystrix)
Flexural involvement	Spared	Involved	Involved	Predominantly involved
Onset	Infancy or childhood	At birth or infancy	At birth	At birth
Collodion membrane	Absent	Absent	Present	Absent
Associated features	Keratosis pilaris, hyperlinear palms and soles, atopy	Cryptorchidism, comma shaped corneal opacity, h/o prolonged labor	Scarring alopecia, ectropion, eclabium, heat intolerance (LE), decreased sweating and heat intolerance (CIE)	Blistering at birth, frequent infections leading to bad odor

Other disorders of keratinization

Keratosis pilaris

It is characterized by plugging of hair follicles, sometimes with perifollicular erythema, predominantly affecting the extensor aspect of upper arms, thighs, and buttocks. It is common in children and adolescents, and in a majority of cases, it is physiological. Keratosis pilaris is often associated with ichthyosis vulgaris and atopic dermatitis. Rarely, a variant of keratosis pilaris followed by atrophy is seen to involve eyebrows, scalp, and cheeks.

TABLE 15.3

Disorders presenting with collodion membrane at birth

Autosomal recessive congenital ichthyosis

X-linked hypohidrotic ectodermal dysplasia

AEC (Ankyloblepharon – Ectodermal defect – Cleft lip and palate) syndrome

Chondrodysplasia punctata

Loricrin keratoderma

Trichothiodystrophy

Neutral lipid storage disorders

Gaucher's disease

Self-healing collodion baby

TABLE 15.4

Causes of acquired ichthyosis

Physiological – old age

Malignancies – Hodgkin's lymphoma; non-Hodgkin's lymphoma; mycosis fungoides; carcinoma of breast, lungs, cervix

Acquired immunodeficiency syndrome

Autoimmune disease – SLE, dermatomyositis, mixed connective tissue disorder

Endocrine causes – hypothyroidism, diabetes mellitus

Bone marrow transplant

Sarcoidosis

Drugs – lipid-lowering agents, clofazimine, butyrophenone, allopurinol, hydroxyurea

Nutritional deficiency, malnutrition, malabsorption states

Treatment

Topical retinoids and keratolytics like salicylic acid and urea can improve the condition.

Darier's disease (keratosis follicularis)

It is an autosomal dominant disorder, though sporadic cases are common. The causative mutation lies in the ATP2A2 gene, which codes for SERCA 2, a calcium transporter.

Clinical features

The disease starts around puberty and is characterized by the eruption of dirty looking, greasy, keratotic papules over face, scalp, ears, neck, upper chest, and back (Figure 15.7). The papules may coalesce to form plaques and may become infected and malodorous. The condition usually worsens in summers. Palms and soles show pitting and nails show characteristic red and white longitudinal stripes with a v-shaped indentation at the free edge.

Histopathology

Histopathology is characteristic and shows suprabasal clefting due to acantholysis. There is abnormal keratinization of individual keratinocytes (dyskeratosis), leading to eosinophilic bodies called corps ronds and grains.

Treatment

Avoidance of sunlight and heat may help in reducing exacerbation of the disease. For limited lesions, topical retinoids like tazarotene and keratolytics like urea are helpful. Oral retinoids are effective in case of widespread disease.

Hailey Hailey disease (benign familial pemphigus)

This is an autosomal dominant disorder due to mutation in the ATP2C1 gene. It is clinically characterized by vesicles, hypertrophic vegetating plaques, and painful erosions over flexures (Figure 15.8). The disease worsens due to heat and sweating. It usually appears in the third to fourth decade of life and as such shows a waxing and waning course. Histopathology shows acantholysis of keratinocytes giving rise to a 'dilapidated brick wall' appearance. Dyskeratosis is usually not very prominent.

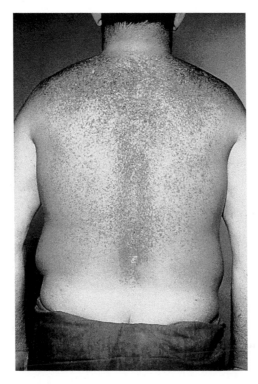

FIGURE 15.7 Brown keratotic papules on the trunk in Darier's disease (from Marks and Motley, 18th edition, with permission).

Palmo-plantar keratoderma (tylosis)

This group of disorders, which are clinically and genetically heterogeneous, is characterized by abnormal thickening of the skin of palms and soles. The thickening may involve the whole of palms and soles (diffuse) or may be focal or punctate. It may occur alone or may be accompanied by skin lesions elsewhere or involvement of other organs of the body.

Pachyonychia congenita types I and II

These are rare autosomal dominant disorders that show plantar keratoderma at pressure points, with occasional blistering and subungual hyperkeratosis. Hair and teeth anomalies may be present. The mutation lies in genes encoding for Keratin 6 (a & b), 16, and 17.

Other genodermatoses

Tuberous sclerosis

It is an autosomal dominant disorder caused by mutations in TSC1 or TSC2 gene encoding for the proteins 'hamartin' and 'tuberin', respectively. The disease is characterized by hamartomatous tumors involving the skin, brain, eyes, kidneys, heart, lungs, and other organs of the body. Cortical tubers and subependymal nodules are often found in the brain. Patients may present with epilepsy, mental retardation, or behavioral changes. Skin lesions are often diagnostic and include multiple 'ash leaf' hypopigmented macules, facial angiofibromas, fibrous plaques on the forehead, and shagreen patch over the lower back or buttocks. Nail involvement is common and is in the form of subungual and periungual

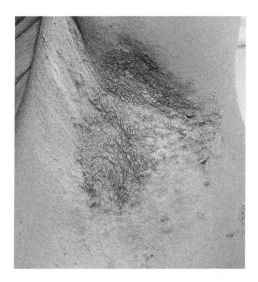

FIGURE 15.8   Hailey Hailey disease showing vegetating plaques and painful erosions affecting the axilla.

fibromas (Koenen's tumors) with resultant longitudinal grooving of the nail plate. Gingival fibromas and hyperplasia with dental pitting are frequently seen.

Neurofibromatoses

These are a group of autosomal dominant disorders, of which NF1 (von Recklinghausen's disease) and NF2 are the commonest. Rarely, segmental NF1 and familial café-au-lait macules without neurofibromas have been reported.

NF1 is caused by decreased levels of neurofibromin, due to mutation of the NF1 gene. The presence of multiple brown macules (café-au-lait macules), axillary and intertriginous freckling, and neurofibromas, which are benign nerve sheath tumors are characteristic of this disorder. Neurofibromas arising from peripheral cutaneous nerves appear as soft, skin-colored, pedunculated masses protruding from the

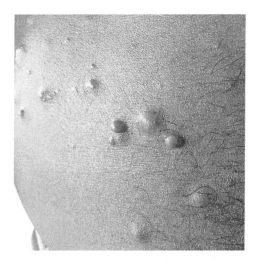

FIGURE 15.9   Neurofibromas: soft, skin-colored, pedunculated masses protruding from the skin surface in a case of NF1.

skin surface and result in significant cosmetic disability (Figure 15.9). Lisch nodules in the iris are diagnostic. Optic nerve tumors and bony lesions like hypoplasia of the sphenoid wing, pseudoarthrosis of the long bones, and scoliosis due to vertebral involvement are common causes of morbidity. These patients are also at an increased risk of developing a variety of neoplasms like pheochromocytoma, rhabdomyosarcoma, chronic myelomonocytic leukaemia, etc.

NF2 is less common and is caused by mutations in the gene which codes for a protein "merlin". This condition is characterized by vestibular schwannomas and a variety of central nervous system tumors.

Anhidrotic/Hypohidrotic ectodermal dysplasia

This rare condition is inherited as an X-linked recessive disorder. The affected males present with sparse and fine scalp hair, frontal bossing, saddle deformity of nose, and peg-shaped or abnormal teeth. The eccrine sweat glands are absent, leading to absent or severely reduced sweating with resultant heat intolerance.

16

Metabolic disorders and reticulohistiocytic proliferative disorders

Soumya Jagadeesan

Porphyrias

Porphyrias are rare disorders caused by defects in haemobiosynthesis. Most of them are inherited and many of them have specific cutaneous manifestations due to the phototoxic effects of porphyrins (haem precursors), which accumulate in these disorders. Traditionally, these disorders are classified into hepatic and erythropoietic forms, depending upon the sites where the defective enzymes are expressed. However, from a clinician's point of view, it is more appropriate to classify them as acute and non-acute forms, depending on the presence or absence of acute neurological attacks. The important porphyrias are summarized in Table 16.1.

Porphyria cutanea tarda

Porphyria cutanea tarda (PCT) is the most common of all porphyrias and results from the deficiency of uroporphyrinogen decarboxylase (UROD) enzyme, the fifth enzyme in the haem biosynthesis pathway. (A schematic diagram representing haemosynthesis and the enzymes involved is given in Figure 16.1.) This results in the accumulation of haem precursors, called uroporphyrins and coproporphyrins, in the blood, stool, and urine. These substances are responsible for photosensitization. This enzyme defect is acquired/sporadic and is seen only in the hepatocytes in the majority of the cases; however, inherited forms where the enzyme defect is present in all tissues also do occur. A wide variety of factors, especially hepatotoxins, are known to trigger the clinical features of PCT, including alcohol, estrogens, iron, polychlorinated hydrocarbons, and viral infections, like hepatitis C and HIV.

Clinical features

The disease onset is usually in the third or fourth decade of life, though it may present earlier in the familial forms. The characteristic features are seen in the light-exposed areas. In the early stages of the disease, blistering and fragility of the skin on the face and backs of the hands are noted (Figure 16.2). The affected areas also develop an odd pigmented and mauve, suffused appearance. Later, increased hair growth occurs on the involved skin and a sclerodermiform thickening of the skin develops. Erosions, crusting, and scarring are also seen in the affected areas. The patients often experience worsening in summer but may not correlate the skin changes with sun exposure as the burning sensation accompanied by severe photosensitivity seen in erythropoietic porphyrias is not seen here.

TABLE 16.1

Summary of the important porphyrias

Disease	Inheritance	Incidence	Age of onset	Clinical features
Porphyrias with cutaneous disease alone				
Porpyhria cutanea tarda	AD, sometimes acquired	Commonest type	Third–fourth decade	Moderate–severe photosensitivity, vesicles, and bullae, milia, hypertrichosis, scarring in the sun-exposed areas
Congenital erythropoietic porpyria	AR	Rare	Infancy or the first decade of life	Severe–very severe photosensitivity, vesicles, bullae, hyperpigmentation, hypertrichosis, mutilation, and scarring
Erythropoietic protoporphyria	AD, XLD, AR	Second most common among cutaneous porphyrias	Early childhood	Pain following sun exposure, urticaria, erythema, oedema, sometimes blistering
Cutaneous disease with acute attacks				
Hereditary coproporphyria	AD	Very rare	Any age	Photosensitivity is rare, blistering can occur
Variegate porphyria	AD	Common in South Africa	15–30 years	Cutaneous manifestations are indistinguishable from Porphyria cutanea tarda. Acute attacks as in AIP
Acute attacks only				
Acute Intermittent porphyria	AD	More common in Scandinavian countries	10–40 years	No skin manifestations. Acute attacks ranging from mild abdominal pain to very severe attacks with bulbar palsy and respiratory paralysis

AD – Autosomal dominant; AD- Autosomal recessive; XLD – X-linked dominant; AIP – Acute intermittent porphyria.

Investigations

The diagnosis is made by finding increased uroporphyrins and coproporphyrins in the urine and stool. A plasma spectrophotometry peak is seen at 615–620 nm. Iron overload is also a frequent, accompanying feature. Histologically, the blistering is subepidermal with festooning of the dermal papillae and, in the long-standing cases, fibrosis develops and deposits of immunoglobulin are found perivascularly.

Differential diagnosis

Other porphyrias like variegate porphyria, hereditary coproporphyria, milder forms of congenital ery-thropoietic or hepatoerythropoietic porphyrias and pseudoporphyrias may mimick PCT. But a careful examination of urine, stool, and plasma porphyrins is helpful in identifying PCT.

Treatment

The objective is to reduce the circulating levels of porphyrins. This is achieved by regular venesection – removing a pint of blood at a time – every 2 or 3 weeks, or by the use of low doses of the antimalarial drug chloroquine orally, resulting in the secretion of large amounts of porphyrins in the urine. Photoprotection plays an important role in controlling the symptoms before specific therapies take effect. Regular monitoring of liver function and regular ultrasounds and alpha-fetoprotein levels is essential to detect hepatic carcinoma at a treatable stage.

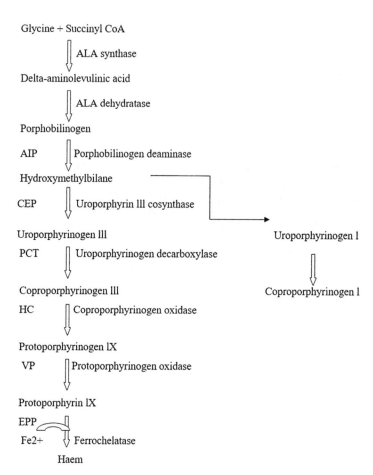

Glycine + Succinyl CoA

ALA synthase

Delta-aminolevulinic acid

ALA dehydratase

Porphobilinogen

AIP   Porphobilinogen deaminase

Hydroxymethylbilane

CEP   Uroporphyrin lll cosynthase

Uroporphyrinogen lll   Uroporphyrinogen l

PCT   Uroporphyrinogen decarboxylase

Coproporphyrinogen lll   Coproporphyrinogen l

HC   Coproporphyrinogen oxidase

Protoporphyrinogen lX

VP   Protoporphyrinogen oxidase

Protoporphyrin lX

EPP

Fe2+   Ferrochelatase

Haem

FIGURE 16.1   Schematic diagram representing haemo-synthesis and the enzymes involved. Haemo-synthesis pathway illustrating the enzyme defects in the various porphyrias. ALA, Aminolevulinic acid; AIP, Acute intermittent porphyria; CEP, Congenital erythropoietic porphyria; PCT, Porphyria cutanea tarda; HC, Hereditary coproporphyria; VP, Variegate porphyria; EPP, Erythropoietic protoporphyria.

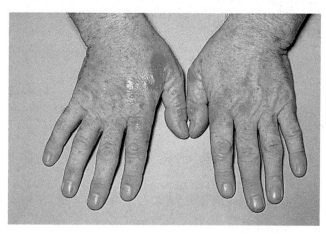

FIGURE 16.2   Porphyria cutanea tarda; note the eroded areas in the light-exposed skin of the backs of the hands (from Marks and Motley, 18th edition).

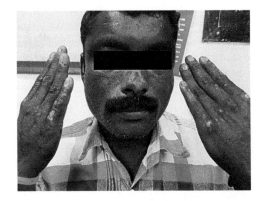

FIGURE 16.3 Congenital erythropoietic porphyria with erosions and scars in the face and hands (courtesy of Dr MS Sadeep, Govt Medical College, Kottayam).

Congenital erythropoietic porphyria (Gunther's disease)

This is a very rare porphyria, causing severe mutilating photosensitivity and haematological disease. It is inherited as an autosomal recessive disorder due to the deficiency of the enzyme uroporphyrinogen III cosynthase. This enzyme is required to form the biologically useful type III porphyrin isomers, and the defect in this enzyme causes accumulation of type 1 isomers (which cannot participate in haem formation) in the erythroid precursor cells, which later leak into the plasma.

Clinical features

The onset is usually in infancy itself, but a late-onset, milder variant has also been described. Affected individuals are extremely photosensitive and shun the light. They develop dreadful facial scarring with hypertrichosis (Figure 16.3). This combination of clinical features has suggested to some that these patients provoked the fable of 'werewolves'.

The eyes and internal organs are also frequently involved. The teeth are almost always stained brown and fluoresce under Wood's lamp (Figure 16.4). There may be osteopenia, pathological fractures, vertebral collapse and resorption of the bones of the digits. The high concentration of porphyrins in erythrocytes results in haemolytic anaemia and marrow hyperplasia. Earlier, the affected individuals used to die by the age of 40, but now, the mortality rates have come down with the improved management of complications. Haematological complications may still be fatal.

Investigations

Red cells and urine contain large amounts of type 1 isomers of uro- and coproporphyrins and feces contain increased concentrations of type 1 isomers of coproporphyrin. Due to the presence of porphyrins, urine shows bright pink-red fluorescence.

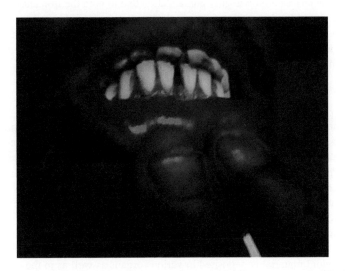

FIGURE 16.4 Erythrodontia in congenital erythropoietic porphyria, reddish fluorescence under Wood's lamp (courtesy of Dr MS Sadeep, Govt Medical College, Kottayam).

Treatment

Management involves strict photoprotection, treatment of haemolytic anaemia by hypertransfusion and prompt treatment of secondary infections. Allogenic bone marrow transplantation from a tissue-matched donor may be considered in the severely affected cases, as it offers a chance of long-term cure.

Erythropoietic protoporphyria

Erythropoietic protoporphyria (EPP) is a very rare, autosomal dominant disorder in which excess protoporphyrins are produced. These protoporphyrins are detectable in the blood, and this forms the basis of diagnostic tests. Clinically, the disorder often presents in childhood as episodes of skin soreness and extreme pain and discomfort when exposed to the sun, unlike other cutaneous porphyrias. Physical signs may be minimal with subtle oedema and minimal erythema. Later, fine pitted scarring is found on exposed sites. Pigment gallstones may develop.

Porphyria variegata

This is a very rare combination of PCT and acute intermittent porphyria (AIP). Cutaneous changes mimic a milder form of PCT and acute attacks ranging from mild abdominal pain to very severe attacks with bulbar palsy and respiratory paralysis, as seen in AIP, may occur. The latter is caused by a deficiency of delta-aminolaevulinic acid synthetase and is precipitated by certain drugs and anaesthesia, among other things.

Pseudoporphyria

It is a non-porphyric dermatosis that clinically and histopathologically mimics PCT, but has normal porphyrin levels in the urine, feces, and blood. The most common causes are photosensitizing drugs, especially non-steroidal anti-inflammatory drugs like naproxen and nabumetone, UVA tanning beds, and hemodialysis.

Haemochromatosis (bronzed diabetes)

There are primary and symptomatic forms of this disorder. In the primary form, there is excessive gastrointestinal absorption of iron, resulting in iron deposition in the liver, testes, skin, and pancreas. Involvement of the skin causes a brown–grey pigmentation due to both the iron and increased melanin in the skin. Diabetes is caused by deposition of iron in the pancreas, and cirrhosis due to liver involvement. The condition seems to be inherited as a recessive characteristic but is much more common in men.

Secondary forms are found in conditions necessitating repeated blood transfusion and in conditions in which there is chronic haemolysis (e.g. sickle cell disease).

Amyloidosis

'Amyloidosis' is the term used for a group of disorders in which an abnormal protein is deposited extracellularly in tissues. Amyloidosis can involve the skin alone, as localized cutaneous amyloidosis or as cutaneous manifestations of systemic amyloidosis. Systemic amyloidosis is divided into primary and secondary forms. The latter develops after long-standing inflammatory disease, including infections such as chronic tuberculosis and chronic osteomyelitis. It may also occur in patients with long-standing severe rheumatoid arthritis. Skin manifestations are rare in secondary systemic amyloidosis. A classification of the amyloidosis affecting the skin is given in Table 16.2.

In primary systemic amyloidosis, the abnormal protein components are synthesized by clones of abnormal plasma cells and the condition is sometimes associated with multiple myeloma. In primary amyloid disease, amyloid material is deposited in various organs as well as in the skin. In the skin, it is deposited in and around the dermal capillary blood vessels, which become fragile and leaky. Swollen

TABLE 16.2

Classification of amyloidosis

Localized cutaneous amyloidosis
Primary localized cutaneous amyloidosis
Papular primary localized cutaneous amyloidosis
Macular primary localized cutaneous amyloidosis
Nodular primary localized cutaneous amyloidosis
Secondary localized cutaneous amyloidosis

Cutaneous amyloidosis due to systemic disease
Non-hereditary systemic amyloidosis with cutaneous involvement
Primary systemic or myeloma-associated amyloidosis
Secondary systemic amyloidosis associated with inflammation or tumor
Hereditary systemic amyloidosis with cutaneous involvement
Familial amyloid polyneuropathy
Hereditary systemic disease with secondary cutaneous amyloidoses
Muckle–Wells syndrome
TNF-receptor 1 associated periodic fever syndrome

---

mauve–purple areas develop around the eyes and around the flexures, especially after trivial trauma. Hemorrhagic blisters, macroglossia and dystrophic nail changes may also be seen.

There are also 'amyloid' disorders that are restricted to the skin, called localized cutaneous amyloidosis. In the type called macular amyloidosis, itchy, 'rippled', brown macular areas appear over the trunk (Figure 16.5). It seems to be more common in women and in patients of Asian origin. Friction and sun exposure seem to play an important role in the development of the lesions. Lichen or papular amyloidosis is another localized cutaneous form of amyloidosis in which brown or pink, firm popular or nodular lesions occur, especially over the shins (Figure 16.6). Histologically, the deposits of macular and papular amyloidosis are seen in the papillary dermis.

Amyloid can be detected in tissue using various histochemical tests. It appears as amorphous

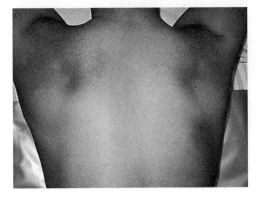

FIGURE 16.5 Pigmented area on the back in macular amyloid. Note the rippled pattern.

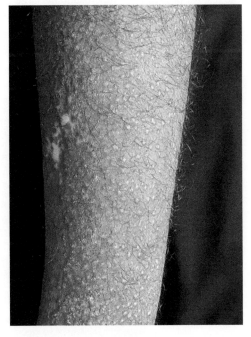

FIGURE 16.6 Papular lesions on the shin in lichen amyloidosis (courtesy of Dr Ashique KT, KIMS Alshifa Hospital, Perinthalmanna, Kerala).

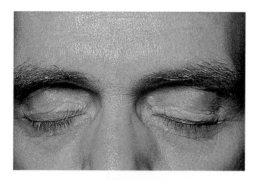

FIGURE 16.7 Yellowish plaques on the eyelids in xanthelasma (from Marks and Motley, 18th edition).

eosinophilic deposits in routine Hematoxylin and Eosin staining. Using Congo red stain, amyloid deposits exhibit the typical 'apple green' birefringence, when viewed under polarized light. They also exhibit fluorescence with thioflavine T and can also be demonstrated by immunohistochemical tests.

Xanthomata

Xanthomata are deposits of lipid in histiocytes in the skin and may be associated with normal levels of lipids in the blood (normolipaemia) or with elevated levels of serum lipids (hyperlipidaemia). The lipidized histiocytes have a characteristic 'foamy' appearance.

Xanthelasma

Xanthelasma is a common form of xanthoma in which lesions appear as arcuate or linear yellowish soft plaques around the eyes (Figure 16.7). The condition is not associated with hyperlipidemia in 60–70% of patients. The lesions can be removed by surgical excision, electrocautery, or by topical treatment with trichloroacetic acid, if the patient finds them to be a cosmetic nuisance. However, they may often recur after treatment.

Xanthoma tuberosum

The lesions of xanthoma tuberosum are large nodules containing lipidized histiocytes and giant cells. The nodules develop around the tendons and extensor aspects of the joints in familial hyperlipidaemia, particularly over the Achilles tendon, the knees, and the elbows (Figure 16.8).

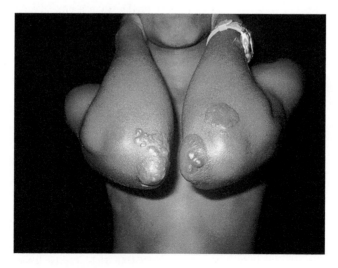

FIGURE 16.8 Xanthoma tuberosum affecting the elbows.

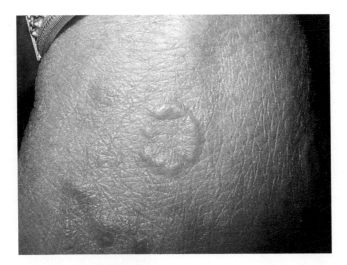

FIGURE 16.9   A typical lesion of granuloma annulare over the dorsum of the hand.

Eruptive xanthomata

These mostly develop in diabetes and any diseases associated with hypertriglyceridemia. Large numbers of yellowish-pink papules develop rapidly over the skin, especially over the extensor surfaces of elbows, knees, and buttocks.

Treatment

The treatment of these xanthomatous disorders is based on the treatment of any underlying disease, diet, and the use of lipid-lowering agents.

Necrobiotic disorders

The term 'necrobiosis' is applied to a particular histological change in which there are foci of damage making the dermal structure 'blurred' and more eosinophilic than usual. The foci are surrounded by inflammatory cells – lymphocytes, histiocytes, and occasional giant cells.

Granuloma annulare

This is not an uncommon inflammatory disorder, often seen in children and young adults, characterized by papules and plaques that adopt a ring-like pattern (Figure 16.9). Lesions develop on the extensor aspects of the fingers, dorsae of the feet, hands, and wrists. Granuloma annulare (GA) tends to last for a few months and then disappears as mysteriously as it came. Treatment is generally not indicated.

There are different types, including disseminated, papular, perforating, subcutaneous, and patch GA. Diabetes is more common in this group of patients.

Necrobiosis lipoidica diabeticorum

This condition is seen in 0.3% of diabetics and is strongly associated with the diabetic state. It occurs mainly on the lower legs as yellowish-pink plaques, which persist and become atrophic. It is characterized by necrobiotic foci histologically.

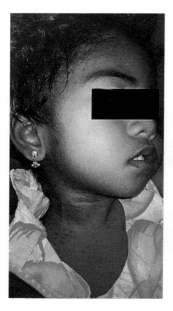

FIGURE 16.10 Seborrheic dermatitis-like lesions with purpura in Langerhans cell histiocytosis (courtesy of Dr Shobhana Kumari, Government Medical College, Kottayam).

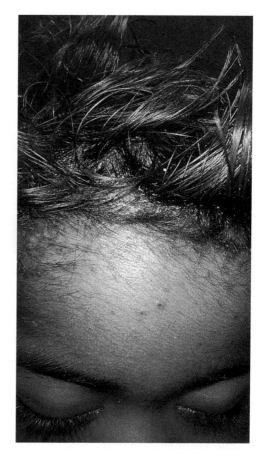

FIGURE 16.11 Seborrheic dermatitis-like lesions in Langerhans cell histiocytosis.

Reticulohistiocytic proliferative disorders

This is a group of poorly understood disorders that includes the proliferation of the cells of the mononuclear-phagocyte system, including the dendritic cells. The major types include Letterer–Siwe disease (LSD), Hand–Schüller–Christian disease (HSCD), eosinophilic granuloma (EG), xanthoma disseminatum (XD), and juvenile xanthogranuloma (JXG).

LSD, HSCD, and EG seem to belong to the same 'family of diseases' in which there appears to be a reactive proliferation of Langerhans cells, grouped together as Langerhans cell histiocytosis (LCH) and the other entities belong to non-Langerhans cell histiocytosis (non-LCH). The revised classification of Langerhans cell histiocytosis by the Writing Group of the Histiocyte Society is shown in Table 16.3.

TABLE 16.3

Classification of Langerhans cell histiocytoses

Single system disease	
Localized	Mono-ostotic bone involvement/isolated skin involvement/solitary lymph node involvement
Multiple sites	Polyostotic bone involvement/multifocal bone disease/multiple lymph node involvement
Multisystem disease	
Low-risk group	Disseminated disease with involvement of pituitary/skin/lymph node/bone
High-risk group	Disseminated disease with involvement of haemopoietic system/lung/liver/spleen

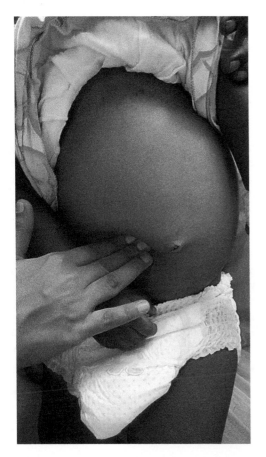

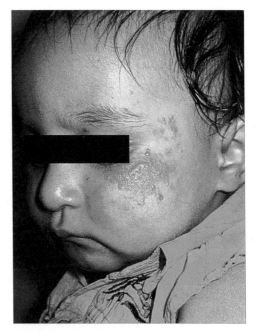

FIGURE 16.13 Yellowish lesions in juvenile xanthogranuloma.

FIGURE 16.12 Hepatosplenomegaly in acute disseminated Langerhans cell histiocytosis (courtesy of Dr Shobhana Kumari, Government Medical College, Kottayam).

LSD is an uncommon disorder of infants and young children, characterized by a papular and scaling eruption of flexures, trunk and scalp, with some resemblance to seborrhoeic dermatitis. Purpuric lesions may also be seen (Figures 16.10 and 16.11). There is a dense infiltrate of cells having the ultrastructural and immunocytochemical characteristics of Langerhans cells. There may be severe malaise and hepatosplenomegaly and some patients succumb (Figure 16.12). Treatment with corticosteroids and cytotoxic agents is required.

In HSCD, abnormal Langerhans cell deposits occur mostly in the lung, pituitary, bone and orbit. In EG, the deposits are, for the most part, limited to the bony skeleton.

Historically, LCH has been described under the names as described earlier: LSD being the prototype of the acute, disseminated, multisystemic form that appears in infancy with an often fatal course and HSCD being the chronic, progressive, multifocal form, usually presenting in childhood and eosinophilic granuloma, the localized, benign form; now this classification is maintained only for didactic purposes and LCH is mainly classified into single-system disease, multisystem disease, and self-healing variants.

XD and JXG do not belong to the same 'Langerhans cell' group of disorders but are characterized by the proliferation of the histiocytes other than Langerhans cells. JXG is the prototype of the non-LCH group of disorders, characterized by isolated or limited numbers of yellowish-pink nodules occur in young infants, which eventually disappear, usually by 5 years of age (Figure 16.13). Solitary, popular, nodular, and plaque forms have been described. Systemic manifestations like ocular and visceral involvement, bony changes and diabetes insipidus are rare in JXG, though not unknown. In XD, many papular lesions develop on the skin, and sometimes mucosae, which often persist for long periods. The lesions may be persistent, self-healing, or progressive. There is an association with paraproteinemias and internal organ involvement may also be seen.

Cutaneous mucinoses

Cutaneous mucinoses are a class of disorders characterized by the deposition of mucin in the skin. They are primarily divided into two groups: (i) primary cutaneous mucinoses, in which mucin deposition is the main histopathological feature; and (ii) secondary mucinoses, in which mucin deposition is secondary only an additional finding. A classification of cutaneous mucinoses is given in Table 16.4. Lichen myx-oedematosus/scleromyxedema is a prototype of idiopathic cutaneous mucinoses and is discussed next.

Scleromyxedema

Idiopathic disorders are characterized clinically by a generalized papular eruption and induration of skin (sclerodermoid appearance) and histopathologically by the triad of mucin deposition, increased fibro-blast proliferation, and fibrosis. The exact pathogenesis is unknown; it may be associated with a monoclonal gammopathy and has systemic implications. The age of onset is between 30 and 80 years. There is no ethnic or sexual predilection. Scleromyxedema should be differentiated from other localized forms of lichen myxedematosus, where the skin is the sole site of involvement. Treatment is usually targeted against the gammopathy and can often be disappointing.

TABLE 16.4

Classification of cutaneous mucinoses

Primary mucinoses
Dermal mucinoses
Lichen myxedematosus
Scleredema
Reticular erythematous mucinoses
Myxedema in thyroid disease
Self-healing mucinoses
Papular mucinoses in connective tissue diseases
Cutaneous focal mucinoses
Digital myxoid cyst
Follicular mucinoses
Alopecia mucinosa
Urticaria like follicular mucinosis
Secondary mucinoses
Epidermal
Dermal
Follicular

17

Hair and nail disorders

Sumit Sethi

Both hair and nails are epidermal structures that originate from invaginations of the epidermis into the skin (Figure 17.1). Hair and nails may develop signs of disorder, such as psoriasis or lichen planus, in the absence of an obvious skin disease. In addition, there are disorders that are confined to either the hair or the nails.

Disorders of hair (Table 17.1)

Hair loss (alopecia)

Hair loss may be diffuse over the scalp or localized to one or several sites on the scalp. The process may be destructive and may be scarring or non-scarring in nature.

Congenital alopecia

Congenital alopecia may occur in isolation or with other congenital disorders.
    Rarely, scalp hair growth is very slow and hair shaft density is low (*congenital hypotrichosis*).

Androgenetic (pattern) alopecia

Definition

This is a common, dominantly inherited, progressive form of alopecia, which is seen mostly in men. It develops symmetrically at certain specific sites on the scalp and eventually causes almost complete scalp hair loss in some patients.

Clinical features

The loss of hair starts in both temporal regions. Shortly after this bitemporal recession, thinning of the hair and then alopecia develop over the vertex. The bald area over the vertex expands to meet the triangular temporal bald areas until almost complete loss of hair results. There is almost always preservation of hair growth in the small area of the occipital scalp. A general reduction in the density of hair follicles also occurs and this may be the main feature of the disorder in women, in whom bitemporal recession and some vertical thinning occur less commonly than in men. The condition may start as early as in the late teens but generally presents in the third decade. Its rate of progress varies and seems uninfluenced by environmental factors.
    Pattern alopecia causes an enormous amount of psychological distress and patients will go to extraordinary lengths to attempt to arrest and reverse the process and/or to disguise its presence. The

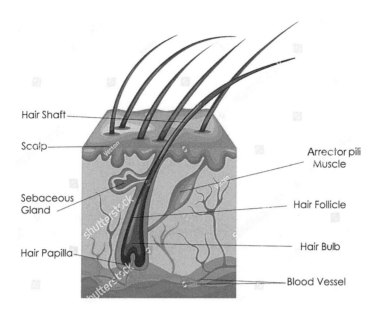

FIGURE 17.1 Diagram of a hair follicle showing the relationship between the hair shaft, follicular epithelium, and sebaceous glands.

TABLE 17.1

Overview of hair disorders

Hair loss	Non-scarring	Diffuse	Ageing
			Telogen effluvium
			Drug-induced
		Localized	Male pattern baldness alopecia areata
			Mechanical causes
	Scarring	Trauma	
		Lupus erythematosus	
		Lichen planus	
Increased hair growth (hirsuties)		Constitutional	
		Androgenization	
		Drug-induced	

condition is firmly embedded in popular mythology with regard to its supposed causes, which range from dietary deficiencies to sexual excesses.

Pathology and pathogenesis

The hair follicles in the affected areas become smaller, sparser, and eventually disappear. Finally, true atrophy of the skin occurs at the involved sites. The disorder is dominantly inherited but requires androgenic stimulus in the form of testosterone and the passing of the years for full phenotypic expression. The disorder can be precipitated by administering testosterone to female patients and is also a sign of virilization in patients with a testosterone secreting tumor.

Treatment

The drug finasteride has been used to treat androgenetic alopecia in men with good results. Its effect is limited to the specific testosterone receptor, which is found only in the hair follicle and prostate gland (the drug was originally developed to treat prostatic hypertrophy). It is well tolerated and its side effects are just higher than placebo; however, a statistically non-significant increase in the incidence of male breast cancer has been reported in men taking the drug. The progress of pattern alopecia in men is halted by castration, but there are few patients who would undergo the operation for this purpose. In women, the use of an anti-androgen–prostagen combination (cyproterone acetate and ethinylestradiol – DianetteR) has been tried and some reduction in the rate of hair loss has been claimed. The antihypertensive vasodilator minoxidil has also been used topically, as increased hair growth was noted as a side effect from its oral use. Although the drug may increase hair growth in 20–30% of patients, hair is lost again when treatment stops, and the extent to which hair regrowth occurs is modest. Finasteride is contraindicated in women at risk of pregnancy – because it would cause feminization of a male fetus and variable results have been reported from studies in which it has been given to women with female pattern hair loss alopecia.

Hair transplantation utilizes hairs from the occipital scalp, which are harvested and reimplanted in other areas. The best results are achieved with transplantation of single or small numbers of follicular units, but typically 2000–3000 units have to be transplanted to achieve a reasonable outcome.

Pattern hair loss in men may be disguised in a number of ways, including:

- Wigs and toupes and hair weaving, in which the remaining hair is woven to cover the defect
- Surgical procedures such as 'scalp reduction', in which an area of bald scalp is excised, or hair transplantation, in which follicles harvested from hair-containing skin in the occipital scalp are transplanted to holes made in the bald area or advancing flaps of hair-bearing skin over bald areas

Alopecia areata

Definition

Alopecia areata is an autoimmune disorder of hair follicles causing loss of hair in sharply defined areas of skin.

Clinical features

Alopecia areata often starts quite suddenly as one or more rounded patches from which the hair is lost (Figure 17.2). The hair loss continues for days or weeks until all the hair from the affected sites has fallen. The individual areas vary in size from 1 cm^2 to the entire scalp (alopecia totalis); rarely, the eyelashes and eyebrows and all body hair are lost as well (alopecia universalis). Affected areas may extend outwards and disease activity can be recognized by the appearance of so-called exclamation mark hairs at the margin of the lesions. The condition occurs over a wide age range but seems particularly common between the ages of 15 and 30 years.

Pathology and pathogenesis

The disorder can be associated with autoimmune disorders, such as vitiligo and thyrotoxicosis, and it has been assumed that an immune attack is launched against components of the hair follicle. When biopsies are taken from an actively extending patch, a dense, 'bee swarm'–like cluster of lymphocytes can be seen around the follicles.

Differential diagnosis

Patches of baldness due to hair pulling (trichotillomania) are bizarrely shaped, not as well-demarcated as alopecia areata, and have no exclamation mark hairs at the edge. Tinea capitis is marked by broken hairs

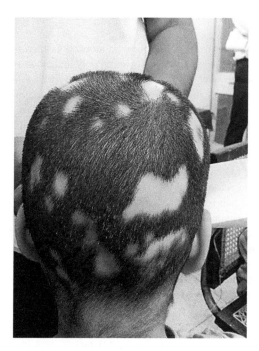

FIGURE 17.2   Multifocal alopecia areata.

and by a degree of redness and scaling of the scalp skin. Disorders that inflame the skin and destroy hair follicles can usually be easily differentiated by the scarring they cause.

Treatment

Patients with a solitary patch or few patches usually do not need treatment. When the patches coalesce to become a problem cosmetically or when there is alopecia totalis, treatment is often required by patients. Intradermal injections of potent corticosteroids (typically 10 mg/mL triamcinolone) are the most effective therapy, although overuse may lead to skin atrophy. It is reasonable to inject the affected skin at 1 cm intervals, and, if necessary, repeat after a period of 3 weeks. Other less effective treatments include potent topical steroids or systemic steroids; photochemotherapy with longwave ultraviolet irradiation (PUVA); dithranol; and allergic sensitization with diphencyprone. Even topical minoxidil has been claimed to be partially successful. All of the preceding have inconvenient side effects and usually work only while they are being given. Allergic sensitization with 1% diphencyprone causes an eczematous response and 'kicks' the follicles back to life in about half the patients. Some patients, having experienced the side effects and frustration of the lack of efficacy of the treatments, decide to cut their losses and disguise their disability with a wig. Sympathy and support are the most useful tools for this depressing disorder.

Diffuse hair loss

This is predominantly a problem for middle-aged and elderly women. It is not a single entity, and its causes include patterned hair loss, hypothyroidism, systemic illness such as systemic lupus erythematosus, and drug administration (particularly the anticancer drugs and the systemic retinoids). Diffuse hair loss is also caused by telogen effluvium (see the following discussion). Ageing results in a lower density of hair follicles, which is more obvious in some subjects than in others.

Having considered the previously mentioned possible causes, there are still some patients with obvious diffuse hair loss for whom there is no adequate explanation. Various deficiency states (particularly iron) have been incriminated, but in the majority of instances, the supposed deficiency appears to have no other sequel, and attempts at its rectification fail to improve the clinical state.

If there is no obvious cause for diffuse hair loss, the only medical treatment available is topical minoxidil, but this is unlikely to give a substantial benefit.

Telogen effluvium

The human hair cycle (Figure 17.3) is asynchronous but can be precipitated into synchrony by childbirth or a sudden severe systemic illness, such as pneumonia or massive blood loss. The stimulus causes all the scalp hair follicles to revert to the telogen, or resting, phase. There is a sudden and significant loss of terminal scalp hair some 3 months after the precipitating event, which continues for a few weeks but then spontaneously stops. Hair regrowth gradually restores the scalp hair to its original state.

Traction alopecia

Repeated tugging and pulling on the hair shaft may produce loss of hair in the affected areas, such as that which occurs when hair rollers are used or if the hair is tied back tightly from the forehead (Figure 17.4). The hair is repeatedly damaged and this may lead to permanent hair loss. Hair loss can also develop in young children due to friction when they continually rub their scalp on their pillow. Youngsters sometimes tug out their hair, producing hair loss in a bizarre distribution over the scalp (trichotillomania, Figure 17.5). The motivation for this strange behavior usually remains obscure; it is an impulse control disorder requiring psychiatric treatment. The main differential diagnosis is alopecia areata and tinea capitis.

Scarring alopecia

Any inflammatory process on the scalp sufficient to cause loss of follicles and scar formation will result in permanent loss of hair in the affected area. Mechanical trauma, burns, bacterial infections, and severe inflammatory ringworm of the scalp can produce sufficient damage to cause scarring and permanent hair loss. In discoid lupus erythematosus and lichen planus, the scalp skin may be characteristically affected by the dermatosis concerned, but it may be difficult to distinguish these two conditions, even after biopsy. Usually, the affected area is scarred and there is loss of follicular orifices – the few remaining being distorted

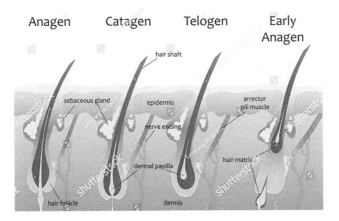

FIGURE 17.3 Diagram showing the various stages of the human hair cycle.

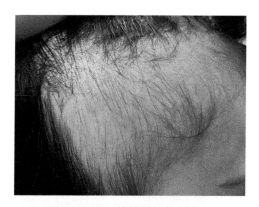

FIGURE 17.4   Traction alopecia due to the tight braids.

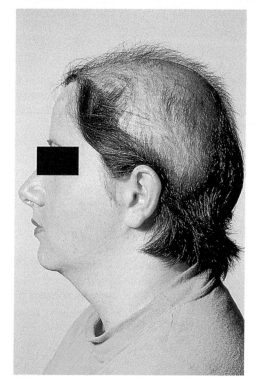

FIGURE 17.5   Trichotillomania: a bizarre pattern of hair loss from the scalp due to constant tugging of the hair (from Marks and Motley, 18th edition, with permission).

and dilated and containing tufts of hair. An odd and unexplained type of scalp scarring known as *pseudopelade* is characterized by small, rounded patches of scarring alopecia without any inflammation and presumably represents the remnants of a disease process which has spontaneously resolved.

Hair shaft disorders

Hair shaft abnormalities may be either congenital or acquired. Acquired abnormalities are more often seen. All long hairs tend to become 'weathered' at their ends due to climatic exposure and the usual washing and combing routines.

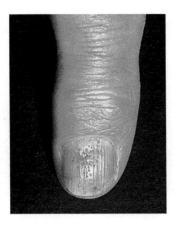

FIGURE 17.6   Thimble pitting of the fingernail in psoriasis. There is also an area of onycholysis (from Marks and Motley, 18th edition, with permission).

Twisting hairs between the fingers, and other obsessive manipulation of hair, results in a specific type of damage to the hair shafts known as *trichorrhexis nodosa*, in which expansions of the shaft (nodes) can be seen by routine light microscopy and scanning electron microscopy. These nodes rupture and leave frayed, 'paintbrush'-like ends. This deformity leads to broken hairs and even to the complaint of loss of hair.

Isolated congenital hair shaft disorders include the condition of *monilethrix*, in which there are spindle-like expansions of the hair shaft at regular intervals, causing weakness and breaking of the scalp hair.

Hirsuties

This is the name given to the complaint of excessive terminal hair growth in women. When hirsuitism is accompanied by acne, early pattern alopecia, and menstrual irregularities, tests for masculinization and polycystic ovary syndrome should be performed. Removal of facial hair is usually by depilatories, waxing, electrolysis, or with intense pulse light, alexandrite, or diode laser systems.

Disorders of the nails

Psoriasis, lichen planus, and eczema may all affect the nails, causing characteristic clinical appearances. Psoriasis characteristically causes 'thimble pitting' of the fingernails (Figure 17.6). Psoriasis causes irregular, deep, and random pitting of nail plates along with onycholysis and subungual hyperkeratosis (Figure 17.7). The nail plates may be thickened, with a yellowish-brown discoloration and subungual debris often making it difficult to distinguish from onychomycosis of the nails. In lichen planus, the nail plate may develop longitudinal ridging and pterygium formation (Figure 17.8). The process may even destroy the nail matrix and cause permanent loss of the nail. Eczema, affecting the fingers, may cause irregular deformities of the fingernails and even marked horizontal ridging.

Paronychia

This term is applied to the inflammation of the periungual tissue at the sides of the nail. In the common form of chronic paronychia, the paronychial skin is thickened and reddened. It is often tender, and pus may be expressed from the space between the nail fold and the nail plate. The eponychium disappears and the nail plate is often discolored and deformed (Figure 17.9) and may demonstrate onycholysis (see the following discussion). There is a deep recess between the nail fold and the nail plate, containing

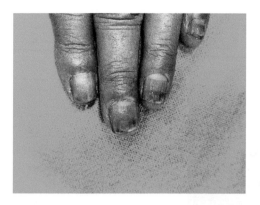

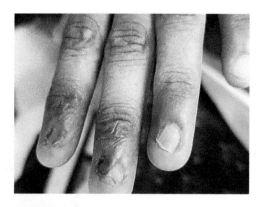

FIGURE 17.7   Fingernails in psoriasis showing onycholysis, subungual hyperkeratosis, and orange–red discoloration of the nail plate.

FIGURE 17.8   Pterygium in lichen planus.

debris and microorganisms, which is difficult to keep dry. The condition mostly occurs in women whose occupation involves frequent hand washing or other 'wet' activities (e.g. cooks, cleaners, barmaids), and it seems likely that the inability of this group of individuals to keep their hands dry contributes substantially to the condition's chronicity. *Candida* microorganisms may contribute to the recurrent inflammation to which the affected fingers are subject, but they are not the cause of the disorder. The cause is compounded by mechanical trauma and overhydration, resulting in microbial overgrowth.

Treatment

The major goals in management are keeping the fingers completely dry and avoiding wet work. Potent steroids combined with antifungal lotions are useful. Acute exacerbations may need to be treated with systemic antibiotics. Provided the advice is taken and the treatment used, patients usually gradually improve.

Onycholysis

Onycholysis is a physical sign in which the terminal nail plate separates from the underlying nail bed. It is observed in psoriasis, eczema, chronic paronychia, the 'yellow nail syndrome' (see the following discussion), thyrotoxicosis, as a result of repeated mechanical trauma and idiopathicity.

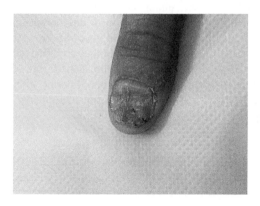

FIGURE 17.9   Irregular, discolored nail plate seen in chronic paronychia.

Brittle nails and onychorrhexis

In older women, the nails may break easily and separate into horizontal strata (onychorrhexis). Probably the single-most important factor causing this problem is repeated hydration and drying, as in housework, as well as mechanical and chemical trauma.

The nails in systemic disease

Onycholysis due to thyrotoxicosis has already been mentioned. In hypoalbuminaemia (as in severe liver disease), the lunulae may be lost and the nail plate turns a milky white. Beau's lines are horizontal ridges due to a sudden severe illness, trauma, and/or blood loss and presumably have the same significance as telogen effluvium. They grow outwards and are eventually lost.

Brown–black pigmentation

Pigmented linear bands along the length of the nail may be due to a nevus or, may be caused by malignant melanoma. Brown–black areas may be due to melanin or haemosiderin from trauma, and the two may be very difficult to tell apart. Uncommonly, *Pseudomonas* infection of the nail plate produces a diffuse black or black–green pigmentation. A yellow–green discoloration is also seen in the *yellow nail syndrome* (Figure 17.10). In this rare disease, nail growth is greatly slowed and the nails are yellowish-green, thickened, and show increased curvature. In addition, ankle and facial oedema, sinusitis, and pleural effusion often accompany this condition, the cause of which is unknown.

Ringworm of the nails (*Tinea unguium*)

Ringworm of the toenails is quite common, but much less common in the fingernails due to their faster growth. The affected nails are thickened and crumbly and are discolored yellow or yellowish-white or black (Figure 17.11). Subungual debris is often present. The differential diagnosis includes psoriasis and paronychia as well as the rare yellow nail syndrome.

Treatment

Treatment is dealt with on pages 26–27.

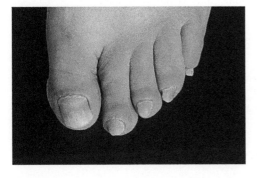

FIGURE 17.10 Nails in yellow nail syndrome. The nails are discolored a yellowish-green and show increased curvature. There is also loss of eponychium (from Marks and Motley, 18th edition, with permission).

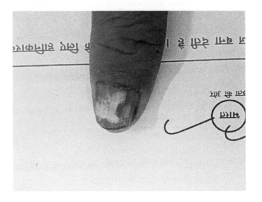

FIGURE 17.11 Discoloration and subungual debris in thumbnail due to ringworm infection (tinea unguium).

18

Systemic disease and the skin

Anupam Das

Skin markers of malignant disease

Some skin disorders are precipitated by an underlying malignancy and almost always indicate a visceral neoplasm. Early recognition may assist in the detection of the underlying neoplastic disease. There are certain disorders that have a strong association with malignancies, while some have a moderate or poor association. However, the importance of recognition of the dermatosis cannot be overemphasized, as this can lead to urgent systemic workup and diagnosis of the underlying malignancy.

BOX 18.1   STRONG ASSOCIATION WITH MALIGNANCY

Acquired hypertrichosis lanuginosa
Acrokeratosis paraneoplastica of Bazex
Erythema gyratum repens
Necrolytic migratory erythema
Paraneoplastic pemphigus
Sign of Leser-Trélat
Tripe palms
Trosseau syndrome

Moderate association with malignancy
Acanthosis nigricans
Dermatomyositis
Neutrophilic dermatoses (Sweet syndrome, pyoderma gangrenosum)

Weak association with malignancy
Acquired ichthyosis
Amyloidosis, primary systemic
Bullous pemphigoid
Dermatitis herpetiformis
Juvenile xanthogranulomas
Multicentric reticulohistiocytosis
Necrobiotic xanthogranuloma
Progressive systemic sclerosis
Scleromyxedema

Disorders with a strong association with the underlying malignancy

Acrokeratosis paraneoplastica of Bazex

It presents with erythematous to violaceous psoiasiform lesions distributed on the ears, nose, cheeks, hands, feet, and knees, along with palmoplantar keratoderma and nail dystrophy, mostly associated with squamous cell carcinoma of the upper aerodigestive tract. Histology shows hyperkeratosis, parakeratosis, lymphohistiocytic infiltrate, basal layer degeneration, and dermal melanophages.

Necrolytic migratory erythema

Clinically, it is characterized by erythematous scaly lesions with centrifugal growth over the groin, perineum, buttocks, lower abdomen, perioral areas, and distal limbs. This is usually caused by pancreatic neuroendocrine tumors (PNETs) secreting glucagons. The skin disorder responds to the removal of the underlying tumor, but usually, a complete removal is not possible.

Histology shows epidermal necrosis, neutrophilic infiltrate, bulla (acute lesion), and psoriasiform lesions (chronic lesion). Blood tests reveal increased circulating glucagon, hyperglycemia, and hypoaminoacidaemia.

Paraneoplastic pemphigus

This unique entity is characterized by intractable painful stomatitis and a polymorphous cutaneous eruption (pemphigus vulgaris-like, bullous pemphigoid-like, erythema multiforme-like, and lichen planus-like), associated with non-Hodgkin's lymphoma, chronic lymphocytic leukemia, Castleman's disease, retroperitoneal sarcoma, etc.

Acquired hypertrichosis lanuginosa

This is typified by the growth of silky and non-pigmented hair around the eyebrows, forehead, ears, and nose. It has a strong association with the underlying adenocarcinoma of the gastrointestinal tract, lung, breast, uterus, etc.

Tripe palms

Clinically, as the name suggests, it presents with thickened velvety palms. In patients with only tripe palms, the most common malignancy is lung carcinoma. However, in patients with both tripe palms and acanthosis nigricans, gastric carcinoma is the most common.

Acanthosis nigricans

Clinically, it presents as a sudden onset of symmetric hyperpigmented, hyperkeratotic, verrucous, and velvety plaques on the intertriginous skin and mucosae and is associated with tripe palms, most commonly with a background of gastric malignancy. Histology shows hyperkeratosis, papillomatosis, and minimal acanthosis.

Acquired ichthyosis

It is associated with lymphomas and leukemias. Other causes of acquired ichthyosis include acquired immune deficiency syndrome (AIDS), sarcoidosis, and leprosy, but if these can be excluded, a neoplastic cause is the most likely explanation.

Sign of Leser Trelat

This is characterized by a sudden onset of multiple itchy seborrheic keratotic lesions, mostly associated with adenocarcinomas of the gastrointestinal tract.

Dermatomyositis

A sudden onset of classical lesions of dermatomyositis is associated with malignancies of the genitourinary tract, mostly ovarian cancer.

Erythema gyratum repens

Clinically, it presents as extremely itchy serpiginous bands in concentric red swirls, referred to as a 'wood-grained' appearance, along with rapid migration of rings, commonly associated with malignancies of lung, oesophagus, breast, etc.

Sweet syndrome

It is clinically characterized by painful, edematous, and erythematous papulo-nodules and plaques over the head, neck, and upper extremities; if associated with malignancies, acute myelogenous leukaemias are the most common.

Pyoderma gangrenosum

Acute myelogenous leukaemias and multiple myeloma are the most common malignancies.

Skin metastases

Carcinomas of the breast, bronchus, stomach, kidney, and prostate are the most common visceral neoplasms to metastasize to the skin. Secondary deposits on the skin may be the first sign of the underlying visceral cancer. The lesions themselves are usually smooth nodules, which are pink or skin-colored but may be pigmented in deposits of melanoma.

Bullous pemphigoid

This subepidermal blistering disorder occurs mainly in those over 60 years of age, who are anyway more likely to be affected by a neoplasm. Nonetheless, there are a few patients with pemphigoid in whom the skin disorder is provoked by the malignancy and remits after the neoplasm has been removed.

Trousseau syndrome

It is an acquired coagulopathy presenting as migratory thrombophlebitis, mostly associated with cancers of the lung and pancreas.

Endocrine disease, diabetes, and the skin

Thyroid disease

Cutaneous manifestations of hyperthyroidism are varied. Skin, hairs, and nails have some important clinical pointers, which can readily serve as clues to diagnose the underlying hyperthyroidism. The skin is soft, smooth, and velvety, along with increased temperature and sweating. Besides, palmar erythema and facial flushing may be seen due to hyperdynamic circulation. Other associations include

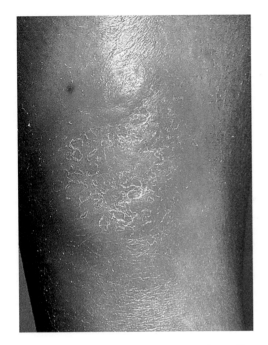

FIGURE 18.1 Plaque of pretibial myxoedema (from Marks and Motley, 18th edition, with permission).

hyperpigmentation, pretibial myxedema, vitiligo, goiter, urticaria, palmoplantar pustulosis, melanoderma, and melasma. Nails typically have a fast growth rate. Besides, soft nails, koilonychias, Plummer's nails thyroid acropachy may be found. Hairs are fine and thin. Diffuse alopecia and alopecia areata have also been documented.

In hypothyroidism, the skin is pale, cold, scaly, wrinkled, and ivory-yellow colored. Palmoplantar keratoderma is frequently seen. Other findings are puffy oedema of hands, eyelids, face; punctate telangiectasias on arms and fingertips; delayed wound healing; xanthomatosis; cutis marmorata; and livedo reticularis. Nails are brittle and striated, with a very slow rate of growth. Hairs are coarse and scalpe. Loss of lateral eyebrows may be found (Hertoghe's sign). Interesting associations include macroglossia, gingival swelling, and oral candidiasis.

Pretibial myxoedema is characterized by reddened, elevated plaques, often with a *peau d'orange* appearance on the surface (Figure 18.1). Histologically, there is a cellular connective tissue with deposition of mucinous material. The serum from such patients contains substances that stimulate the growth and activity of fibroblasts *in vitro*.

The condition is almost always a sign of Rebreak thyro-toxicosis and is accompanied by exophthalmos. It occurs in 5% of patients with thyrotoxicosis. It is persistent and difficult to treat, although treatment with PUVA is sometimes successful. Rarely, there is diffuse infiltration with the similar mucinous connective tissue of the hands and feet and finger clubbing in the condition of *thyroid acropachy*. Patients with thyrotoxicosis have warm, sweaty skin, and some complain of pruritus. There is a diffuse loss of scalp hair in some patients.

In myxoedema, the skin often feels dry and rough and may have a yellowish-orange tint, as carotenaemia may accompany the disorder. In addition, there may be coarsening of the scalp hair, hair loss, loss of the outer third of the eyebrows, pinkish cheeks, but a yellowish background color – the so-called peaches and cream complexion.

Skin manifestations of diabetes

The manifestations may be classified as under:

1. *Dermatological lesions associated with diabetes*: pruritus, granuloma annulare, necrobiosis lipoidica, diabetic dermopathy, diabetic thick skin, acanthosis nigricans, diabetic bulla, perforating dermatoses, lichen planus, vitiligo, bullous pemphigoid, skin tags, eruptive xanthoma, dermatitis herpetiformis, psoriasis, xerosis, keratosis pilaris
2. *Cutaneous infections in diabetes*: candidiasis, dermatophytosis, rhinocerebral mucormycosis, furuncle, carbuncle, necrotizing fasciitis, malignant otitis externa, intertrigo, erythrasma, gas gangrene
3. *Cutaneous lesions due to vascular abnormalities*: distal ischemic changes, with shiny, atrophic skin, hair loss, nail dystrophy, cold toes, and ischemic ulcers, pigmented purpura, erysipelas-like erythema, periungual telangiectasia, splinter nail hemorrhages, pterygium inversus unguis, diabetic rubeosis, wet gangrene of foot, diabetic dermopathy, etc.
4. *Changes due to diabetic neuropathy*: diabetic foot ulcer

5. Dermatologic complications of diabetic treatment:
   - Due to oral hypoglycemic agents: pruritus, maculopapular rash, phototoxic rash, erythema nodosum, exacerbation of porphyria cutanea tarda
   - Due to insulin: pruritic nodule, localized induration, ulceration, abscess and scar formation, keloid, lipoatrophy, lipohypertrophy, insulin oedema
6. Miscellaneous: chronic fluctuating dermatoses, annular figurate erythema, erosion, and bulla

Necrobiosis lipoidica

More than 50% of individuals who present with this disorder will already have insulin-dependent diabetes. Many of those who do not have diabetes when they present will develop diabetes or have a first-degree relative with diabetes. It starts as a firm dull-red papule and progresses to develop into yellowish, atrophic irregular plaques with a glazed porcelain appearance and comedo-like plugs on the lower legs and around the ankles (Figure 18.2). Uncommonly, lesions may occur elsewhere and there may be areas of atrophy, telangiectasia, hypohidrosis, hypoesthesia, and ulceration. These plaques are persistent and quite resistant to treatment.

Histologically, there is a central area of altered and damaged collagen in the mid-dermis, surrounded by inflammatory cells, including giant cells.

Granuloma annulare

This disorder has some superficial resemblance to necrobiosis lipoidica, both clinically and histologically, but in its common form, has no association with diabetes. However, there is a rare, generalized, and 'diffuse' form that is strongly related to diabetes. The lesions in this diffuse generalized form are not annular and not raised and plaque-like.

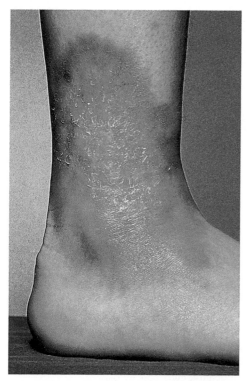

FIGURE 18.2   Necrobiosis lipoidica on the ankle (from Marks and Motley, 18th edition, with permission).

Ulceration of the skin in diabetes

The neuropathy of diabetes can result in neuropathic ulceration due to the failure of the so-called nociceptive reflex, in which the limb is rapidly withdrawn from a painful stimulus. Deep 'perforating ulcers' may develop on the soles and elsewhere around the feet.

Atherosclerotic vascular disease is more common in people with diabetes and the resulting ischaemia may also contribute substantially to the ulceration of the feet or legs. There is also a depressed ability to cope with infections, and infection of the ulcerated area usually complicates such lesions in diabetic people. The resulting ulcerating areas tend to be moist, contain slough, and be purulent. Wounds in people with diabetes also tend to heal more slowly, turning any minor injury of the foot into a serious health risk.

Diabetic dermopathy

It is characterized by asymptomatic multiple, bilateral, annular/irregular, erythematous papules and plaques, and atrophic hyperpigmented macules, which clear within 1–2 years with residual atrophy, mostly on pretibial areas, thighs, and forearms.

Xanthomata

Xanthomata is due to deposits of lipid within dermal histiocytes. Their clinical appearance and lipid composition depend on the type of lipid abnormality. In diabetes, there is usually mixed hyperlipidaemia in which both cholesterol and triglycerides are elevated. When the lipid levels are very elevated, eruptive xanthomata may develop in which numerous small, yellow–pink papules appear anywhere, especially on extensor surfaces (Figure 18.3).

Skin infections and pruritus

As mentioned earlier, people with diabetes appear particularly susceptible to skin infections. Monilial infection is a particular problem and monilial vulvovaginitis and balanoposthitis are common. These are 'itchy disorders,' and it may be that this is how it came to be believed that diabetic patients can develop the generalized itch. In fact, there is little evidence that diabetes is responsible for generalized itch.

Cushing's syndrome

The cutaneous signs of Cushing's syndrome are the same regardless of whether they are caused by an adrenal tumor, hyperplasia, or the administration of corticoids.

Clinical features

The most consistent clinical feature is skin thinning. The underlying veins can be easily seen and the skin has a 'transparent' quality (Figure 18.4). The thinning is due to the suppressive action of glucocorticoids on the growth and synthetic activity of dermal fibroblasts and the epidermis.

The dermal thinning also results in rupture of the dermal elastic fibres and the formation of striae distensae. These are band-like atrophic areas that develop in areas of maximal stress on the skin. A certain number is found on the upper arm, the anterior axillary fold, the lower and mid-back, and occasionally elsewhere in normal adolescents. They also occur in most pregnant women on the thighs, breasts, anterior axillary folds, and lower abdomen. It is thought that both tissue tension and the level of circulating glucocorticoids are important in the production of striae.

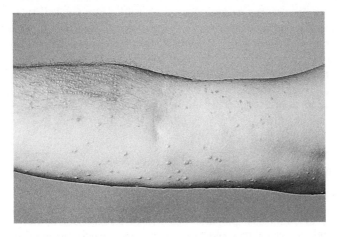

FIGURE 18.3 Numerous yellow–pink papules due to eruptive xanthoma in a patient with diabetes (from Marks and Motley, 18th edition, with permission).

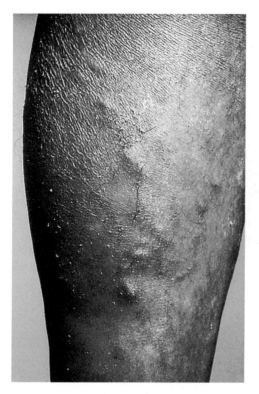

FIGURE 18.4 Skin thinning in Cushing's syndrome (from Marks and Motley, 18th edition, with permission).

Acne papules occur on the chest, back, and face in most patients with Cushing's syndrome. Steroid acne lesions are more uniform in appearance than adolescent acne and consist predominantly of small papules with few comedones. This type of acne is more resistant to treatment than ordinary acne.

Skin infections are also more common and more severe in patients with Cushing's syndrome. Pityriasis versicolor is often present and often very extensive.

Addison's disease

This disorder, due to the destruction of the adrenal cortex from autoimmune influences, tuberculosis, and amyloidosis or metastatic neoplastic disease, results in weakness, hypotension, and generalized hyperpigmentation (Figure 18.5). The increased pigmentation may be particularly evident in the major flexures and on the buccal mucosa and in the palmar creases.

Androgenization (virilization)

This disorder of women may be due to androgen-secreting tumors of the ovaries or the adrenal cortex, but it is usually due to polycystic ovaries in which there is an abnormality of steroid metabolism, leading to an accumulation of androgens. Patients present with acne and increased greasiness of the skin, or hirsutism. Increased hair growth is also a major complaint of patients with androgenization. Vellus hair on forearms, thighs, and trunk is transformed to pigmented, thick, terminal hairs. A masculine distribution of body and limb hair develops.

The appearance of beard hair is usually the reason for patients attending the clinic. In clinical practice, the most common problem is to distinguish hirsuties due to androgenization from hirsuties due to non-endocrine causes. It is not generally recognized that the presence of some terminal hair on the face or limbs of some otherwise healthy women is normal. This is particularly the case in dark-complexioned women of Arab, Asian, or Mediterranean descent. The tendency for 'excess hair' is also familial. Thinning of the scalp hair and pattern alopecia are also quite common and very distressing to women with virilization.

In authentic virilization, the following features help distinguish the condition from 'non-endrocrine' hirsuties: the excess hair growth is recent in onset and progressively becoming more noticeable, the hirsuties is accompanied by other physical signs including acne and seborrhea and there is a significant menstrual disturbance.

In most cases, extensive investigation is not appropriate and plasma testosterone and abdominal ultrasound are all that is required.

Nutrition and the skin

Marasmus

It is characterized by dry, thin, lax, purpuric, and wrinkled skin; monkey facies; baggy pants; and diminished axillary fat. Hairs are thin and brittle with excessive lanugo hair. Nails show impaired growth.

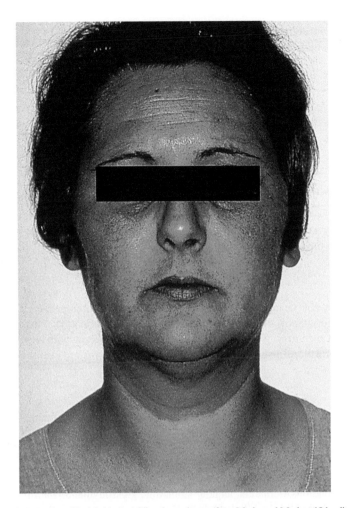

FIGURE 18.5   Hyperpigmentation of facial skin in Addison's syndrome (from Marks and Motley, 18th edition, with permission).

Kwashiorkor

This is referred to as 'wet' protein-energy malnutrition leading to a sugar baby appearance. Important findings include generalized dermatitis, flaking enamel paint appearance, etc. Hairs show alternate bands of normal pigmentation and reduced pigmentation, known as Flag sign. Mucosa is characterized by cheilosis and angular stomatitis. Systemic findings are anasarca, bloated abdomen, hepatomegaly, and irritable child.

Essential fatty acid deficiency

The skin is dry, scaly, leathery, and erythematous along with intertriginous erosions. Besides, alopecia is an important finding.

Vitamin A (retinol)

Retinol is a vital, lipid-soluble vitamin found in dairy produce and liver, and is also obtainable in the form of beta-carotene from carrots, tomatoes, and other vegetables. It is essential for growth and development, resistance to infection, reproduction, and visual function. In deficiency states, it causes follicular hyperkeratosis and roughening of the skin (phrynoderma). When excessive amounts are ingested, pruritus, widespread erythema and peeling of the palms and soles, and liver damage occur. These symptoms and signs are similar to those of retinoid toxicity.

Nicotinic acid

This is a water-soluble B vitamin found in grains and vegetables. Its deficiency causes the condition of pellagra, resulting in diarrhoea, dementia, and photosensitivity dermatitis. The photosensitivity dermatitis develops a characteristic post-inflammatory hyperpigmentation and is often very marked around the neck.

Vitamin C (ascorbic acid)

Vitamin C is a water-soluble vitamin found in fruit and vegetables. Deficiency results in scurvy, which causes a clotting defect and poor wound healing. A characteristic rash seen in patients with scurvy consists of numerous tiny haemorrhages around hair follicles.

Zinc

The inherited form of zinc deficiency is known as acrodermatitis enteropathica. Clinically it presents with acrally and periorificially distributed pustular and bullous dermatitis. There are patchy red dry scales with exudation and crusting over the face, flexors, and groin along with angular cheilitis. Chronic lesions acquire a psoriasiform pattern. Alopecia and thinning of nails are also seen.

Selenium

Deficiency leads to leuconychia and Terry's-like nails along with hypopigmentation of skin and hair (pseudoalbinism).

Iron

Deficiency leads to aphthous stomatitis, angular stomatitis, glossodynia, and atrophied tongue papillae. Nails show thinning, flattening, and koilonychias. Hairs are lusterless, brittle, and dry.

Senile osteoporosis

In this disorder of faulty bone mineralization due to vitamin D deficiency, bone thinning, and multiple fractures, the skin becomes 'thinner' and is almost transparent, with the veins being abnormally prominent. The thinning can be demonstrated by ultrasound – using a simple pulsed A scan device.

The skin and the gastrointestinal tract

There are numerous interrelationships between the skin and the gastrointestinal tract, and only the more important ones fall within the scope of a book of this size.

Buccal mucosa

Erythema multiforme is a widespread inflammatory disorder accompanied by severe mouth ulcers.

Behçet's syndrome causes marked orogenital ulceration, ocular inflammation, and other problems, including arthropathy.

Dermatitis herpetiformis

This itchy, blistering disorder is strongly associated with an absorptive defect of the small bowel. Small-bowel mucosal biopsy using a Crosby capsule or endoscope demonstrates partial villous atrophy in some 70–80% of patients with dermatitis herpetiformis. There are also some functional absorptive abnormalities in most patients, which can result in serious clinical consequences such as anaemia or osteoporosis. This gut disorder is, in fact, a form of gluten enteropathy (as is coeliac disease) and can be improved by a gluten-free diet.

Peutz–Jeghers syndrome

This is a rare, autosomal dominant disorder in which perioral and labial pigmented macules occur in association with jejunal polyps. Pigmented macules also occur over the fingers.

Gardner's syndrome

In this autosomal dominant disorder, epidermoid cysts and benign epidermal tumors occur in association with colonic polyposis.

Hepatic disease

In severe chronic hepatocellular liver failure, hypoalbuminaemia occurs, which results in the curious sign of whitening of the fingernails (Figure 18.6). Severe liver failure may also cause multiple spider naevi to develop over the arms, upper trunk, and face. These vascular anomalies consist of a central 'feeding' blood vessel ('the body') with numerous fine radiating 'legs'. Their cause is uncertain, but they may be related to the plasma levels of unconjugated oestrogens.

In biliary cirrhosis, severe pruritus develops, resulting in excoriations and prurigo papules. In addition, Jaundice and a generalized dusky pigmentation are seen.

In hemochromatosis, the findings include greyish pigmentation, black keratin cysts, black stasis dermatitis, and porphyria cutanea tarda.

Wilson's disease is characterized by blue lunulae and pretibial hyperpigmentation.

Cutaneous manifestations of hepatitis B virus infections are urticaria, serum sickness, angioedema, erythema nodosum, erythema multiforme, polyarteritis nodosa, etc.

Cutaneous manifestations of hepatitis C virus infections are mixed cryoglobulinemia, porphyria cutanea tarda, polyarteritis nodosa, nec-rolytic acral erythema, urticarial vasculitis, lichen planus, etc.

Systemic causes of pruritus

End-stage renal failure (uraemia) often causes a persistent, severe itch. The itch is accompanied by a dusky, grey–brown pigmentation.

Obstructive jaundice from any cause results in intolerable itching.

Thyrotoxicosis sometimes causes itching, but this does not seem to be due to the sweatiness or increased warmth of the skin experienced by such patients.

Itching is sometimes a complaint of patients with hyperparathyroidism and other disturbances of calcium metabolism.

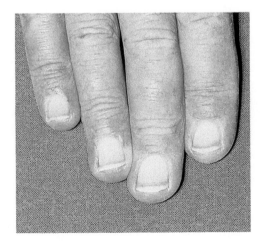

FIGURE 18.6 White fingernails due to liver disease (from Marks and Motley, 18th edition, with permission).

The symptom of an itch is occasionally a sign of Hodgkin's disease or, less often, of another type of lymphoma. Rarely, the itch is a presenting symptom of the neoplasm.

Itch is a well-known disabling complaint of patients with polycythaemia rubra vera. For some curious reason, the itch may be a particular problem when these patients have a bath.

It has often been claimed that patients with diabetes have pruritus, but if this is the case, it must be extremely rare. People with diabetes are prone to candidiasis, which causes perigenital itch, and it is possible that this is how the idea began.

19

Disorders of pigmentation

Rashmi Sarkar
Anupam Das

Melanin pigment is produced in melanocytes in the basal layer of the epidermis. The degree of racial pigmentation does not depend on the number of melanocytes present, but on their metabolic activity and the size and shape of their melanin-producing organelles – the melanosomes. Melanocytes account for 5–10% of the cells in the basal layer of the epidermis. They are dendritic but appear as 'clear cells' in formalin-fixed sections.

Melanin synthesis is controlled by melanocyte-stimulating hormones and is influenced by oestrogens and androgens. Melanocytes are also stimulated by ultraviolet radiation (UVR) and by other irritative stimuli. Melanin is a complex, black–brown polymer synthesized from the amino acid dihydroxy-phenylalanine (L-DOPA). Two forms of melanin exist: 'ordinary' melanin, known as eumelanin, and a reddish melanin synthesized from cysteinyl DOPA, known as phaeomelanin.

Melanin synthesis is initially catalyzed by a copper-containing enzyme known as tyrosinase, which also catalyzes the transformation of L-DOPA to tyrosine. Melanin is produced in melanocytes, but 'donated' via their dendrites to neighboring keratinocytes. The melanin granules then ascend through the epidermis in the keratinocytes. Melanosomes go through several stages of melanin synthesis during their melaninization (stages I–IV). Mature melanosomes aggregate into melanin granules and it is these granular particles within keratinocytes that give protection against damage from UVR.

Melanin in keratinocytes is black and absorbs all visible light, UVR, and infrared radiation. It is also a powerful electron acceptor and may have other uncharacterized protective functions.

Excessive pigmentation is known as hyperpigmentation and decreased pigmentation is known as hypopigmentation. Both may be localized or generalized. Non-melanin pigments may also cause skin darkening.

Hypopigmentation

The etiology of hypopigmentation is diverse and can be broadly summarized as in Table 19.1.

Generalized hypopigmentation

Oculocutaneous albinism

There are several varieties of genetically determined defects in melanin synthesis, the most common of which is recessively inherited oculocutaneous albinism. Affected individuals have a very pale or even pinkish complexion with flaxen, white, or slightly yellowish hair, and very light-blue or even pink eyes. Albinos are also subject to nystagmus, either horizontal or rotatory. In addition, they are photophobic and often have serious refractive errors. They are extremely sensitive to the harmful effects of solar irradiation and in sunny climates often develop skin cancers.

Albinos have a normal number of melanocytes in the basal layer of the epidermis, but lack tyrosinase and are unable to synthesize melanin. If the hair is plucked and incubated in a medium containing L-DOPA, the hair bulb does not turn black, as it does normally.

TABLE 19.1

Classification of hypopigmentation

- Genetic and nevoid: oculocutaneous albinism, Hermansky–Pudlak syndrome, Chédiak–Higashi syndrome, Piebaldism, Waardenburg syndrome, phyenylketonuria, vitiligo, tuberous sclerosis, incontinentia pigmenti, hypomelanosis of Ito, naevus depigmentosus
- Disruption of melanoblast migration to target tissues during development: Waardenburg syndrome, piebaldism, Cross syndrome
- Disruption of melanin synthesis: oculocutaneous albinism
- Disruption of melanosome formation: Hermansky–Pudlak syndrome, Chediak–Higashi syndrome
- Disruption of melanosome transport: Griscelli syndrome
- Post-inflammatory and infections: pityriasis versicolor, leprosy, post kala-azar dermal leishmaniasis, pinta, syphilitic leucomelanoderma, onchocerciasis
- Endocrine: hypothyroidism, hypopituitarism, hypogonadism
- Chemical factors: monobenzylether of hydroquinone (rubber factories), monomethylether of hydroquinone, p-tertiary-butylphenol, p-tertiary amylphenol, chloroquine and hydroxychloroquine, topical steroids, arsenic
- Physical factors: heat, freezing, X-ray, ionizing radiation, UV radiation, laser light
- Nutritional: Kwashiorkor, selenium deficiency, copper deficiency
- Neoplasms: melanoma-associated leukoderma, halo nevus
- Hypopigmentation with vascular cause: Bier spots, Woronoff ring, cutaneous edema, anemia
- Miscellaneous: pityriasis alba, mycosis fungoides, sarcoidosis, lupus erythematosus, scleroderma, idiopathic guttate hypomelanosis, lichen sclerosus et atrophicus

Mutation in the TYR gene, P gene, TYRP1 gene, and MATP gene leads to OCA-1,2,3 and 4, respectively. Ocular albinism is a distinct variant wherein only ocular symptoms are present without any cutaneous lesions.

Management

Albino patients must learn to protect themselves against UVR with sunscreens and avoid sun wherever possible. Regular checks to detect early changes in skin cancer is also important.

There are several other types of albinism, most of which are recessive. In the Hermanski–Pudlak syndrome, there is an associated clotting defect due to a platelet abnormality. Patients have a bleeding tendency, interstitial pulmonary fibrosis, and granulomatous colitis. This is 'tyrosinase positive' and hair bulbs turn black after they are incubated with L-DOPA. Chediak–Higashi syndrome is characterized by severe immunodeficiency and silvery-white hair, and the histology is classical, showing giant melanosomes within melanocytes. Griscelli syndrome, on the other hand, is a severe immunological disorder with hemophagocytic syndrome in addition to having silvery-white hairs and pigmentary dilution of skin. Waardenburg syndrome is a distinct entity manifesting as achromia of skin, hairs, and eyes, heterochromia iridis, congenital deafness, broad nasal root, and dystopia canthorum. The hallmark finding in piebaldism is white forelock and the presence of normal skin within the depigmented patches.

Vitiligo

Definition

This is a common skin disorder in which there is focal failure of pigmentation due to the destruction of melanocytes that is thought to be mediated by immunological mechanisms.

Clinical features

Sharply defined areas of depigmentation appear (Figure 19.1). The depigmented patches are often symmetrical, especially when they are over the limbs and face. Nascent patches of vitiligo are more

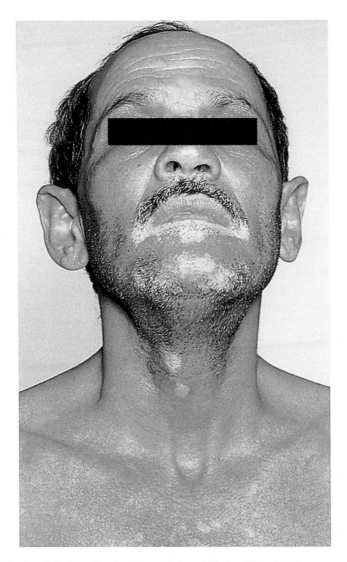

FIGURE 19.1   Vitiligo in a dark-skinned patient (from Marks and Motley, 18th edition).

easily identified if the skin is examined with UV light illumination. UV light may also enhance the appearance of follicular pigmentation within patches of vitiligo. The melanocytes associated with follicles are often unaffected and act as the reservoir from which repigmentation may occur.

In some patients, vitiligo shows a propensity to develop at sites of skin trauma (the Koebner phenomenon). Based on distribution, vitiligo can be focal, segmental, acrofacial, generalized, universal, and mucosal. Vitiligo may occasionally be associated with regression of pigmentation in malignant melanoma and it is wise to examine the entire skin surface of patients presenting with the condition. In *halo naevus* (Sutton's naevus, Figure 19.2), the depigmentation of vitiligo begins around one or a few compound naevi. This may also be associated with a regressing malignant melanoma – although it is usually a benign phenomenon in children and teenagers. Clinical variants include trichrome, quadrichrome, pentachrome, and confetti type.

Vitiligo is more noticeable in summer when the surrounding skin is tanned. It is a serious cosmetic problem for darkly pigmented people.

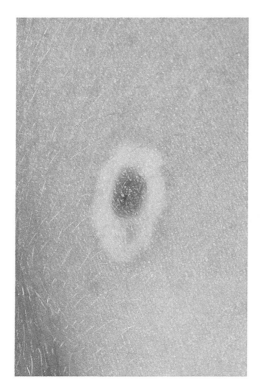

FIGURE 19.2   Halo naevus (from Marks and Motley, 18th edition).

The condition often starts in childhood and may spread, ultimately causing total depigmentation, or persist, with irregular remissions and relapses.

Pathogenesis and epidemiology

Vitiligo occurs in 1–2% of the population and is more common when it has already occurred in other members of the family. It is also more common in hyperthyroidism, hypothyroidism, pernicious anemia, Addison's disease, alopecia areata, and diabetes, and appears to be due to an autoimmune attack on melanocytes.

Treatment

Treatments with topical corticosteroids – 0.3% tacrolimus – or photochemotherapy with long-wave ultraviolet irradiation (PUVA) is sometimes effective in stimulating repigmentation, but the response is irregular. Reassurance and cosmetic camouflage are helpful in many patients. Where the vitiligo is stable, of limited extent, and in a cosmetically sensitive area – such as the face or dorsa of the hands, it may be possible to transplant autologous melanocytes using epidermal skin grafts from unaffected skin. The epidermis is removed from the area of vitiligo – either by dermabrasion or laser ablation – and a thin epidermal skin graft is raised from an area of pigmented skin – either by creating a large blister in the skin – and taking the roof of the blister or by the use of a mechanical dermatome. In some circumstances, areas of vitiligo may be camouflaged by tattooing the skin; however, the normal skin may alter in color in response to sun exposure and the tattooed skin then becomes conspicuous again due to its different pigmentation.

Other causes of localized depigmentation of skin

In many countries, the fear of leprosy makes the differential diagnosis of a 'white patch' an urgent and vitally important issue. The classical lesion of leprosy is a hypopigmented hypoesthetic patch along with peripheral nerve thickening. Examination in long-wave UVR enhances loss of epidermal pigment (as in vitiligo) and helps identify areas of developing depigmentation. It may also detect a yellow–green fluorescence in some cases of pityriasis versicolor, which is otherwise clinically seen as round-to-oval, centrally coalescent hypopigmented macules with furfuraceous scales.

Tuberous sclerosis is characterized by the presence of 1–100 hypopigmented macules, present since birth or early neonatal period over the posterior trunk. The pigmentation can be polygonal, confetti-type, segmental, or thumbprint-like. Hypomelanosis of Ito is identified by the typical whorled patches of hypopigmentation along the lines of Blaschko. Nevus depigmentosus manifests as a circumscribed area of depigmentation on the posterior trunk.

Pityriasis alba manifests as a hypopigmented patch with powdery white scales on the head and neck region of pre-adolescent children.

Hyperpigmentation

Hyperpigmentation, similarly, has a wide range of causes and they have been tabulated as follows:

Congenital

Circumscribed

- Nevus of Ota
- Nevus of Ito
- Mongolian spot
- Dermal melanocytic hamartoma
- Lentiginosis (generalized, zosteriform, eruptive, centrofacial)
- Café-au-lait macules

Diffuse

- Incontinentia pigmentii
- Linear and whorled nevoid hypermelanosis
- Dyskeratosis congenita
- X-linked reticular pigmentary disorder
- Naegeli–Franceshetti–Jadassohn syndrome
- Dermatopathia pigmentosa reticularis
- Dyschromatosis hereditaria universalis
- Reticulate acropigmentation of Dohi
- Reticulate acropigmentation of Kitamura
- Dowling–Degos disease
- Familial progressive hypermelanosis

Acquired

Circumscribed

- Freckles
- Fixed drug rash
- Post-inflammatory hyperpigmentation
- Becker's nevus
- Nevus of Hori
- Riehl's melanosis
- Erythema dyschromicum perstans
- Flagellate pigmentation

Diffuse

- Endocrine: Addison's disease, Cushing's syndrome, Melasma, pregnancy, diabetes, acanthosis nigricans
- Nutritional: Kwashiorkor, pellagra, vitamin B12 deficiency
- Metabolic: prophyria, cutanea tarda, hemochromatosis
- Physical: radiation, trauma
- Drug induced: clofazimine, amiodarone, zidovudine, antimalarials, minocycline

TABLE 19.2

Non-melanin causes of brown–black discoloration

Haemosiderin – from broken haem pigment in extravasated blood

Homogentisic acid – deposited in cartilage, in particular, in the inherited metabolic defect known as alkaptonuria

Unknown pigment in thickened stratum corneum – severe disorders of keratinization such as lamellar ichthyosis

Drugs and heavy metal toxicity – dark pigmentation of the skin and mucosae seen in silver, gold, mercury, and arsenic poisoning; amiodarone and phenothiazines cause slate-grey, dusky skin pigmentation in exposed sites; minocycline may cause patchy pigmentation in exposed or other sites

---

- Toxin mediated: arsenic
- Neoplastic: mast cell disorders, melanoma
- Miscellaneous: onchocerciasis, erythema ab igne, prurigo pigmentosa

It has to be determined whether the pigmentation is due to melanin or some other pigment (Table 19.2). Generalized melanin hyperpigmentation is seen in *Addison's disease* due to destruction of the adrenal cortex from tuberculosis, autoimmune influences, metastases, or amyloidosis. Pigmentation is marked in the flexures, sites of trauma, scars, and sun-exposed areas, but the mucosae and nails are also hyperpigmented. The pigmentation is mediated via activation of the melanocortin-1 receptor. The diagnosis is supported by hypotension, hyponatraemia, and extreme weakness. The hyperpigmentation is due to an excess of pituitary peptides resulting from the lack of adrenal steroids. After bilateral adrenalectomy, pigmentation may be extreme (*Nelson's syndrome*). This is associated with an enlarged pituitary gland, elevated fasting plasma ACTH level, and neurologic symptoms. Pheochromocytoma is characterized by Addisonian pigmentation due to ectopic ACTH and MSH production. Carcinoid syndrome manifests with diffuse hyperpigmentation due to an MSH-secreting tumor; along with pellagroid dermatitis.

Generalized hyperpigmentation may be part of *Acanthosis nigricans* (see p. 254), which is much more marked in the flexures and is accompanied by exaggerated skin markings and skin tags.

A 'bronzed appearance' is seen in *primary haemochromatosis* (bronzed diabetes), in which iron is deposited in the viscera, including the pancreas (giving rise to diabetes) and the liver (causing cirrhosis). The increased pigmentation is caused by both iron and excess melaninization in the skin. The pigmentation is more pronounced over sun-exposed areas, genitalia, and scars. Increased pigmentation is also evident in secondary haemosiderosis. Generalized hyperpigmentation is also seen in cirrhosis, particularly primary biliary cirrhosis, chronic renal failure, glycogen storage disease, and Gaucher's disease. Biliary cirrhosis and renal failure are usually accompanied by severe pruritus.

Drugs can cause generalized diffuse hyperpigmentation, patchy generalized, or localized hyperpigmentation. Classic examples are due to the rare heavy metal intoxications. Arsenic ingestion causes a generalized 'raindrop' pattern of hyperpigmentation, and topical silver preparations cause 'argyria', producing a dusky, greyish discoloration of the skin and mucosae.

Modern drugs can also produce darkening. Minocycline (Minocin®) can cause darkening of the scars of acne; it can also produce dark patches on exposed areas. The pigment is a complex of iron, the drug, and melanin, and the condition is only partially reversible but can be successfully treated with Q-switched frequency-doubled Nd:YAG and ruby lasers. Amiodarone, an antiarrhythmic drug, causes a characteristic greyish color on exposed sites. Phenothiazines, in high doses over long periods, produce a purplish discoloration in the exposed areas due to the deposition of a drug–melanin complex in the skin. Chlorpromazine is particularly prone to doing this.

Carotenaemia produces an orange–yellow, golden hue due to the deposition of beta-carotene in the skin. It is seen in food faddists who eat large amounts of carrots and other red vegetables. Beta-carotene is also given for the condition of erythropoietic protoporphyria (see p. 235). Systemic sclerosis can also lead to diffuse hyperpigmentation, without elevated MSH.

Canthexanthin is another carotenoid that produces a similar skin color and was sold for this purpose to simulate a 'bronzed' suntan. Pigment crystals were found in the retina of patients taking the drug and it has been withdrawn for this reason.

Transient skin discoloration is seen in methaemoglobinaemia and sulfhaemoglobinaemia due to dapsone administration.

Localized hyperpigmentation

Mongolian spots, the naevus of Ota, and the naevus of Ito are large, flat, grey–brown patches and can be confused with bruising and other conditions (Figure 19.3). The bluish color is attributed to the Tyndall effect. Hori's nevus, otherwise known as ABNOM (acquired bilateral nevus of Ota like macules), *café-au-lait* patches are part of neurofibromatosis (von Recklinghausen's disease, see Chapter 12). Numerous flat, light-brown macules, which vary from 0.5–4 cm^2, are present all over the skin surface – and characteristically in the axillae alongside the neurofibromata (Figure 19.4).

Not dissimilar brown macules are found on the lips and around the mouth and on the fingers in Peutz–Jeghers syndrome, accompanied by small bowel polyps, and in Albright's syndrome, in which there are associated bone abnormalities.

A very common type of localized hyperpigmentation is chloasma or melasma. This facial pigmentation may be part of the increased pigmentation of pregnancy or may occur independently. The cheeks,

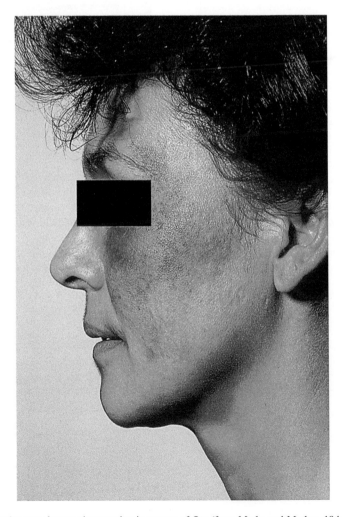

FIGURE 19.3   Macular grey–brown pigmentation in naevus of Ota (from Marks and Motley, 18th edition).

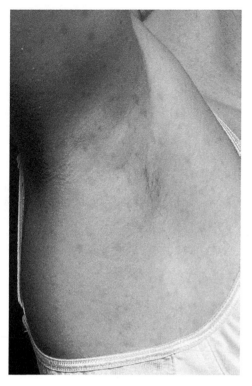

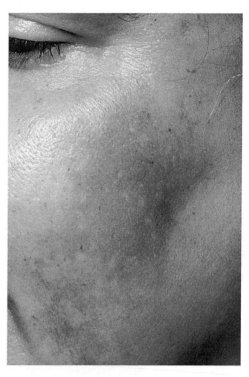

FIGURE 19.5   Diffuse brown pigmentation of the cheek in chloasma (from Marks and Motley, 18th edition).

FIGURE 19.4   Axillary freckling in a patient with von Recklinghausen's disease (from Marks and Motley, 18th edition).

periocular regions, forehead, and neck may be affected in this so-called mask of pregnancy (Figure 19.5). Riehl's melanosis (pigmented cosmetic dermatitis) is frequently seen over the forehead.

Post-inflammatory hyperpigmentation may be due to melanocytic hyperplasia occurring as part of epidermal thickening in chronic eczema, particularly atopic eczema. This is transient and of no real consequence.

It may also be due to the shedding of melanin from the damaged epidermis into the dermis, where it is engulfed by macrophages. This 'tattooing' may last many months. It is seen in lichen planus and in fixed drug eruption.

Index

Note: *Italicized* page numbers refer to figures, **bold** page numbers refer to tables.

A

ABNOM (acquired bilateral nevus of Ota-like macules), 259
acanthosis nigricans, 243, 258
ACE inhibitors, 66
aciclovir, 90
acitretin, 65, 130
acne, 134–43; aetiology, 140–1; chloracne, 138; clinical
course, 137–8; clinical features, 134–6; conglobata,
138; cosmetica, 138; cystic, 134, *135*; definition, 134;
drug-induced, 138, *139*; epidemiology, 138;
excoriated, 139; infantile, 139; mechanica, 139;
neonatal, 139; nodulocystic, 134; occupational, 138;
pathogenesis, 140–1; pathology, 140–1; prevalence,
134; rate variants, 139–40; sites affected, 137; special
types, 138–9; treatment, 141–4, **144**; antibiotics, 143;
antimicrobials, 142, 143; basic principles, 141;
hormonal therapy, 144; isotretinoin, 143–4;
macrolides, 143; systematic, 142; tetracyclines, 143;
topical, 142; tropical, 138
acne conglobata, 88, *90*
acne fulminans, 134
acquired bilateral nevus of Ota-like macules
(ABNOM), 259
acquired hypertrichosis lanuginosa, 243
acquired ichthyosis, 216, **218**, 243. *see also* ichthyosis;
keratinization disorders
acquired immune deficiency syndrome (AIDS). *see* HIV/AIDS
acrodermatitis continua, 122
acrodermatitis enteropathica, 249
acrokeratosis paraneoplastica of Bazex, 243
actinic keratosis, 187–8, *188*. *see also* non-melanoma skin
cancers
acute generalized exanthematous pustulosis (AGEP), 75
acute intermittent porphyria, **223**, 226. *see also* porphyrias
acyclovir, 60
Addison's disease, 15, 248, *249*, 258
adenoma sebaceum, *172*, 179
adipocytic tumors, 158
adnexal structures, 6
AIDS. *see* HIV/AIDS
albinos, 253–4
Albright's syndrome, 259
alitretinoin, 102, 130
alkaptonuria, 15
allergic contact dermatitis, **97**, 109–11. *see also* dermatitis
(eczema); clinical features, 109; definition, 109;

diagnosis, 110; epidemiology, 109–10; natural history,
109–10; pathogenesis, 111; pathology, 111;
treatment, 111
alopecia; androgenetic (pattern), 233–5; areata, 235–6, *236*;
congenital, 233; diffuse, 236–7; scarring, 237–8;
traction, 237
amiodarone, 258
amoxicillin-clavulanate, **31**, 32
amyloidosis, 226–8, *227*, **227**. *see also* metabolic disorders
anagen, 7
androgenetic (pattern) alopecia, 233–5; clinical features,
233–4; definition, 233; pathogenesis, 234; pathology,
234; treatment, 235
androgenization (virilization), 248
androgens, 138
angioedema. *see also* immunologically mediated skin
disorders; angioneurotic, 57; in drug eruptions, 75;
drug-induced, 57; hereditary, 58; idiopathic, 57; without
wheals, 57–8
angiokeratoma, **172**, 183
angioneurotic angioedema, 57
angiotensin (AT) II antagonists, **119**
angiotensin-converting enzyme (ACE) inhibitors, **119**
anhidrotic/hypohidrotic ectodermal dysplasia, 221.
see also keratinization disorders
animal scabies, 48
annular erythemas, 61–2, *62*
anogenital warts, 41
anthrax, 34
anti-p200 pemphigoid, **80**, 81. *see also* blistering skin
disorders
antibiotics, 61, 143
antigen, 111
antihistamines, 59
antimicrobials, 102, 142, 143
antiretroviral drugs, **91**
apocrine hidrocystoma, **160**, 166, *166*, **166**. *see also* tumors,
benign
apocrine sweat glands, 8
aquagenic urticaria, 57. *see also* urticaria
argyria, 258
arterial ulcers, 153
arthritis, psoriatic, 121, *122*
arthritis mutilans, 121, *122*
asteatotic eczema, 105–6, *106*
ataxia telangiectasia, **93**
atopic dermatitis, 96–102, **97**; aetiopathogenesis, 100;